# Angels "See Our Needs"

*Healing of body, soul and spirit*

"Remember, each person on this earth shall reach his Father in a different way. No two souls upon your earth are identical; no two spirits upon your earth are identical, and no two mortal bodies upon your earth are identical. Each body must be fed its own fruit; each soul must be fed its own fruit. And above all, if the body and the soul are fed the proper fruit, then the spirit shall grow, and therefore, the immortal body shall climb your ladder as three."

*(Spiritual messengers of God, Aka, September 14, 1970)*

# The Health Readings

*by Aka, the spiritual messengers of God*

And now we should give thee a task. In the readings, as in the name we have given you, was the Association for the Spiritual Philosophy of God. [Note: In1974, the name became the Association of Universal Philosophy.]

Therefore, you should separate these readings. Separate the philosophy from the medical readings; separate the life readings from the medical readings; but combine all three into one writing, yet make yet three writings. Can thy understand of which we speak?

*(Spiritual messengers of God, March 5, 1971)*

# *An Introduction*

The spiritual messengers of God, Aka, arrived in 1970 and began speaking through the unconscious Ray Elkins, who had given up his life again, as he had before, so that they may come and speak through his body to us. At first, Ray really didn't understand what was happening to him. He only knew he had less pain. By going into trance the severe headaches he'd experienced since his injuries in 1965 improved for the first time. That's why he continued to do it. As he walked up a ladder or stairway to stand with God he felt much better. This was the only thing that helped him.

It was a gift the Messiah had given to him when Ray passed on, before he chose to return to life again. "It" could more appropriately be called, the spiritual messengers of God. They were linked to his soul as a new life. Ray truly had been given life back and more. He received a greater Life beyond his understanding. Some people may call it, eternal life. Others may remember Jesus' words in *John* 3:1-10, "Unless you be born over again you cannot see the kingdom of heaven." But it has been given throughout time to many, for our Father sends those who know Him best to remind His children that we know Him.

But whether you call them angels, or cherubim – or by whatever name you know them – they stand as close to our Father as His eyes, His ears, and His heart. The miraculous gift for us to know is that they also come to man – in this case, Ray, that he (and so also we) may receive healing and know our Father better. Soon after, Ray began to see with their eyes and hear with their ears. He began knowing how to heal the sick and to see our needs.

With our Father's eyes, the spiritual messengers of God can look into each body, soul, spirit and immortal body and see. Yet they are always respectful of our free will. They can do nothing without our permission. The many who came for healing, as Aka spoke and worked through Ray from 1970 to 1989 in trance, always asked for their help. Often their questions were written.

In this collection of health readings you will find suggestions made by the spiritual messengers of God (and perhaps a few consultations with doctors or wise healers who'd passed on who chose to serve God). They gave wise counsel or provided healing of the bodies and minds of thousands of individuals.

They offered healing of "the body, the soul, the spirit and the immortal body." Healing is not for just one part of a person, but for the whole. And that is a very big whole when you include all that the Father would give unto man and woman.

The author has attempted to place the guidance for spiritual healing into other books: the parables, the philosophy, and the life readings. This book contains the health readings, that offer healing of the body and sometimes the soul (mind).

To the spiritual messengers of God, each person is an unique individual with his or her own needs. What is medicine to one may be poison to another. So the reader is advised not apply guidance given to someone else for healing to what may sound like the reader's own needs. The spiritual messengers of God looked directly into an individual's body and soul; they spoke in a personal and loving way, meant only for this one, as they saw their needs.

No two people are alike. There is no one else just like us. Our Father loves us especially in this way, for who we are. And so do those He sends to guide and give us healing.

Hopefully, this is the precious view you will see as you read these health readings – for they are given through angels' eyes.

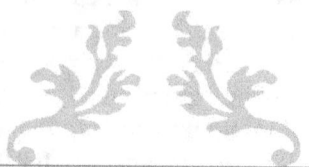

# THE HEALTH READINGS

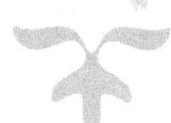

## A Gift from One with More Love in His Eyes than Anyone

All the words you see typed in bold in this book are transcribed just as the spiritual messengers of God, Aka, spoke them as they were being tape recorded. They arrived in 1970 with the brightest light in the heavens of the century, Comet Bennett. As it (and they) passed over Earth, God's messengers hovered over and entered into the body of a dying man to speak. The man who'd passed on, Ray Elkins, was given a choice, to remain with all those who gathered before one who was seated in their midst, or to return back to his body. As Ray returned to life, he was given a gift by "One who had more love in his eyes than anyone he had ever seen." Ray didn't know what the gift was; he only knew the love in which it was being given. He was told to give this gift freely to others in the same manner of love it had been given to him, asking nothing in return. Each evening Ray's voice was recorded from 1970 to 1989 after he left his body to again stand with God, the spiritual messengers of God entered it and spoke to us.

This gift speaks to you here, through these words. The spiritual messengers of God announce, "We are here to prepare a way for the coming of the Messiah."

# Contents

# 1970 Health Readings

The first time the voice was recorded with Margaret's mother's hand-held tape recorder, already, the spiritual messengers of God, Aka, were seeing Ray's needs. Margaret (Ray's wife's) questions are typed in italics. In bold are Aka's answers.

April 3, 1970: *"How can we help his body?"*
**Rest. Rest, relaxing of his nervous system.**
*"How?"*
**Massaging the lower and upper part of his back and neck, using vibration, not as has been used before — the vitamins....**
[Editor's note: As these words were spoken, the tape ran out on the small recorder. She rewound the tape to the middle, recording over some of the message to get these instructions on how to wake Ray up.]

By April 6, 1970, the second time the spiritual messengers of God spoke, already they were seeing the needs of others around Ray. In this case, it was his wife's aunt, far away in another city. Then Aka spoke of the needs of Margaret's mother in Yuma. And her father. And Ray's best friend. Then Ray. And then a friend in Yuma.
And so this continued for the next 19 years, speaking not only of health needs but answering anything they were asked. They planted seeds, as fishers of men, seeking a place in each person's heart for the Messiah, for whom the Father sent them to prepare a way upon the Earth.
This is a collection of the health readings.

April 6, 1970: *"What did you want to tell me the last time about my aunt?"*
**Of this soul — house, now deep rug, walking, walking — inflammation of kidney.**
*"Which aunt?"*
**M_____.** [Editor's note: To respect the privacy of each individual, the names are not written.]
*"Should she see a medical doctor?"*
**Yes.**
*"Any particular medical doctor?"*
**Beranton, name doctor. Mostly problem — Ray must go deeper in trance.**

*"How shall he go deeper?"*
[After a long pause, he says:] **Soul.....I come through, now, stronger. Ray, deeper in trance.**
*"Is this safe for Ray?"*
**Very safe for Ray.**
**M_____, aunt, soul, inflammation of left kidney.**
*"Is she aware of it?"*
**Awareness, I do not know — psychological block on her part.**

April 6, 1970: **Conscious mind plane [unchanged].**
*"Are you speaking of D_____?"*
**Yes.**
*"What of my father?"*
**Father must rest.......**
*"Ray?"*
**I have not finished D_____.**
*"I'm sorry."*
**D_____'s health not good because of neglect of body. Psychological block. To prepare and eat Jerusalem artichoke — have told Ray — results negative.**
**Through with soul D_____.**

April 6, 1970: *"Anything of my Father?"*
**Soul B\_\_\_ — good soul, B\_\_\_. Sometimes selfish, otherwise, good soul. Preparing in thought and action to purchase certain items — cause chaos. Father — health not good, needs higher altitude. Heart murmur, faint; needs electrocardiograph. Needs change diet. Needs physical exercise. Needs chiropractic treatment of upper neck. Needs different glasses, better correction — present not good. Needs more spiritual guidance, more study. When Ray awakens, he'll have message and more extent knowledge on subject.**
**Now finished soul W_____.**

April 6, 1970: *"Does your coming hurt Ray's body?"*
**No. Shall improve Ray's body and mind. I am he and he is I, for I was reborn at time as he. For we are one.**

April 6, 1970: *The vitamins that he's taking, you said he was allergic to them?"*
**Allergic to alfalfa which vitamins are extracted from.**
*"What kind of vitamins should he take?"*
**Simple, vitamin without as much alfalfa in same. "Nutralite," as you call it, vitamin good. [There] are many others. Needs more fish in diet.**
*"Any particular kind?"*

Some are better than others.
*"Can you tell me one that is better? I don't know fish."*
**Names different in my time than in yours.**
*"What is in the fish that he needs? Is it a certain substance in the fish?"*

**Yes.**
*"What?"*
**Sulphur, for one.**
*"Does he need more iodine?"*
**Iodine, yes; natural salt which comes from sea food.**
*"Would it help if he drank sea water?"*
**No. I shall give better reading on Ray at different time. I'm not here now to speak of Ray.**

April 6, 1970: **You have thought of soul J____.**
*"Yes."*
**Have message, but must have permission from soul to give same.**
*"How is permission gained?"*
**Ask.**
*"Can you tell me of J____?"*
**Mother has not heard bidding of Ray; thinks daughter to play with Devil. J____ could learn to become close to God, only through lessons from Ray. Must listen or soul is lost again, or she will dream forever of houses, which are her soul. Unless she heeds, her mother shall die. Must not play with power unless believe in God, her creator.**

**Many messages. Many souls. You may ask questions of any subject as long as permission is given from the soul. Only way to give details is if soul has permission and really needs help — both mental for the soul and physical for the body.**

**Am growing weak; is time to awaken Ray from his slumber.**

April 11, 1970: **Now I have a reading for soul [4-3-70-002].\* She must discontinue the drinking of coffee because her body chemicals are changing, as they change and have changed since the beginning of time in all men. Her body chemicals are changing so that she may receive the insight of God, as yours are changing.**

**Remember also, you have talked of diet. This is good.**

**In soul [4-3-70-002], she has a problem of an old back injury. I see a vertebrae which is tilted; it should be fourth from the bottom. She should see, not a chiropractor, but an osteopathic doctor to make these adjustments.**

*\*Editor's note: Numbers have been substituted for names and personal information to respect the individual's privacy.*

April 11, 1970: **I see that thy group should change the water that** thy drink, and drink of distilled water. There is a strong acid content to this water, also another foreign chemical called "salicyscope" which has contaminated the water of this area.* If this chemical is not used again for eight months, the water shall have a chance to cleanse itself, and then it will be good again, except for the acid content. Therefore, the purchasing of water from another area, which has been, then been distilled, would be good. Do not distill the water from here because you have not the means of cleansing it, and it would be too costly.

Now, you have other questions which I shall answer, if I am given permission.

*"Yes, I — I have become interested in the last few days in distilling this water. Do you mean that we could not get the chemical out by distillation?"*

No, not unless thy run it through carbon filters after the distillation.

*"Thank you very much."*

The carbon filters must come, could come, from the carbon which can be extracted from what thy call thy *"mesquita."*

*"Mesquite?"*

Yes. If, by burning at one — no, at 560 degrees Fahrenheit, and then re-burning at the same temperature, three times, then using the carbon extracted from this as filter, after the water has been distilled, then it could be made purified.

*"Where should we buy water from?"*

The water which comes from the Safford area is fair, but not good because it has a large sulfur content, a sulfuric acid content.

*"How about Wilcox?"*

Wilcox has — and shall come to pass — the chemicals of [oil] leaking into its water; therefore, it is not too good. But yet, in the San Simon Valley at — at the Shainty place.

*"Shainty?"*

It is known as the Shanty place, and it is an artesian well which flows.

What other question?

*"What about the purified water such as 'Cascade' or — "*

[Rod turns to ask Ray's wife, Margaret], *"What other purified water in place of this?"*

She answers him, *" 'Triple A' "*] —

*" 'Triple A?' Will the purified water from any of the commercial companies be good?"*

Yes, your "Triple A" would be fair; they use carbon filters in their distilling process. It is not perfect, but it's better than what you would normally find.

*"The water from the artesian well at the Shanty place is very good, isn't it?"*

Very good; once distilled, would be perfect.

*"All right."*

It is almost in a pure form now.

There is one other place; it is a place in Arizona called Agua Caliente.

*"Uh huh."*

That water could be very good. But also it should be filtered.

*"Not distilled, but filtered?"*

Yes, that's true — because it is picking up a very, not strong, but a fairly strong iron content. There is one other well, and it is pure in its present form. This well has been capped for ten years. It is owned by what you call a railroad company. It is located in the town known as Coolidge, Arizona. Ray, soul Ray, which at that time was known by his family as soul Ammie, knew of this well. He has blotted this memory from his mind, but when he awakens, I shall place this thought in his mind, and he may tell you about it.

*"Why? Will it be easy to get the water, or will the railroad give us trouble?"*

They will give a slight bit of trouble, but I think — I must ask for permission, will thy wait?

*"Yep."*

Permission has been granted.

You should write a letter to the Southern Pacific Railroad Company, to "Care of the Division Engineer's Office, Tucson, Arizona," asking for permission to take water from their railroad well at Coolidge, Arizona. This water is also high in chemicals which are very good for the teeth and the preservation of the teeth. If this water is drunk, none of thy group shall ever have cavities in thy mouth and shall have teeth, all of them, to the day that thy pass into my plane.

---

\*Editor's note: The U.S. Forest Service sprayed "Agent Orange," which had recently been used in the Vietnam war to defoliate forests, on mountainsides near Globe, Arizona, to increase water runoff. Later it was found to cause cancer and birth defects. Aka may have been speaking of "Agent Orange" in the drinking water, or of another chemical that seeped into the ground water from local copper mining.

---

April 11, 1970: *"Do you have any more specific information on the diet or hygiene or the care of Ray's body?"*

Yes. He must also seek osteopathic treatment. He has nerve pressure in the joint between the neck bone and where the collar bones connect.

He also needs, as I said before, more fish in his diet. He also needs rare beef, not pork, but rare beef in his diet, at least once a week, and very rare, almost to the warming of the meat and serving it to him. At least once a week, feed him a fish which is high in iodine, in sulfur, in calcium. These fish can be had locally. Or (chuckle) with his desire to fish let him catch his own; they are there. (Chuckle) it's also good for his soul

(chuckle.)

Also, to relieve the pressure that we have built on his mind, it would be good for at least every third day, and if thy can, every other day, put him into trance state. We do not mean, this you must realize, with [the injury, the hemorrhage] of his brain, new tissue has grown and been replaced. This tissue has helped the changing his body chemicals so we may pass through more easily. But we also had to build a barrier, that only spirits of our kind and not of the lost spirits could pass through him. We had to do this that he could maintain his sanity. As a result, the headaches he has are as pressure from this barrier of other spirits trying to come through, but also partially from the pressure of our presence.

His body chemicals will change even more rapidly, so that farther awakening knowledge may come to him. Bear with him — it will be harder for him — for he will know things that we would want him to know. And I say, "of we," I speak of the spirits of God.

Now, that will do at this time. Also feed him spinach, as you call it (chuckle). Feed him as many raw vegetables as he will eat. Avocados are good for him. This will build a vigor. This is also high in what thy call the vitamin B, and D, which he needs at this time. These vitamins are better to come in their natural form than any other way. Sometimes in the processing of vitamins they have used too much heat, therefore, killing the effect of the vitamins that are needed for the human chemicals.

But remember, your chemicals are changing. Your diet must change with it. Each of you, diet is, as individuals, the individual choice. Answer your urging, for as the body of man is similar to an animal, think thee of the animal's instinct for certain foods. Your body tells you if you will listen. These same urgings, heed them.

April 13, 1970: **You have a reading from a small child. This [worries me] very much, for this is an essential.**

*"This is on [4-13-70-002]?"*

**This is true, on soul [4-13-70-002].**

*"All right."*

**Ask, and this reading shall be granted.**

*"And [4-3-70-002] has asked that a general health reading be given on [4-13-70-002]."*

**Normally, through [4-3-70-002]'s request, this could not be granted. This request comes from the child's mother, and the mother has explained to the child; therefore, all souls are in accord. There shall be [no] mental block on the soul [4-13-70-002].**

Her biggest problem at this time is that the child's body is developing far beyond her age in numbers. Her time for menstrual is about to start. Her mother — it is hard to believe this because of the years — the child needs very definitely to see a good gynecologist. Therefore, it would be suggested that there is a doctor in Tucson,

Arizona, who we would recommend, not because he is so much greater than others, but he would be practical in their small budget for medical needs and be sympathetic, both toward the child and the parents' financial needs. His name is Doctor Scott. He was connected a few years before with a Doctor [Bernard]. He is very good and should be consulted.

Next, with this child, since they did not ask for, only a medical reading and not a life reading on this child, the other information on the child's lives cannot be given at this time. But the child's diet should be changed — very definitely.

Next — first, I should finish with the diet. I must seek some information on this; if you would wait for a moment I should have it.

*"All right."*

Yes, now we have the full information. The child's diet consists of too many starches; therefore, she should have more protein in her diet. Should this be done with a rare meat, the child should have the liver of beef. The child should have, not of the black olive, but of the green olive, more of this. The child should have a more regulated diet, in other words, three meals a day, for fasting for this child is not good because she is developing so fastly that her body is eating up all of the energy.

Second, there are certain vegetables the child should have more of in her diet. One, the child is a slight diabetic; therefore, in the preparing and eating, at least once a day, of Jerusalem artichoke, this will be very necessary in her diet. This is the reason, one of the reasons, for the, oh, child feeling as though she doesn't care. Next, parsley, more of this should be served [to] the child. More okra would be very good. Second, the child should have more fish in her diet, at least once a week.

Now, as I have told your group, this child should stop drinking the water from this area at this time. The water is contaminated. It is affecting the child's nervous system very, very harshly. They should purchase their drinking water.

Third, the child has, and should have, by her mother preferably, the child has certain desires of a physical nature. They are interfering with her religious state, with what [she's] being taught, that these things are wrong; therefore, she feels herself, for feeling these urges, deeply in sin. This is wrong. Teach not a child that the natural things of the body are sin! Teach her of her waiting, but of the wonders God has placed in the body. This does not come from the Devil, as some have thought, but from the Lord, our God, our Father.

Now, the child's spiritual need should be fed. But as soon as possible, get her to a medical doctor — if not the one I have suggested, then another, but soon. The child's health is deeply in danger.

That is all of the reading on soul [4-13-70-002].

*"All right. While [we are on] this particular vein...."*

One other thing, this child should have readings as she progresses. There will be certain changes in her chemical makeup of her body that she should heed, so her readings should be often.

*"Once a week?"*

At this time that would do.

*"All right.*


April 13, 1970: *"We have so many important questions I don't know which one to ask next."*

Ask thee of the second reading thy had in mind.

*"[4-7-70-002] has requested a reading on her headaches."*

Her headaches, as we have given this information to soul Ray in his awaking, partially are from the lack of calcium in her body, secondly, from the need of more rest, thirdly, the chemicals of her body are greatly in danger at this time. You were given [these] two suggestion by soul Ray. One you have heeded, the second you have not. Get her the other substance which Ray, soul Ray, has suggested. Then, she needs more of vitamin B. This [could] build. If she could think of her soul at peace, her headaches would go downward.

First — have I her permission to give a medical reading?

*"Yes,"* [she says.]

*"Yes."* [Rod, the hypnotist and her husband, says.]

Then, with this in mind, we will take it step by step.

In your hypnosis, it's too fast, too swift; there's not enough time. You are crowding it, too swiftly.

*"With [4-7-70-002]?"*

Yes. Take her in slowly and out very slowly. Leave her there for longer periods of time. Do not, and I repeat — and I repeat, do not try to suggest away any of the pains of her own body. These pains are there for a reason. Should you suggest, the mind shall take the suggestion, but the warning which her body is sending out, you are disguising. Therefore, she needs the hypnosis for the rest and the comfort of her soul.

Secondly, she still has an injury of her back which she received as a small child, of the pelvic. Before, it was suggested by soul Ray that she see a chiropractor. Now, it is my suggestion that she see an osteopathic doctor for certain corrections of her pelvic region. This should be done immediately for [her] preparation for the birth of her child.

I have warned you before of her diet. Put more fish in her diet, [put] — with her it would have to be cooked down quite a lot, yet, it would not really be necessary. But you could get the same thing from the soy bean as you could from the beef, and probably in her case it would do more good. Uh, you will find that you already have this information in a diet book by soul Cayce. Heed this. Remember, though, that her soul is an individual soul with individual needs. If you should go ahead, getting two — the one you have, [and] the one you haven't — of [the] substances suggested by soul Ray, her health shall improve quite definitely.

That is all for this time on soul [4-7-70-002].

*"The other substance was more calcium, is this correct?"*

**This is true.**

*"Thank you."*

**And, some will laugh, but with the combination of the substance you already have and the substance known as Lydia E. Pinkham, which can be purchased in the same store which you purchased the last, this will greatly improve.**

*"Use the combination, you say?"*

**Yes.**

*"All right."*

**But you should have regular readings on her so that her count on certain substances does not rise beyond the control.**

*"Once a week suitable with her too?"*

**Yes.**

*"All right.*

April 13, 1970: *"Do you have an osteopath that you would suggest for [4-3-70-001], [4-3-70-002], and [4-7-70-002], and anyone else who should, who would be sympathetic towards this work, and also practical in the monetary end?"*

**Yes, there is one in Tucson and there are several in Phoenix. At this time, it has been suggested that this should come from thy free choice. This choice is suggested for this reason, because, as I have said before, your body chemicals, all of you, are changing so acceptance of this work may go on. With this in mind, it is time now for you to pick one for yourself.**

**If you are in doubt, then there is an osteopath on McDowell Street, the number is thirty, six [306]. Yes, I think that is what I read. It is close to the downtown area. If I think right, it is off of 3rd Street, off of McDowell. It, ah, the name, this Doctor Jennings — [Jones] — [Howell?] — I must check this again.**

*"Check."*

**If you will give me a moment [I'll go and] look.**

*"You have it."*

**Yes, now [we] have it; Dr. Jensen would be very sympathetic to your work.**

*"All right."*

**But as I said before, try on some things to pick up yourself because, for what is good for one [will] not always be good for all.**

*"All right.*

April 13, 1970: *"Well, I have a couple of other questions here, but I think possibly our visitors have some questions. One, a soul named John [4-13-70-003], [who] was here last night, asks the question, 'Who am I, past and present?'"*

John, soul John is himself. All he needs to do is find himself. He needs help. Give this to him. Bring him here that I might speak with him.

*"All right."*

One thing else. I shall say this much. The reason for his frustration is from another plane. It's something he must learn. Once he has learned this, then the knowledge of his previous planes we will be glad to have known to him.

This is all on soul John at this time.

*"All right."*


April 15, 1970: **Also, if the things that I have suggested are done our time will grow longer.**

Now you have asked the question of the group, how may they cleanse thy soul and body? This I shall answer. The body is pure within itself; it is only sometimes our diet that makes it unpure. Then I tell thee the same — take thee of the root of the sage, fast, eat one meal per day.

Now this cannot be done with all, for certain of your group must have three meals per day, every day. Soul [4-7-70-002] must have three meals per day, but leave out the starches. With the substance we have already given her, she would be inclined to gain too much weight. It bothers me that she has not complied with our last reading.

*"In what way?"*

The substances that we have suggested, she has not taken regularly, and not all of them. This is needed, not only now, but in the future, for a preventative of any female trouble in her body. Should she take the things we have suggested, her body shall be whole for the bearing of children, all of her female organs shall mature and be everlasting.

*"We have had a problem obtaining one or two of the items. Our water has not come, and the calcium has not come; it is ordered. There is a question on 'Lydia Pinkham,' and the 'SSS,' of just how this should be combined. You said it should be in combination, and as to the dosage we have a question."*

For one week, take the prescribed dosage on the bottle. After the second week, drop it into one-half dosages. At that time ask for another reading, because her body chemicals are developing quite rapidly, and at that time the — at that time, we can take another reading.

*"How should these be combined?"*

Taking as prescribed on the bottle. If necessary, these may have an ill taste to her, I would suggest that they be disguised some in some type of either fruit or vegetable juices, but not a citrus fruit.

*"All right. Ah, yes, we were going to ask about the citrus fruit."*

The citrus fruit, preferably. This does not have to be because other substances come from the same as citrus, but preferably a certain amount of citruses for your climate should be eaten daily. This is the reason God placed them here in this climate. Now, I shall have — no, that will wait for another time. Ask thy other question.

*"[4-7-70-002] asks, how can she take these substances without throwing up?"*

I have already told her.

*"By disguising them, and by laying off the starches. [4-7-70-002] also asks, she would like to know about a pinching on the inside of her chest cavity."*

Is she not to bear a child? Her body is readying itself for this. There will be many changes in her body. Therefore, there will be certain cramps, [for] which we have prescribed certain medication that will take care of these. The next is more rest.

April 15, 1970: *"All right.[4-20-70-001] has requested a general health reading."*

Yes, we have soul [4-20-70-001] in our mind. Soul [4-20-70-001] suffers from slight inflammation of the kidneys and slight infection of the uterus. Also she needs a change in diet to improve and help her eyes. She needs a change of her lens; this, in itself, would help correct her eyesight.

First, with the diet — the eating of more carrots, celery, and okra in her diet would greatly improve this area.

Now we see she has something like (chuckle) a corn which bothers her on her foot. Well, there are many very good corn removers now.

Also, she needs to see a good medical doctor, and then, in her case, it would be advisable to see a chiropractor for straightening out certain things in her back. We see, somewhere she has a slight fracture of the left upper part of the leg. But if she does the others, this will take care of itself because it mended a little out, not quite right; it would not be suggestible for re-breakage.

Now, these baths I have suggested would be very good for her.

Also, we see she has sinus condition, almost of asthma. It would be suggested that she eats three times a day a honey from the mesquite, putting three drops in each of her — drops of vinegar, in each — would you wait and let me check that? Yes, now it is better — three drops of vinegar, of the pure apple, mixed in her honey.

Now, we also see that she must either cut off, shorter, her hair or wear it in such a way that it is not serve such a pulling of the scalp. Now, if she should decide that she does not want to do this, then it would be suggested that she use a hot olive oil treatment on her scalp. This should be done by first applying the olive oil into the scalp, and then rubbing very, very vigorously until her scalp becomes warm; then taking hot towels, wrapping her skull in these, as hot as she can stand, repeatedly.

If she does this — there is one other thing (chuckle) — I think, for the taking of what is known as Lydia E. Pinkham, It would help her vitality and preserve her female organs. Otherwise, should she become pregnant again, and, for some reason, I think she might, she would have a rather hard time carrying this child. That is all.

April 15, 1970: *"Is 'Lydia E. Pinkham' a friend of yours? (Laughter)."*
No. There are some here who think that more should be done for the preservation of the female organs. This substance, not only, if taken regularly, would improve the whole female — I won't say improve, but preserve what organs there are of the female, even to the more maturing of the breast, keeping it firm.
That is all.

April 15, 1970: *"How much time do we have?"*
We have time left. Ask thy question.
*"How often should* [4-20-70-001] *take this? Just as prescribed on the bottle?"*
As prescribed on the bottle.
*"Ok.*

April 15, 1970: Now, I have something else for you. Thy teeth have bothered thee. I would suggest that thy get immediate attention, because not all of thy teeth shall have to be extracted. Save those that thy can save! Also, thy must get more rest. Now, at a later time I should give a more complete reading on you. We must study this.

April 15, 1970: Now, there is one among you who has requested a health reading. We do not have the name, only that it is, there is a troubled soul — and this permission has been granted. If this person should take — first, using a very good cleansing cream upon her face and hands; then second, by using a compound made of soda and water, placing this almost like a mud pack upon her face; then with the use of olive oil — first, between there, there must be the use of an alcohol base, after this has been taken, the soda has been taken away — then the use of an olive oil rub; and then, with hot towels, as hot as she can stand them, her complexion will clear. But only if she should cleanse her soul, for there is the biggest reason for her problem.

April 15, 1970: Now, you have one more question; ask this question.
*"Well, it seems that, uh, I would like very much to have my teeth repaired, but there is a little problem, called money."*
There is a dentist in the town of Miami; if thy go to him this will be taken care of.
*"I see."*

April 15, 1970: **Now thy have another question, not thy, but [4-3-70-002] has another question, soul [4-3-70-002.].**

*"Soul [4-3-70-002], she asks (chuckle), 'Why sometimes do I become frustrated and almost afraid?'"*

**This is normal. Seek a peace within thyself. Also, be patient with thyself, for thy chemicals are changing. Do not drink too many hot beverages, nor neither real cold.**

April 15, 1970: **Now thee have a question. Let it be known.**

*"I?"*

**Yes.**

*"I have, hmmm, a thousand."*

**Then, thy have a soul in thy group tonight known as [4-6-70-003]. Let her ask her question.**

*"Just a minute."*

"Aka?" [the woman asks.]

**Yes.**

"It is my husband's health I am concerned with."

**I realize this. Then soul [4-7-70-001] shall ask and receive from thee a health reading, but for some reason, permission has not been given from thy husband. This should be obtained from him as soon as possible. And come back and this shall be given. But it would be suggested that also a life reading should be given upon him that certain other information can be handed down.**

April 20, 1970: **And permission granted. Now, you have a reading from a soul [4-20-70-001].***

*"Yes."*

**This permission has been granted.**

**For the first proportion of this, we shall say, there is certain information which might be harmful to him if he thought others knew; therefore, this information will be given at another time and only to him. Now, he is, he has, for one thing, a very deep-seated guilt complex. We shall go in that, as I said, at another time.**

**But to the physical body — first, it would be good for him to have the baths that were suggested, as before. Also, it would be good for him to drink of the sage root for the cleansing of his kidneys. This would be also for the cleansing of the soul; it is also a good tonic for the cleansing of his kidneys. Because of the drinking of alcohol, he has a slight case of what is known as uremic poisoning and inflammation of the liver. This man should not drink any alcoholic beverages under any condition at all because it is killing his body functions. When we speak of the body function, the body in itself is a pure source of energy, and usually in birth — unless from some past life is carried through — is usually in perfect working order.**

Now, this soul needs lens, corrective lens.

Also, it would be suggested for osteopathic treatment for an injury he received as a child. This injury has affected a proportion of his mind.

Once this work was done, I'm sure his mind would be a great deal clearer.

Now, we see a problem of a collapsing of arteries. He should see a good medical doctor and a check be taken of this. There are natural herbs he could take. But for some reason we feel as though he would feel better taking medicine from a doctor, and prescribed by a doctor. There is no great urgency; this is a gradual process and shall really not affect him until his later years.

We see a slight arthritis of the left knee and cramping of the fingers also, arthritis there. The arthritis is growing in the body. We would suggest the baths for this would be very good. Also, there is a cactus in thy region known as the Night-Blooming Citros [Cereus].

*"Night-blooming what?"*

Citros. The digging up of the part of this plant and the eating of it in its natural form, though it would have a bitter taste, would be good for this. Do not boil this plant, and be careful with it, because it contains certain poisons and also a certain alcoholic content to it. Therefore, use it in its natural form, in very small quantities.

*"How much and how often?"*

Oh, we would say the chewing of a quarter-by-one inch — in thy measurements — per day would be sufficient.

*"Just chew it?"*

Yes, in its natural form.

*"And spit the pulp out?"*

Right.

*"Ok."*

*Editor's note: Numbers are substituted for names to respect privacy.

April 20, 1970: *"Yes, I have it written down. It was stated that at a later date this reading could be given, and I would ask at this time, if possible, to give both health and life readings."*

Yes, we have the soul, [4-3-70-001], here. We also have his body. It would be suggested that you also should seek certain — no, that is not right. It has been suggested that thy seek, first, dental care. This is poisoning thy whole system, and if it was not done soon, shall cause a great amount of trouble of the gall bladder and of the liver area. These both, in their working, were meant to extract the poison; you are overloading these.

Now, it would be suggested, — and there is doubt in your mind of where to get the root of the sage. It grows in great quantities a short distance from you, wild. The cultivated does not have the mineral that we seek in it. Now, it would be suggested, in your case, of the drinking of this three times a day, approximately one-half pint, without sugar, as a tea form. If this is not compatible, even the chewing of the root would help, but not give you what we have desired from this.

Also, it would also be suggested that you need an osteopathic doctor from an old injury of the right knee, of the right shoulder, and of the upper proportions of the neck. Also, there are a definite amount of straightening to be done in the back area — this would also be suggested — a very definite amount. This would help in thy seeking of sleep more readily.

It would also be suggested that thy get more rest.

Also, it is suggested, the eating of soy bean, prepared, as the religion of a — known of thy plane as the Seventh Day Adventists prepare this — very good. Now, the more eating of okra in thy diet would be good, of radish, of carrots, of celery. The lessening of salt in thy diet would also be good. This is suggested for the purification, and the help of the purification, of the blood.

It is also seen that in later years, unless certain precautions are taken, that you shall have what is known as a hardening of the arteries.

Now, also, eating of the pulp of the Night-Blooming Citros [Cereus] would be suggested in the quantities of, a little larger of that, maybe an inch by an inch in your case. This would also help in the prevention of any arthritis in the body.

Now we see a lesion from improper diet as a child. This lesion is centered around the left kidney area. It would be suggested there — by using hot castor oil packs, as hot as you can stand it, very, very hot — use this in, on cloth and use it in three layers — no, no, this isn't right, four, four would be better — as hot as can be applied to this area. Keep this on, if you can, for, oh, 12 to 24 hours, and then another reading should be taken after this.

Also, you have a scalp problem — unless it is corrected, could cause the falling of the hair. This problem and the tightening of the scalp could be relieved with hot olive oil treatment — rubbing very, very brisk — vigorously into the scalp area, and then using, as hot as you can stand it, hot towel treatments. Then, after this is over, using a good natural shampoo on the hair would be good. Now, this would do for the body at this time of soul [4-7-70-001].

Now for the soul in itself. The need for more belief in mankind would help thy soul tremendously; less doubt. There was words spoken once before in the time of David — "For who but a fool should speak that there is no God? And the belief of him would only bring foul and foolish things."

There was something else spoke — "How many times shall my Lord forgive thee of thy sins? And thy Lord spoke back and said, 'FOREVER.'" But the Lord shall shed for each of these times a mighty

tear, and He should cry for thy soul* — as He cries for all thy souls and
spirits, for He loves thee so.**

Now, you have a great question, and permission has been granted
upon this. As we have told you before that no money, as thy call it, or
material needs may come from these readings, only when they are to help
thy spirit, thy soul and thy family. In this case, permission also has been
granted for it.

*Editor's note: The voice is sobbing deeply.
**Such love is heard in the voice.

April 20, 1970: **This information is of [4-7-70-002]. Soul [4-7-70-
002] — it cannot be given at this time until permission has been given by
herself.**

*"We have her permission."*

*"Well, what other information did he ask?"* [Editor's note: Rod, the
moderator, seems to be speaking to someone else in the room.].

*"Okay."* [She answers him.]

*"We have her permission."*

**Permission still has not been given; there is a psychological block
there. It would be suggested that this be brought up at a different time.**

*"What is the nature of this?"*

**It is in *her* mind. Until this matter is cleaned up in her own mind,
no further information may be given to her, or about her.**

April 24, 1970: **Now, ask thy other questions.**

*"Aka, you said last week the health reading on soul [4-13-70-002]
should be continued."*

**Yes, we have soul [4-13-70-002]. We have her body here.**

**The advice given in the last reading has not been totally included
at this time. It was told at that time that the eating of Jerusalem
artichoke, Jerusalem artichoke at least once a day and the preparing of
it.**

**Also, the water that she is drinking is causing great harm to her
body. It would be advised that the purchasing of water, or water taken,
as I have told before, in the location and the streams of the Young valley,
filtering in the proper process, would greatly improve her health.**

**Also, she should be taken to a good gynecologist. There is no
definite threat right now, but there shall be in the future. Soul [41370002]
shall go and grow into her teens. As she approaches this time, without the
help needed from [your] gynecologist, her whole mind and attitude shall
change. With that help, her mind will stay normal and progress along the
plans of God.**

**If these things are done, when she is 19 she shall wed — and she
shall have three children, a boy and two girls. At that time, if she is
taught and coached properly, her mind will be developed to where she**

shall become, as you'd call it, a psychic, but this will come slowly and should not be pushed. But do the others, first, and then you shall look beyond.

*"We are having trouble acquiring the Jerusalem artichoke."*

If thy would go to the food stores in Phoenix, Arizona, there thy would find the needed plant. Also, thy could have it ordered from thy Safeway Store here. If this is not advisable, then it would be advisable at this time to have her see a good medical doctor who would prescribe certain insulin in a very mild form for her. It would be better, the Jerusalem artichoke [would] make her body normal; putting her on insulin [would] continue her being a diabetic as long as she lives. The artichoke would stabilize her body, and gradually, she will become at a point to where she will not need it. This is why it was suggested.

*"Very good."*

If these suggestions are taken, the wounds of her body will heal very rapidly.

April 24, 1970: **Now it is time,** [Editor's note: his breathing deepens] — now is the time that thy guide comes to thee and shall speak through I to thee. Listen and thy shall hear thy guide.

"Margaret, I come to thee, for I am one of thee. Thy have known me before, for I walk with thee and sometimes try to talk to thee, but thy do not listen."

Now, in thy meditation, think thee of Linda, and she shall come to thee and guide thee and walk with thee in thy daily life. She shall teach thee love and compassion, and she shall teach thee all things that thy must know. Now think of her, and she shall come through I. [Editor's note: another voice spoke through the body of Ray; it sounded higher with different intonations, and it was dramatically different than the one that had been speaking.]

"Margaret?"

*"Yes."*

"I am Linda. I come to you because the Council has let me speak. Thy must learn to love. Thy must learn to give of thyself. I must go."

*"I must what?"*

Now you have heard from her. She shall come again to you.

April 29, 1970: [Rod asks Ray's wife and the group]:

*"Are any of these, uh, in a real rush — anything drastic here?"*

*"We have three readings. But first, I would like a regular weekly reading which was advised by yourself on [4-7-70-002]. Any corrections in her diet and this sort of thing?"*

Her diet is going along fairly well. There are a few changes. One of these that would be suggested, that consuming a little more, as you would call it, radish, in her diet would be helpful. Also, as we have suggested before — the seeking for osteopathic treatment as soon as advisable would be suggested. We have noticed that as the changes come into her body, it would be advisable at this time for her to increase the intake of calcium by at least 10 milligrams a day.

*"This is in addition to what she's taking now?"*

**Yes.**

*"All right."*

**With this, we should take another reading at a different time.**

*"Is it time to change the Lydia Pinkham's and the SSS dosage?"*

**Yes. Cut it now down to one-fourth for one week. The present intake — the body is consuming far too much of this right at this time. After one week it would be suggested that you take a further reading. Also, it would be suggested that the taking of the sage root for her once a week would be suggested.**

*"Uh, one cup full of the tea?"*

**Yes, one cupful of tea. This should be watched to see that there are no offensive reactions to her body. If there is, stop it immediately.**

*"All right."*

**If she should break into a rash of the chest it would be suggested that this be stopped.**

*"Uh, what is the sage tea for?"*

**One, for her soul; the other, for cleansing of the body.**

*"Anything else?"*

**This is all at the present time.**

April 29, 1970: *"We have a reading for* [4-29-70-001]*...He's in school."*

**Repeat the name.**

*"[4-29-70-001.]"*

**And the suggested reading?**

[Rod says to Ray's wife]: *"Uh, health reading?"*

*"Health reading."*

**At this time we shall give a fraction of that. Because one, in this case, would not be any good without the other — because the boy's mental balance is deeply affecting his body at this time. Also, for his diet, [it] should be changed — with more fish in his diet, at least twice a week if this is possible — the more eating of raw vegetables. The present type is good. But it would greatly improve his mental attitude with the eating of okra in his diet, which he is not now receiving.**

**Also, the child should see a dentist. There are a problem in his molars, which is also affecting his mental attitude.**

**There are certain psychological blocks caused by the death of his father of this plane. It would be advised that this child be told that his father is at complete rest, and loves him very dearly. It would also be suggested — that more outdoor recreation, more outdoor exercise for this**

child. And at the present time do not push the child into crowds of people. Let him go back gradually. This will satisfy his own need for companionship.

Now, the child needs certain corrective shoes at this point. And, it would be suggested that the taking of calcium because of certain bone deficiencies in his body.

Yes, also — no, not now, but in the near future — it would be suggested that he be taken to a good medical doctor.

At this present time the boy has a slight case of the flu. Now, as I have suggested before, for the prevention of certain diseases in the body and viruses of the body, that the drinking of the sage tea would be recommended. Also, in this child's case, the eating of the Night Blooming Citron [Cereus] would also be suggested in the quantity of a quarter-by-a-quarter of an inch.

*"Chewed or eaten?"*

**Chewed.**

*"Ok."*

Now, the baths that I have suggested before would be good with the sinus condition of this child.

Also, it would be recommended that the mother of the child spend more time with the child, and that the child seek more food for his soul. It would be suggested, as soon as possible, the family in itself return to church, and therefore, by attending together, it will grow together.

This is all at this time on soul [4-29-70-001].

*"On soul [4-29-70-001]?"*

April 29, 1970: *"We have two other readings here. If they are urgent you might — one is a [4-28-70-002], the other is [4-28-70-003], all of the same family. If there is anything urgent here, we'd like to have it, otherwise —"*

On [4-29-70-003], soul [4-29-70-003], it would be suggested — one moment, please.

*"All right."*

This child is deeply affected at this time. The child has a very bad sinus infection. It would be suggested that if the baths that we have suggested before are not available, that the taking of salt water for this child, boiling it very slightly, that the water becomes slightly to a boil; using a towel above the child's head for a vapor, and letting her breathe of this would be very good. And if sea water cannot be obtained, using the pure sea salt in the pint of water, after the water has been boiled, and then left to cool and then placing the salt in it, and brought to a slow boil again. [it] would be very helpful to her.

The other child has a mastoid condition. This should be taken care of by a medical doctor as soon as possible. The rest will be taken up at a different time.

*"All right.*

April 15, 1970: *"The little girl, [4-13-70-002], that a medical reading was given on last time, her mother has requested the life reading."*
First, take the steps that were suggested in her medical reading. Then come back, and thy shall be given her life reading. If these steps are not taken, there shall be no life to read.

April 20, 1970: Now we have (chuckle) as I have said before, a need for other help. He has asked for a life reading. In his case, a full life reading at this time cannot be given.
The suggestion has been made that he might seek employment at a different job. It would be suggested, rather than quitting his present job, that he ask and receive permission from his employer to be — as a leave of absence might be granted there. If it was done in this order, and then the waiting until the changing of his employer at the job in which he holds, he might find a great improvement there.
Ordinarily, readings of this type, for material gain, is not given unless we feel that it would affect his physical and mental body — also for the good of his family. That is the reason this information has been given.
It would also be suggested, as soon as possible, that he come here and speak with us in person. He has a great reluctancy on his part for this, for he fears the knowledge that we know.
That will be all on the time on [4-20-70-001]. He should have regular readings.

May 1, 1970: Now, there is a soul, which is not among you, which has asked and wanted a reading for health purposes. This soul has a non-malignant growth in the arteries which is wrapping itself around the arteries leading to the upper proportion of her head. It would be suggested that surgery be done as soon as possible. This may be detected by a physician very easily through x-ray. There may be — yes, this should be done preferably with what thy has known as a laser beam, so that it may be totally destroyed. Yet, if this is not done, it will — yes, three operations will be needed for the removal of all of the foreign matter.

May 1, 1970: *"Now we have a request for a follow-up reading on [4-13-70-002]."*
Yes, we have soul [4-13-70-002] here, and her body. There have been certain suggestions given before which have not been taken care of. If this child does not start with the eating of Jerusalem artichoke, she shall go back again. It would be suggested that if this cannot be done, and is not practical, that the child be put on a mild form of insulin. We do not

care for this at all, for once she is put on this, she will be inclined to take heavier doses the rest of her life. Also, her diet needs more vegetables. Since this seems to not be the thing to do at this time it would be necessary that the child to be given a very good natural vitamin and mineral supplement. It would also be suggested — one moment, please.

Yes, yes, now —

Yes, it would be suggested that taking of SSS, a tonic, known — yes — one moment — yes — that this should be given in not full dosage, but half dosage at this time.

*"Half the adult dose?"*

Yes. One moment — yes, yes — this also should be, uh — no — yes, this is correct. It also would be suggested that for the next 30 days, the child should not be sent anywhere alone without supervision, and this means the supervision of her parents, no one else. She should not be entrusted to the care of anyone. This is all on soul [4-13-70-002] at this time. It should also be suggested, that as soon as possible, that she be taken to a good gynecologist.

*"Can she go to school by herself?"*

This, this is all right — yes — For it is within the mind of someone else close to them, "an eye for an eye and a tooth for a tooth."

*"Mi_____'s mother would like to ask a question, if it's all right at this time?"*

Yes, let her come closer.

*"Aka, [4-13-70-002] was planning on having an overnight trip to [a] church activity with some other children and ladies during this 30 days. Should she be kept from this?"* [Mi_____'s mother asks.]

Yes, I think she should. One moment.

Yes.

She should not go; very definitely she should not go.

*"Very well."* [The mother answers.]

*"Any more on [4-13-70-002]?"* [The moderator, Rod, asks.]

This is all on soul [4-13-70-002] at this time.

May 1, 1970: *"And [4-3-70-002] has asked about a dream and about her general and, well, physical and mental health at this point."*

Yes, we have soul [4-3-70-002] and her body here.

Yes.

To begin with, she should stop taking the vitamins which she has taken, and instead go to a good natural form vitamin and mineral. These are one thing which is interfering with her health. But [these] should be taken regularly.

Secondly, it would be suggested that — yes — because of a certain problem in an ovary, it would be suggested that the taking of Lydia E. Pinkham at this time, in prescribed amount on the bottle.

Yes. Second, she should stop drinking the water of this area. It is having a very bad effect on her nervous system.

Now, also, information shall be given to soul [4-3-70-002]. We are preparing a block in [4-3-70-002] so no outside spirits or souls may enter. This will be the necessary for us, using soul Ray. Because of our usage, as I have said before, there are other spirits other than ourselves, and lost souls, who would do her harm. They will use all powers they can to stop our work here. This is why we shall build a block into her.

Now, we see soul [4-3-70-002] has a slight case of what thy call the flu. This is a virus attacking her system. It would be suggested, for one, in her diet, the eating of more fish, of the fresh water type, with using of salt of the natural state.

Now, we see from an old injury of soul [4-3-70-002], of a laceration — no, of the third — no, of the fourth vertebrae of the back area. Yes, this, this is true. It would be suggested, as soon as possible, that she see a good either osteopathic doctor or chiropractor.

Yes, ah — oh, yes — we see, ah, soul [4-3-70-002] also, from an injury received in the last two weeks, that the upper proportion of the neck is bothering the nervous system too. This should be straightened out at the time — yes, yes — this should be done.

It would help soul [4-3-70-002] a great deal if she could start each day with a prayer for guidance. Also, her dream. Yes, these dreams, as I have said before, are because of the coming of foreign souls to her.

This is all for soul [4-3-70-002] at this time except, as we have said before, the drinking of any liquids that are too cold or too hot for her would highly affect her nervous system. Within a short while, after she changes her drinking water, then she may go back to her old habits. That is all on soul [4-3-70-002] at this time.

May 1, 1970: *"[4-3-70-002] has asked about some information on this food supply."*
One moment, please.
Yes, there is a suggestion here for soul [4-20-70-001]. Change his drinking water immediately.
Yes, there is one who would speak to soul [4-20-70-001].
"I'm here." [Soul Bill says.]
*"Here is soul Bill."* [Rod says.]
[*"Utinte he sckmehat."*] [Editor's note: Here something was said in an unknown language, sounding like an American Indian dialect.]
Aka is here now.
*"Do you want to say anything to [4-20-70-002]?"*
No, message has been granted and given.

May 1, 1970: *"I have some red spots on my body. I would like for any pertinent information on these."*
(Chuckle.) Yes, your red spots are from a reaction from the

drinking of thy water. Your body is still not cleansed. If thy would do as had been suggested before, the gathering of the sage and drinking of the root of the sage, this would help considerably.

May 1, 1970: *"On [4-15-70-002], who was given a reading last time, had asked for information on her going to church, if she should continue with the Catholic, or if she should change? If so, she would like any suggestion that you have as to where she should go."*

Yes, it would be suggested that soul [4-15-70-002] either attend what thy call thy Lutheran church of this area or Episcopalian church of this area. These are close to the same religion which she knows of now. But it would also be good for soul [4-15-70-002] for the drinking of thy trough too.

*"Of the same water?"*

Yes, only there are many things for thee to learn too.

*"Yes, any suggestions?"*

Yes, take her thoughts, [4-7-70-001]. You were told before to study Paul, but do not study of his arrogance, nor of the times of his life plane; study of his devotion to God.

*"Whose?"*

Paul's — devotion to God. This would help thee considerable. If this was done, it would help thee to accept God. God is close to thee. All thee must do is accept Him. By accepting Him, then thy would accept this work and thy task in this work.

Now, soul Ray is growing very tired. It is time to awaken him, for we are growing very weak.

May 21, 1970: *"[5-21-70-002] wants to know, Aka, if you have a message for her tonight?"*

Yes, I, I should have, yes, I would have a message. [He exhales deeply.] One moment, please. [He exhales deeply again; then he exhales once more.]

Aka's voice: Yes, we have a message here for [5-21-70-002]. There are certain things on her mind that we are not allowed at this time to answer. It would be advised for her to have a life reading, both on herself and her child.

We have a problem here. We have a problem, Yes. It would be advised that she should seek medical help as soon as possible. So far, this growth is not malignant, but it could become malignant if neglected. Yes. Of her left breast, this should be taken care of *immediately*.

We also see that she has a problem with her slumber. This, we are sure could be handled if she would seek a greater peace of mind. If she should awaken in the morning with a prayer to God for guidance, her own controllers, then, would come through to her in her daily toil. There is important work for her here. This shall be taken up at a different time.

It would also be suggested that she seek chiropractic treatment for the adjustment of the back area and the neck area. We see she has a great deal of trouble and has had an old injury, with her tail bone. We believe that this could be taken care of here. Also, the drinking of sage tea would help immensely. Also, it would be suggested for her the taking of Lydia E. Pinkham. And also, we see that she is a slight diabetic; the eating of Jerusalem artichoke would help immensely.

Yes, yes. We also see [she has] a slight infection in the uterus area. This infection is leading down into the area of the womb; it should be taken care of — antibiotics immediately. This also — yes, yes — in her case, the boiling of the leaf of the sage and drinking it would be good too.

Oh, yes, we have a problem here of passing off the waste. It would be suggested the eating of more of what thy would call the cantaloupe or the watermelon would be good for her, it would help regulate her diet, her waste problems too.

Yes, yes. We have her, nervous headaches. Yes. This problem, should she change her drinking water — seek a more purified form of drinking water — you will find that I have described this in prior readings.

Yes, we — yes. The other things cannot be told at this time because of psychological block.

*"Thank you, Aka.*

May 21, 1970: "[4-13-70-005] *wants to know, 'Would you please tell me how my mother is doing? Am I helping her by sending her love and prayers?'"*

Yes, you're helping. And she shall help you. She has a — your mother has a slight problem. It would be suggested that pray that thy mother should look at the light, turn and look at the light. This would help her immensely. It would help if all your groups should pray this, and soul [4-13-70-005].

Yes, we see, yes . We also have her body here.

Yes. We have a problem here in the intestine, almost tied in a knot, crowding — yes. Yes. It would be suggested that the eating of the Night-blooming Cereus, this should be done as soon as possible — taking the Night-blooming Cereus and the sage root and bringing them barely to a boil, and sipping; three ounces of this daily will greatly help the stomach area. Yes, we, we also see a great amount of trouble in the bowel area. There is — can be done; this is going to take a long time because of neglect of this area over so many years. Yes. This is a karma that you must, ah — yes — we are not allowed to give that information at this time. Yes. It would be suggested, then, that she should seek in the desert area what thy call thy [nutrair serra, nutra cereus, nutra sierrias], of the cactus family. In thy plane, thy would know it as the flat leaf cactus. Boil the pulp from this cactus, add a little ginger to this; sweeten it very slightly. This should regulate and help this; this will have to be done over a long period of time. Yes, without now — yes, she should have more rest, very definitely, and dwell not so much on what has been, but what shall be. It would also be suggested that this subject use Lydia E. Pinkham — in the present dosage.

It would also be suggested that this subject soon have some osteopathic or chiropractic treatment. She has a problem of an old laceration of the 6th vertebrae. Yes, this could be straightened out. It would also be suggested for her the constructing of a bar approximately six inches above her reach, that she hang from this each day with her hands. This would stretch that area and let it slowly go back in place. Even after this area is put in place, because of the long neglect of this area, it will not stay there without this.

Yes. Yes. We see an infection of the mastoid, caused from the sinus. Yes. We have suggested — we have suggested before that certain baths be taken. This should be done in her case as soon as possible. She has an arthritic condition which will bother her worse as time goes on. And this would also help control her sinus condition.

This would be all on soul [4-13-70-005] at this time.
*"Thank you, Aka.*

June 6, 1970: [Editor's note: The voice changes back to the previous one, with a resounding depth, and without the drawl of Edgar Cayce who was speaking before]: **Aka is here. As it has been said before, there are thoughts in thy mind. Thy thoughts are very clear to us.**

**Thy, the two brothers, both have asked the same question, "How may I meditate?"**

**It would be suggested in both their cases that one should study first the works of John, that the other should study first the works of Peter. Then, if in thy mind before thy sleep at night, thy would think upon us and think of thy word, Aka, relate it with God and His works, thy answer shall come. And we shall send a messenger to thee — for there is waiting for each of you an entry, you would call it (chuckle) your guardian angel.**

June 6, 1970: **Now, there is in the mind of [6-6-70-001]'s wife, "Should my children be baptized into this church?"\* And I would answer you this way, the temple of God is in man. Only with the consent of the soul that dwells within thy temple can there be true baptism.**

June 6, 1970: **Now, thy have medical readings for certain souls.**
*"[6-6-70-002], [4-6-70-002]'s sister, has asked for either a medical or life, whichever is most important to her right now."*

One could not be given without the other. Yes, we have soul [6-6-70-002] here, and her body, yes, yes, yes. I think, at this time, let her finish with what she's doing and then we shall disturb her. Go to the next reading and then back to her.

June 6, 1970: *"All right.* [4-6-70-001] *has asked if there are any special health messages for him?"*

Yes, we see here, yes, we have soul [4-6-70-001]'s body and soul here, yes. Soul [4-6-70-001] has an infection of the lymph gland, yes. It would be suggested for soul [4-6-70-001] to have a complete physical examination by a doctor as soon as he can. There is no real rush here.

Then, oh, yes, we find here a karma. Certain things have been suggested for soul [4-6-70-001] before. He has been reluctant to overcome this karma.

Yes, we also see that in a short time corrective lenses shall be needed. These would not be needed if he would start certain eye exercises at this point.

Yes, we also see, yes, a infection, yes, of the pelvic area. Yes, this was caused from lesion. Yes, it would be suggested, as we have suggested before, the baths that we have suggested, yes — if this was done it [would] help a great deal.

Yes, we also see a lesion above the right, yes, above the right eyebrow — yes, yes — there is permanent damage which will cause, in later years will cause him a great deal of trouble here. It would be suggested that during his meditation he should increase his circulatory system in thought patterns here. He can do this if he really wants. Yes, but we find very lazy, yes. Then, one moment, please. Yes, the baths, it would help the circulatory system, but, ah, acetic acid, yes, would help, a few drops of this each day. It would be suggested that the, uh, eating of what thy call the flat cactus, taking of the, yes, taking of the fruit from this, the fruit of the Night-blooming Citros [Cereus], taking of the fruit of the sigar [saguaro], blending in equal parts, of the root of the sage, bringing this not to a boil but to a simmer, yes, then cooling this as fast as possible. Yes, this would help in the healing process. This would also help in the prevention of arthritis.

This soul should also be more careful in his own personal hygiene. We see, oh, yes, he should be a little more careful in his choice of mates. We see an infect — a slight infection here of the penial area, yes.

We also — yes, yes — this subject fell when he was very young, striking the head and also an old lesion of the temple area. Yes, this is causing headaches. Yes, we would suggest this subject should have — sometimes my colleagues forget what plane we are talking on. You will have to wait a moment while we translate. Yes — yes, he has a sinus condition here. And, it would be suggested that this subject should take of the eucalyptic [eucalyptus] tree, the leaves of the eucalyptic tree, boiling them, forming a tent over the boiling pot. This would help a great deal in this case.

Yes, this is all on soul [4-6-70-001] at this time. Oh, yes — it would also be suggested he have certain dental work done. Yes, this would help, but also to help settle his nervous system.

Yes, this is all on soul [4-6-70-001] at this time.

June 6, 1970: *"At this time, Aka, can you give a health reading on [4-6-70-002]?"*

Yes, we have soul [4-6-70-002] here. We have his body. We find old injury of the left foot, in the templic (?) area, yes. It would be suggested for this subject, that first, as hot as he can stand it, the soaking of the foot in either hot olive oil or hot castor oil. It would also be suggested that this subject, the rubbing in of all joints of the body, as hot as he could stand it.

Yes. It would also be suggested — yes, we have a slight heart murmur here. This is caused by clotting of the arteries, yes. This is not good. It would be suggested that this subject get a great deal more rest. He does not have to sleep to get this rest. Yes, one moment — yes, (sigh) yes — yes, before further, yes, yes, before further readings should be given that as before he sleeps tonight he should think upon our name, the word, Aka. As he thinks upon this name, in his own way he should pray to God that we may come through to him and heal his body, and as we heal his body his life shall be dedicated to our work, and for as long as he lives he shall have good health.

Now soul Ray grows tired, and we are growing weak.

June 6, 1970: *"Aka, before you leave, I have one question that I feel is important. Ray has been complaining of pains in his chest. Should this, is this anything serious?"*

We have made certain adjustments to take care of this. How much longer we can build up these areas we don't know, not at this time; only God knows this. (Sigh) he must have more rest, or no matter what we may do, he will destroy our lives — for as I have said before that "as we are Ray and Ray is I," yet we cannot control his awakening hours, only up to a point. He's a very stubborn person to the point of being stupid and bullheaded (sigh).

Yes, we have — (sigh) it would be suggested that he continue meditation of healing that he's taking at this time. Yes, of the tea — one moment — yes, as soon as possible, it would be suggested, take of the sage root, take either of the Night-blooming Citros [Cereus] or the sagar [saguaro] bloom. Boil these together and let, and drink this, oh, we will say, at least an ounce in morning and the afternoon.

Yes, one moment, yes, this should also be suggested for soul [4-6-70-002]. One moment, yes — it would be suggested that in four days from now another reading be taken on soul [4-6-70-002]. We are going to make some adjustments here.

June 9, 1970: **Now, soul B\_\_\_\_ — yes, we see much improvement** here.

**Now, thy have information for thy son, P\_\_\_\_, that he may walk in thy footsteps. Let him think of the story of David. Read upon this; learn from the scripture. It will help thy inner thoughts. Can thy understand this, son of Peter?**

*"Yes, Aka."*

June 9, 1970: **Therefore, we see much improvement with soul \_\_\_\_'s physical health. As we have suggested in other cases, for the purification of thy body, in this locale at this time, we see a virus which most of you think is a sinus growth. It is affecting both man and beast. This virus was started by chemicals used near here, which has infected thy water, even the water at the depth that thy are now taking it. We realize at this time that it would be impractical for you to drill to the depth of the pure water. Therefore, it would be suggested, find the root of the sage, boil it and drink at least one ounce both morning and evening, if possible. In your locale, it would be suggested to purify your water where you are. Drink, each of your family, of the sage.**

**But for their own personal drinking water, build thy slough, as thy would call it. In your case, build it 36 feet long. Build it in a one-foot cube, placing baffles every six inches. Drilling holes — the baffles should be made preferably of oak; if not, pine would do — oak would be better — drilling the holes in one-eighth diameter. Drill 50 holes in each baffle, at the last baffle placing carbon, either from the mesquita or it can be purchased locally. It would do as well. Then, in front and in back of the carbon, placing, as thy would call, the fiberglass back, wrapping this fiberglass in cloth of a close-knit nature, making a compartment where this fiberglass can be changed at least once a week. Therefore, this would purify thy water.**

**But still, at this time, to cleanse the growths that are starting in thy bodies, drink of the sage root, each of thy family.**

June 9, 1970: **We find in soul C\_\_\_\_, we have her, both body —** yes, **we find a great deal of trouble she's having with her feet. It would be suggested that thy would take what thy call the greasewood. Boil this, not once, but three times. Bring it to a boil, and let it cool. Bring it to a boil and let it cool again. Bring it to a boil a third time and let it cool. As thy do this, thy will find a substance coming from this would turn almost into a jelly. Take what is commonly known as soda, placing in this substance. Then take — yes, one moment, please — yes, apply this to the whole feet area twice daily. After this, it would be suggested taking hot olive oil,** first, rubbing the olive oil very vigorously into the foot area, yes, then placing the towels, as warm as she can stand them, over this area. This would greatly improve, yes.

Now we find a problem which was created by birth. This problem eventually, if not taken care of, is going to cause a great deal of trouble. Yes, we find infection in this area, the uterus area — yes, ah, yes, we find the — it would be suggested in this area, there are many very good baths for this area which could be purchased or a good vinegar solution, washing this area twice daily would help, yes, in this case. But we still find of the female organs, problems here. We would also suggest for this, this subject, that the taking of Lydia E. Pinkham as prescribed on the — would be suggested, yes.

Yes, this would also improve the blood area.

Thy have problems here.

Yes, we also see, yes, we find a slight problem in the third valve of the heart area. There are — yes, yes — yes, more rest of one form, and exercise of another form. Yes, we find, yes, rest would be needed of the rest, which is not sleep, just rest. Normal sleep would be suggested for this subject. Also, it would be suggested that this subject purchase a good electrical vibrator, placing this once a day over the heart area. Vibrations in this area would greatly improve the function of this heart. There are — at this time, we could suggest slight shock treatment, but this wouldn't — no, I think we could do without this at this time. Now, this also would help in the heart and blood area. We would suggest, as thy call them, the sauna baths for this subject. This would help the circulatory system.

Now, we find that this subject — less salt in the diet, more vegetables in the diet, more meat in the diet — fish, one of the fresh water, one of the salt water at least once a week. Also, the eating of more liver in the diet would help. Because of past karmas, it would be suggested this subject eat less pork. Yes, it would also be suggested for this subject that the eating of certain foods that she is doing at this time is causing her a great deal of gastrial areas, both of the stomach and the pressure upon the heart. This should not be done.

We also find that the subject — yes, we find the problem; this subject has a back injury, at one time. It would be suggested there is a good chiropractor in the town of Blythe. It would be suggested that this subject go there for treatment. Oh, wait — yes, we find this subject with her various attitudes seems to not — well, then go to a good osteopath or find another chiropractor. Either. Let this be to her own discretion. Yes.

(Sigh) Yes, we find this subject also has a scalp problem (sigh), and she is also worried about losing her hair, but she's not. But it would be suggested that the rinsing of her hair — washing her hair more regularly, rinsing it in vinegar, then rinsing it in good clean water, and then placing a good olive oil, rubbing very vigorously into the scalp, and then placing hot towels into this area as hot as she can stand it, would greatly help this area. And then leaving the olive oil on, oh, let's say for 35 minutes afterward, then washing the hair with any good shampoo would do. Yes.

Yes, also we find this subject has a problem with a rash. This is from her own nervous [tension] condition. The drinking of the sage tea would be necessary here. It would really help this area. Yes, yes, it would take, relieve some of the nervous tension here. Most of the nervous tension she could really relieve with prayer into herself, in her own way. Yes.

Now, we find this subject has a denture problem. This could be corrected very simply by going to her local dentist.

Yes, we also find a lesion of the muscular area, of the left upper portion of the [plamic? practic? pectic? thighatic? sciatic?] muscle. Yes, we could suggest castor oil packs for this area, very hot, leaving them on for at least an hour at a time. It would help this area. Exercise, more exercise, yes. At a later date we will give more specific exercise for this subject. And we should go deeper into the diet.

This is all on soul C_____ at this time, yes.

June 9, 1970: Now, for the good of soul Ray's mind, we will give a reading upon the little soul who in her own way, of Cinder. [Editor's note: Cinder was Ray's dog.] Give this poor animal purer drinking water, each day. Because of the drinking water, she has formed a growth. Now, we shall try through the spiritual mind of soul Ray to help this animal, and it would be suggested giving this animal more vitamins. Get her a good vitamin, with fish — yes, more liver in her diet. Change, yes, change, the, ah, food completely if you can. Mix your own mixture of food for a while. Give bone meal. Also in the food pour two ounces of the sage in her food. Cut down on the amount; feed her at least twice daily only in smaller quantities. Yes, a little rare beef in her diet, yes, for you see, even in the animal which was God's creation, it must have nourishment. On this animal [was] placed much love; that must be in her diet too.

June 9, 1970: Now, for the son of P_____, we should answer because the time goes slowly. We would suggest the same information given for the feet of his sister be used on the son. We shall improve upon this as time goes forward.

This, our information, could also be used on the daughter of soul M_____.

June 12, 1970: *"When we last talked with you, you told [4-6-70-002] how to purify his drinking water and the water for his family. [Prior?] you described a similar method to us. You have told us to put sand in the baffles. Was he also to use the sand?"*

(Chuckle). Sometimes, in the translation from our plane to yours, yes, it is sometimes confusing.

Yes.

But we would say this. In the first baffle, place crushed rock — better of granite for the first baffle; of the second baffle, sand, and then again crushed rock. Can thy understand this?

*"Yes, then do we alternate?"*

Can thy understand this?

*"Yes, Aka."* [4-6-70-002 answers.]

June 12, 1970: Now, there is a question in the mind of [4-20-70-001]. His first question we would answer this way. Only after the reading did these things happen as they did. We warned you earlier of caution. Remember, we can only suggest. You have your own free will to be born again or to choose the direction that thy would take upon this earth plane.

Now, the next question, "What can be done now?" We would tell you — nay, we would say this then. You had been offered a job already and you are thinking this over. Soon, you shall make a trip, and [there] you shall be offered another job. And when you return you shall be offered a third position.

Now you say, "Of which of these shall I choose?" Then we should answer you this way. Be thy own mind. Make thy own decision. Do not chase after the leader goat, for may not this take thee to the slaughter? Therefore, of the positions that shall be offered to you, the one in thy travels would benefit thee the best materially. The one that thy are thinking of would benefit thee both spiritually and materially.

Now, we have a third, "And where should it go?" For the third, as man, you will have to make up your own mind on this one.

June 12, 1970: Now, we ask your friend, yes, usually this can not be granted because permission from the soul involved here has not been given. But — one moment, please.

Yes.

Yes, it has been suggested that this information shall be given.

First, the soul involved is highly affected with the chemical that was sprayed not far from here, the seepage into the water. We also find here an acid, a very strong acid in the body. Yes, we also find that this has attacked the whole nervous system and caused a very irregular growthage in this area. Yes, at this time we would suggest that this soul be given — first of all, the changing of your drinking water, then a very, heavier bombardment of antibiotics. The physician in attendance at this time has knowledge of this.

Second, at this time, [emissive fields] shall be necessary for a short period here.

One moment. If, if this soul could at this time be given of the sage tea, of the root of the sage, in quantities of four ounces three times a day, this might help to neutralize this area.

Yes.

Yes, (sigh) we also find other problems here. We find that the liver and kidney area at this time, if they could be relieved by what is known at this time as a kidney machine, therefore, helping to relieve some of the poison being thrown off in this area, this would help.

Yes.

Yes, we also find — oh, no. We would suggest, before we continue at this point, that this whole group should pray for this soul. Each pray in his own way, that the words may mean something to you. Pray for this soul. Pray for the deliverance of this soul. And we shall pray.

June 12, 1970: **Now, for Peter's wife [5-21-70-003], we would say this. Do what is in thy mind. This is a personal thing, and therefore, we shall not discuss it in front of others. But do what is in thy mind, and it should be right. Can thy understand this?**

*"I think so."*

June 12, 1970: **Now, if thy have other questions, ask. Our time grows short.**

*"We are all preparing to take trips. Is there any reading, or [anything] there any of us should do to take special precautions in our trips?"*

**Yes, for the [4-20-70-001] family, it would be suggested that they purchase a spare tire and wheel for their trailer. And do not let any of the children ride in the trailer at any time, or any grown up.**

**For the [4-6-70-002] family, thy should beware there too.**

**For soul Ray's family, we shall be there.**

**And to all, we would say, if thy would carry the thought of us with thee, then we shall be there also.**

June 12, 1970: **Now, speak thee, soul [4-3-70-002], what is in thy mind.**

*"[J__] has asked if there is anything about money which she could know at this time?"*

**This shall come later; speak thee what is in thy mind.**

*"I would rather not."*

**I think thy should for thy peace of mind.**

**Then we should answer you. As we have told you before, we have chosen you, and each of the disciple's wives, therefore, to work with them. Therefore, as [my] mate, of soul Ray, think thee of God, of the mental block that we have placed there in the mind, that others may not enter. Therefore, only thyself may enter. But even we cannot enter without thy permission. Does this answer thy question?**

*"Yes."*

June 12, 1970: **Now, we should talk of soul [4-13-70-002]. Yes, we have soul [4-13-70-002]. The first thing thy have asked [for] — the plant that thy have now is not the same as Jerusalem artichoke. That plant may be purchased, as you are thinking of it, right here locally. Therefore, buy Jerusalem artichoke and feed it to the child.**

**We can only tell you — can only suggest to you. It is up to you to either take our advice or reject it. As we have said before, if this is not done, and done soon, then take the child to a doctor and start her on mild insulin. But when she has started this insulin, the dosage shall vary.**

**Now, we have suggested before that the child is rapidly developing. We have suggested to you that, suggest to this child of the waiting, not of the sin of the body.**

**We can also see, yes, we would suggest that the child go back to the eating, not of the black olive, but of the green olive.**

**It has also been suggested before — yes, this can wait.**

**We see the child has taken a fall within the last week. She is complaining of headaches. The reason for this is a pinched nerve in the back area, of the fourth vertebrae. This should be taken care of.**

**Also, the child, we see, has a dental problem; this should be taken care of too.**

**We should take another reading on this soul at a different time. This is all at this time.**

**We would suggest that the child be taken to a good osteopathic doctor, or — yes, a good osteopathic doctor.**

**We would also suggest that there are other children of thy family who need help.**

**What other questions would thy ask?**

*"No others."*

**Therefore, we are growing very weak now; it would be suggested at this time that soul Ray should be awakened. It would also be suggested that, as we would come to you, if thy are in accord, it is easier for us to come through.**

*"Relax, Ray."*

June 16, 1970: **Now we see that an urgent reading is necessary on the peril of [5-13-70-001]. Yes, and all, all is in accord here; we have the body, and the soul, yes, and the spirit. We see from mutilation of the body, a problem there.**

**First, we would say, for those who have sinned against this body and soul shall sin no more, for they have lost their soul, but worse, they have lost their spirit.**

**Yes, we would say, yes, this, this soul shall soon have an operation. The problem that they shall find will not be the one they seek. We find thyroid tumors in the vagina area. Yes, we also find a cyst-type**

growth here. Yes, these should be removed. We also find that if this soul becomes pregnant again it may cost her her life unless certain corrective measures are taken here.

Yes, we also find, this patient, yes, the appendix area, quite swollen. This should be also taken care of, of the bombardment [with] antibiotic. This should be done before the operation; otherwise the infection here shall spread. Then we — [from this] sharp, tubular area to the valve we also find infection. We would suggest the antibiotic cause of immunity [that] built up the system to be changed and increased. There should also be tests run on the heart before, before this operation is performed. The equipment should be on hand for electrical shock treatment if it were necessary for the heart.

Yes.

Yes, this soul very definitely should have no intake of alcoholic beverages at this time. We find inflammation of the liver area. It would also be suggested that her drinking water be changed.

We find — yes — sinus infection here. We find — at this time it shall not be found, but a small growth forming in the sinus glands and also the pituitary glands.

Yes, we also see that the — that this soul should have corrective lenses at this time.

June 16, 1970: **Our time is growing short; ask thy other questions.**

"[6-16-70-001] *asks, is there anything that can help her* physical *and mental problems so that she can have children?*"

Yes, bring her here to us that we may speak to her and a message shall be given to her. Do this as soon as possible. Yes, yes. I'm sorry, let her come here that we may speak with her.

June 16, 1970: "[6-9-70-004] *has asked, what can she do to improve her psychic ability? Have you already answered this in her studying of these tapes?*"

Yes, but we would suggest that for her, if she would — yes — if she would pick a time for meditation, spend fifteen minutes each day, preferably the same time each day. At the beginning of her meditation clear everything from her mind, all material things, and if she would think on us, her wish shall be granted, but only as long as this is used for God's work. If it is ever used for material gain, we should take it from her, and by taking it from her, we should cut of her right hand. Can thy understand this?

**Can thy?**

"*Yes, Aka.*"

June 18, 1970: "*Thank you for waiting.* [6-16-70-001] *has come to talk with you tonight, Aka. Do you have any information for her?*"

Yes, we have information for her. We see here all is in accord. We have here the body, and the soul, and also the spirit. This is good. All is in accord.

Yes, first we would answer the question. She has what is known as a tilted uterus. Yes, it shall be necessary before each time of birth that she should visit a good physician, preferably a good gynecologist. And the knowledge is already there. Each time before a planned birth, it would be necessary that she take what is known at this time, as you would call it — one moment, please, yes, this is better — that she should take, as thy would call it, birth control pills, preferably three months before. We see also a slight problem in the blood here. We would suggest at this time, and also that after the first birth of the first child, that the organs continue to function as they should, the taking of what thy would call as Lydia E. Pinkham. We also find calcium is lacking in the diet. Yes, we find in this subject a problem of the menstrual period, yes. We find cramping, very hard cramping here, yes. It would be suggested that thy change at this time the washing that thy have done of the vagina, yes. Change to a milder substance here. Yes, there are many good [kinds] of this product on the market.

Yes, we see also that soul has suffered injuries in her youth, and also, she has suffered injury to the back area and the pelvic area. We would suggest that she consult either a good osteopathic doctor for adjustments here. If this is done and treatment carried out, it may not be necessary — if done correctly, it may not be necessary — this could be, if it was done correctly — in working, the adjustments to be made in the pelvic area and the lower sciabic [sciatic?] part of the pelvis should be worked in an upward position, therefore, relieving the nerves in the central nervous system from the back area.

Yes, yes.

At the same time, working upward, we find both the sixth and seventh vertebrae here, pinched nerves in this area, yes. Yes, we also find a mastoid problem here. This also could be relieved if this area was straightened out.

Yes.

Yes, we also see this patient has, one moment, please — yes — a skin problem here we would not need to go into at this time. This, you already have treatment for this in other readings.

We also find that this subject is a borderline diabetic. We would suggest the eating of Jerusalem artichoke. Also, we would suggest at this time, eating not of the black olive, but the green olive, as much as she would want, to satisfy her desire for this, yes. Do not force this, but eat what you want. Your system will tell you the amount it needs.

Yes, we also see headaches, yes. She is entirely wrong in her belief in the source of these headaches. Once the back area has been relieved, if it is done properly, these will go away.

Yes, yes, most — yes — your other problems you have taken care of already.

Yes, we see this. Yes.

Now we would tell you of this — that as God has said and as the one known as Jesus said — fear not that man might harm thy body. Fear not, for he cannot destroy thy soul. He cannot destroy thy spirit. These are things that only you may destroy. And by your destroying them, then you have nothing for either God or Lucifer.

Now, you have another problem, another question in your mind. To this, we would say, nay. Can you understand this?

*"Are you still talking to* [6-16-70-001]*?"*

Can you understand this?

*"No, Aka. We do not understand this. Are you talking to* [6-16-70-001]*?"*

Yes, we are talking to soul [6-16-70-001]. Can you understand this?

"No, Aka," [she answers.]

*"She said that she did not understand it."*

You are in fear of losing someone very dear to you. This shall not happen at this time if caution is used. Now, can you understand it?

*"Yes, Aka."*

June 18, 1970: Now you have another question in your mind; ask it, soul [6-16-70-001].

"What about Rick? Is he the one I will be married to?"

It would be suggested, since you are out of our field at this time and that we cannot hear you, but only feel your vibrations, that you would convey the message to the conductor, and therefore, the message be conveyed to us.

*"One question she wanted to know, Aka, was, could* [6-18-70-002] *correct her back?"*

He could do a great deal of good here, but we would suggest that thy journey to the osteopathic hospital in Tucson, Arizona. There is also a very good one in what thy would know as Los Angeles, California, very good. And there, let them have a complete examination. This would help them, yes.[6-18-70-002] is good, but it would also be suggested that, that, — one moment, please — yes, yes, yes, yes — yes, start the treatment here, then ask for another reading. If the reading, if the adjustments are not made according[ly], then we will — we shall place a message there, yes. Start them.

*"Thank you, Aka. Then the treatment she was to use for her complexion problem, is that the soda and olive oil that you have recommended?"*

Yes. In her case we find it has been, one moment — yes — we find that in her case — yes, yes — yes, in her case we would suggest that the use of a raw egg in the soda, the white of the raw egg, be used to dampen the soda with, therefore, making what thy would call a mask. After this has thoroughly dried on the skin, washing the skin with a very good, clean water. Yes. Yes, it would also be suggested, yes, then the applying of the olive oil and then a good — either alcohol or a good substitute therefore. But, we also find another problem here. Upon the — it would be suggested at this time that she change her drinking water. The chemicals in the water that she in now drinking are affecting two things, her blood flow and her denture problem. It would be suggested to, for her to purchase more purified form of drinking water, yes. Yes, this will be all on soul [6-16-70-001]. What other question?

*"She also asks in Rick is the person that she should marry?"*

(Laughter). Now you ask as a child. Look into your own heart. There the truth shall be known to thee.

June 18, 1970: Now, we have a message for Peter. If he would think of us, three days from now we would come to him and give him the blessing that he needs at this time, for his heart is heavy.

July 1, 1970: *"Aka, is Ray safe?"*
Soul Ray is safe with God.
*"All right. It's been quite a while since we talked with you. Is there any* [kind of] *information you would like to give us at this time?"*
One moment, please.
For soul Peter, we would say, thy have done well.
For soul John, and we shall call him John now, for he has found his way, we will say, do what is in thy heart, and by doing what is in thy heart, thy will come closer to God. And by doing this, the things that thy should seek will be there, but only as raindrops, a little at a time.

July 1, 1970: Now, we have here soul J____. Yes, we have here the spirit, the soul, and the body; this is good. Therefore, the information which she seeks shall be given.

The adjustments that are being made are slightly incorrect. As we have said before, the correction of the pelvic area, this must be done in a downward motion, then by working up to the vertebrae area. He has corrected one, but not the other; the seventh is still not right, or true.

Yes, now this is better.

Still we find she has not complied with the suggestions we have given her for improving of her complexion; therefore, it would be useless at this time to give any further information on the subject.

If — it would be suggested that a recording be made from the tapes that thou now have in [your] possession and send to her, that she may follow the rest of her reading.

And we would say to her for her other problem, there is a time for waiting and a time to act. But now in not the time to act. Wait. Be patient. The things that thy seek shall come to you.

Now, we are through at this time with soul J____. It would be suggested, before any other readings be given upon this subject, if she would place herself in a better position it would be easier for us to give these readings.

July 1, 1970: **Now we see — yes, soul E____. Yes, we have here her** body, her spirit, and her soul. Yes, all is in accord here. Therefore, the information that she seeks shall be given her.

You ask for a physical reading. We would suggest that some of the medication that you are taking at this time is incorrect. It is way, very far too, too heavy a dosage.

We find here menopause, yes. It would be suggested to see a good gynecologist, and therefore, the necessary medicine should be prescribed. There are very good, widely known medications for this. And you ask, "Why, since I have had most of the other elements in this removed?" And we would say, thy are still a woman. Thy chose to be this and thy will remain such until the day thy die. Therefore, there are other organs in thy body which need tending to. If you would do this, you will find that the problem that you have at this time will vanish.

Now, we also find here problems of the upper neck area, yes. Yes, we find, in what you would call neck [boner] area, which is known as the brainstem area, we find here pinched nerves. This could be corrected very simply by a visit to a good osteopathic doctor. Should this be done — there are many good osteopathic doctors; there are — [is] a very good osteopathic hospital in the area in which you live at this time. Then, yes, we see a deterioration here from an old lesion in the back area. We would suggest that a bar be erected which would be precisely two inches above thy reach, that thy might grasp this once a day. Do, do not strain yourself to do this; do it a little at a time each day. Build up to it. This will straighten this area out. It will not cure it, but will keep it separated and functioning properly.

Yes. Yes, we see the problem of the feet area. Yes, we would suggest that the eating — your problem mostly from not healing, you are a diabetic, therefore, the eating of Jerusalem artichoke. You will find there a natural substance that would feed thy body and take care of its needs. If thy do not care to do this then consult thy doctor, a good medical doctor, having the necessary tests run for this, and they will probably find that at this time two grams of insulin daily by pill form will take care of this matter. Yes. But the artichoke, eating it in its natural form, either — even in its natural form or placing it in a salad will not harm it, you will still get the necessary element from this. It would stabilize the area. Yes, this is good.

One moment. Yes, yes, yes. But at this time we also suggest

soaking of the foot in very warm water — in what thy would call Epsom salts — would help to extract some of the poisons from the area.

Now, we find here over the body in various places arthritis. We would suggest, also for slight circulatory problem here, we would suggest that what thy would call, sauna baths, be taken. This would help. Go into these very gradually; do not overdo it. Let your body regulate itself to this. If you would do this once a day, the poisons that are now in your body would be extracted from it. The heat there would help increase the circulatory system, also relieving the arthritis tremendously.

Now, we also find the problem here, and to this we would suggest, if you would use eye exercises here — finding two objects approximately 20 feet apart, looking as far over to one side as possible to one object and then casting your vision back to that object at the other side — doing this at first, five minutes per day, then finding an object as high up as you can see and an object as low as you may see, casting your vision downward. The whole exercise in the beginning should not exceed five minutes; two even would be sufficient. Yes, yes. If you would do this, gradually working this exercise up, trying to do it at the same time each day.

Now, for your other problem, and you, yourself, know of this problem which we shall not speak of at this time, we would say this. If thy would meditate first — one moment, please. Yes, yes, this is must better. Yes, in your meditation do not exceed in the beginning over five minutes. Do it quite simply in the beginning. Think of God wherever you are. Do not think of Him as someone else would think of Him, think only of what He means to you. Think of Him and talk to Him of the things that mean something to you. By reciting what someone else has thought or said, it means nothing to you; therefore, if it means nothing to you, it can mean nothing to God.

A more extensive reading on this soul can be given at a different time, should it be asked for. It would not be necessary at any time that she journey here for this reading to be given. We may give it no matter where she is.

At this time, we would not give a life reading. Later this can be done.

Now, this would be all on soul E____ at this time.

July 1, 1970: **Now you have other questions, ask them.**
*"At this time is there anything that, that we should know?"*
**We have come to R____. All she must do is think of us each evening and we will be there. It does not have to be evening; at any time, day or night, we are there, for you must realize, from where we come there is no day or night. Can you understand this?**
*"Yes."*

July 3, 1970: **Now, soul John, we see, has a problem. And we** would say again, as has been said before to soul John, have thy no faith — at least a drop enough that thy may catch the blood from thy wound? Must thy always be as Thomas?

Quit doubting yourself. We call thee John because in thy heart thy are John.

Thy want to know from which thy came. We could give you this, all but one life — this thy must realize thyself, the one life.

July 3, 1970: **And now, we would speak again of soul E____. Yes, we have the spirit, the body, and the soul of E____ — this is good; all is in accord here.**

Thy ask first, in what part may you play in the groups that we have asked? We would say this, speak of what you have seen, and what you have heard and what you have felt here, for when you leave you shall have a better knowledge. You shall have God within thee to walk with thee for all thy days. And if thy should choose to walk in His path, thy shall never be alone. Thy shall always be happy, for thy shall know that God may be with you in thy daily life on this plane.

We would say, your other question in this way. If thy would wait one moment, and we would ask permission.

Yes, permission has been given; therefore, we should answer your question. The one thy loved would say this — birth has happened again; therefore, this soul thy asked about has entered again on another plane. At this time he is very happy. But we would say this to you, thy shall meet him again, but not as a he, but as a she. Can thy understand this, soul E____?

Nay.

*"She said, yes, Aka."*

She does not fully understand [of] what we have said. Then, we would answer you in this way. It would be suggested that if thy would listen to the tapes that the group already has, thy would understand [of] what we have said.

Now, thy ask, [of that] what you are taking too much of. We have suggested that by the use of meditation it would allow you to reduce the number of sleeping pills that thy are now taking. This is necessary. Now we would make this suggestion also that thy return back to thy art. Try using thy hands again. Use them for the creation of writing. The ability is there. If thy would write of this work, your mind would be too busy to think of the small quibblings of man. Can thy understand this?

Nay, then we should place in soul Ray's mind a message for you.

July 3, 1970: **Now, ask thy other question.**

*"This information we realize possibly cannot be given, but David has asked for information of his Father."*

This would be suggested, that on the next reading, this

information can be given because the soul, himself, has requested it. Therefore, we would give this information. But do — as we have said before, our time is growing short here, tonight; it would be better that it be given at a different reading.

"All right."

Now, we would say this, from the one who asks from the Valley below the Sea [Yuma, Arizona] — how may she improve what she is doing at this time? We would say this to her, let her come here. If she cares to make the journey, then we would speak to her. Can you understand of whom we speak?

"Yes, Aka, I understand."

Therefore, it is time to waken soul Ray from his slumber.

July 5, 1970: [Editor's note: The transcript could be checked from here on.]

Now, for the wife of Bartholomew, walk tall by this man, and by walking tall thy should be a disciple within thyself, and always a disciple to others. Does this answer your question?

Yes."

July 5, 1970: **Now we would say to soul E_____ who has so many doubts of herself, we have no doubt in thee; why should thee doubt thyself? We know of thy soul, thy spirit, and thy body. We find no sin there, why should you?**

**Now, we have told thee of this, look toward the east for the Cherub. Look through thine eyes to God. Therefore, thine shall see and thy shall hear.**

**Thy have asked the question, "What should we write of?"**

**And we would say, you are right. In writing of your brother, you are writing of this work. But remember, write of it, not to make him a bigger man in man's eyes; write of it as you see it, as it is, and always have truth before thee. Therefore, with truth, which we see in thy heart, thy have nothing to fear, for remember, man may cast stones at thy body, and may kill thy body, but he cannot kill thy soul or thy spirit. Can you understand this, soul E_____?**

"Yes, but that is not the question I asked."

**We know this. We would take, as thy should say, a step at a time. Now, we would go on — one moment, please. We find the question that thy ask is in thyself, the answer to. Therefore, if by the end of this reading thy still do not understand, we shall answer your question.**

July 5, 1970: **Now, we have the body, the soul, and the spirit — yes, all is in accord now of soul W_____ I___. Yes, we find this. And as finding it, we find the choice of soul Peter, yes. Thy cannot understand this, soul Peter. We would try to explain it in this manner. Thy choose thy** father and thy mother. Think thee of this.

Now, as we have said before, we find the body, the soul of soul W_____ I____, yes. Yes. We find in the feet area, on the third toe of the right foot, a problem here. Yes. We would suggest for this that if he would soak this area, first, by taking what is known as castor oil and warming it, and applying this in packs to the area, this would greatly improve this. We also find a rash on this area. This rash is, is of his own making. We would suggest, wear the lighter, as thy would call them, socks. Also, for a short time, we would suggest the wearing of sandals. This would allow more air, and natural healing to the area.

Yes, now we fid over the whole body, arthritis. Now, we would suggest the [diet? baths?] we have suggested before, yes — also of the eating of the Night-blooming Citros [Cereus], the root, in quantities of one-inch-by-one-inch per day.

We also find, this soul, too, is a very slight, slight — it would be good, the eating of the Jerusalem artichoke. We find his diet, there, should be completely regulated — less of the rich, more of the lean; therefore, more vegetables in the diet, more [fruits? fish?] in the diet.

Yes, we would also suggest at this time, a good natural vitamin be taken daily for a period of time. There is a tonic known as the S.S.A., or one other that is known as "S.S.[S]." Yes, either of these would be good. These will be rather difficult for him to purchase in the location which he is now. We would suggest that these should be found in the store of the compounds known as the Central Drug in Miami, yes, Arizona, yes.

Now we find here a kidney problem. Yes. Now we would suggest for this soul the drinking of wine, preferably of the black grape, in the quantity of, oh, four ounces per day would be sufficient; a little above this or below would still be sufficient.

Yes, we find here a back injury. The back area, that whole back area, is very much in need. Yes. Therefore, we would suggest a good osteopathic doctor or chiropractic doctor. Yes, we would suggest this as soon as possible; this would greatly relieve the problem he is having of the ear[s]. Yes. We find pinched nerves; we find, oh, many things here. It would be suggested this be done right away. Also, work in this area in a downward fashion, up to the area of the rib area, and above the ribular area working in an upward position.

Now, as we move upward, we find old lesions, yes. Yes, for these — yes, we find that there are pains of the heart, pressure of the heart, gastroid trouble here. Yes. We would suggest for this, ah — one moment, please. Yes. We would suggest of the flat cactus, the cactus of the flat leaf. Can thy understand of which we speak?

*"Yes, Aka."*

Therefore, we would say, gather the blooms from these. Boil these and make a tea. Drink of this tea, as much as thy can, [as] this soul, can take at one time. Do this for a period of 10 days; therefore, by flushing of the kidney area, therefore, relieving the gastro pains.

Now, we find other problems here. Some of these problems are caused from very, neglect of the body; others, as thy would say, from getting, as he thinks, old. This is not good. We would say, keep thy mind and thy body busy; therefore, the body would stay as young as the mind.

Now, we also find certain growths, or you would call them non-malignant tumors. These are very small at this time. These are caused, in this case, from falls taken at different times in his lifetime. We would say, for these, the drinking of the sage tea, the leaf of the sage, would help in reducing in this area.

Yes, now we also find, yes, of the left ear drum, a slight infection in this area. We would suggest, at this time, there are many good washes for this. Wash this area daily; this would clean this area up. Yes, continue to take the medication prescribed.

We find, yes, yes, we also find here — do *not* overtax this body at this time. Yes, we find — yes — we find other growths here. We would give a further reading on this subject at a different time.

This should be all at this time on soul W_____.

July 5, 1970: **Now we find that soul M_____ has a question; let her ask of it.**

*"Aka, as I feel I am coming closer to God, my divorce bothers me."*

(Chuckles). Now thy think as a child. We have said before, we have given each soul, free choice, both of the woman plane and the man plane. Let this not bother you, for yesterday was yesterday, and today is today, and tomorrow shall be tomorrow. Can thy understand this?

*"Yes."*

Then, as God enters you and you reach out for Him, take each, as thy would call them, raindrops, to thy heart and love them. Fear not from where they come, for there is love in each drop. Can thy understand this?

*"Yes."*

Then fear not, my child, for God has blessed thee.

July 5, 1970: **Now we see in soul T____, a problem. And we would say to thee, if thy would think of us for three days — and as each night, as thy should sleep, we should come to thee — and as each day unfolds into another, more of us shall be with you than in the day before. And by us coming to you, God will be with thee, and thy will know from [which, whence] thy came. Remember, God loves thee. God loves thee, for thy are a very important soul to God. Can thy understand from which we speak?**

*"Yes."*

You say, yes, but you truly do not understand. We would say, when you think of us, then we should try and let you understand this.

July 5, 1970: **Now, for soul Peter — yes, soul Peter, you have done** well. And God has come to you upon this day and shall dwell forever in thy heart, thy soul, thy spirit, and thy body.

And for Peter's wife, we would say — yes, one moment, for there is [work, word from another]. Yes, yes. We would say, forgive those who would offend thee, and do not doubt those who have offended thee, for they shall offend thee no more. God is with thee now, shall walk with thee through all the days of this plane. Thy shall never look backward, for thy shall always walk forward.

July 5, 1970: **Now soul Ray grows weak. Wait one moment.**

**We would say unto soul Luke, God has looked into your heart. God loves thee and blesses thee, and therefore, we call thee, soul Luke.**

**And now thy must look for Matthew. And Matthew shall come to you very soon, for thy know of him.**

**Now soul Ray grows tired, and we grow weak.**

*"Shall I awaken him, Aka?"*

July 11, 1970: **Soul Ray is with God.**

*"Is he safe?"*

**He is safe.**

*"We have a very important question that* [7-3-70-001, Bartholomew] *wants to ask."*

**We know of soul [7-3-70- 001]. Yes, all is in accord here.**

**Therefore, we would say, you are needed — through thy arm of thy wife — first, we sent the message and it was not, at that time, taken. We came to you again, and still, again. This you must remember — as we have said before, as thou should think upon us, we shall come to thee. And in that hour of need, we shall come to thee.**

**For — one moment — yes, this is better. Now, as we have said before, we shall come to thee and lead thee. And for all thy days thy shall walk in the path of God, for God shall walk with thee. And in His footsteps and through His eyes thy shall see thy God. This has been done.**

**You worry, now, of thy wife; worry not, for as we have said before, for those who should work, there shall be a block placed; therefore, none but the soul and the spirits that shall work through God shall enter. Can thy understand this?**

*"Yes."*

July 11, 1970: **Now — yes — now we see the soul, the body, and the spirit of [7-3-70-001]. Yes.**

**We see here that certain suggestions that we have made have not, at this time, been complied with. We would suggest that this, the suggestions that we have given, be done as soon as possible.**

**Also, we plead with this soul to rest — for Matthew, you are needed here! Can you understand this?**

Nay. Nay. Then think of thyself, and study the works of Matthew, and thy shall know of which we speak.

July 11, 1970: **Now, we have here, the body, the soul, and the spirit of soul** [7-1-70-003].
**Yes, yes.**
**We [see] here many, yes, many problems.**
**We find here headaches, severe headaches. We find here blacking out. We would say at this time, we find that some parts of this reading might embarrass this soul, but if she would take it as part of God's work, therefore, we shall give the information. At this time the soul is passing through what is known as menopause. This shall linger on for a number of years; therefore, we would suggest that thy consult a good physician and the necessary medication shall be prescribed for this.**
**We also find a scalp problem here. The scalp in itself is tightened. This is causing this soul great discomfort. Therefore, we would suggest the use of the hot olive oil packs, as hot as this subject can stand them. First, massaging the area very, very briskly. Then it would be necessary that this soul, yes, that these hot, that these packs be placed as hot as possible.**
**We also find that corrective vision at this time is needed, very desperately, and that these should be worn at all times. This would help relieve the nervous tension of thy body tremendously.**
**Now, we find glandular trouble in this area.**
**Yes, yes.**
**So that thy may understand of which we speak, we shall say, of the third gland of the right side of the neck area. Can thee understand this?**
*"Yes."*
**Therefore, it would be suggested that this area, that a good osteopathic doctor may relieve the nerves an the third vertebrae, therefore, relieving the pressure of' this glandular area.**
**Now, we also find that, as a child, a fall here. Yes. We find, yes, a fall from a chair, striking of the left kidney area. We find lesion here of this area. We find dislocation of the spinal area here. It would be suggested that the drinking of a little wine would be very good for this. This may sound at this time to you very foolish. You will find that if you will try this, it is not so. This, also, with the drinking of what is known as the sage tea will relieve the gall bladder area. Therefore, your kidney area shall be flushed and a cleansing of such.**
**We also find here arthritis. We would suggest that the baths in which we have suggested before be taken. If possible, these baths should be taken for a period, short periods at first, building up, we would say, to 15-minute intervals. But do not exceed two minutes to begin with; this would be dangerous.**

We also find here — yes, yes, we find this — we find as a small child, falling, scaring, causing concussion of the head area. Yes. We believe that at this time the proper, either chiropratic or osteopathic treatment of the whole back area and upper neck area would greatly relieve this.

Now, we also find, yes, at this time we would suggest — you are having a problem of the digestive tract. This is causing pains in the upper atrum [atrium?]; therefore, we would suggest — yes — a very simple, a good, simple physic; therefore, putting you on a normal — yes — daily regularity. Can you understand from which we speak?

Nay.

*"Yes."*

Nay. Then we would say, consult your physician on this subject. Therefore, we find here a lack of diet — yes. For this we would suggest a more complete diet, more vegetables of this diet — yes — more fish, more — less of the rich in this diet; this is not good, too much of this is poisoning the system. More, less pork, more beef.

At a different time we would suggest another reading on this soul be given. Can thy understand this?

*"Yes."*

This will be all on soul [7-1-70-003] at this time.

July 11, 1970: *"[4-6-70-003] wants to know if there is anything she can do to help her stepfather with his kidney stones?"*

If permission is given from the soul, information shall be given.

Now, soul Ray grows tired; we grow weak. Before our leaving tonight, before two days of thy calendar have passed, another reading should be taken as soon as possible. There are [is] other information which is urgent at this time.

Now we would suggest that they should awaken soul Ray from his slumber.

*"Thank you, Aka."*

July 12, 1970: Now, for soul Matthew — thy say, "Why me?" Why should we reach down and pick this soul? We would tell you, think of a life before, when you were not father and son and daughter, when you were all brothers of a kind, when you all walked by the sea of Galeah [Galilee], and therefore, all loved the same. If thy could think of this in thy heart and if thy could think of us for three days — each night, as thy go to bed at night and sleep for slumber, if thy could think of God first and then of us, we shall come to you in a way that you shall know of yourself, and therefore, believe in thyself.

Remember, there is great work here.

July 15, 1970: Now, we would say to one of thee, God is with thee.

God loves thee. God has known of you many times before. Stay in the light of God, and permit God to walk with thee, for God loves thee, my son.

Now, we should say of one in the valley below the sea [Yuma, Arizona] who asks, how may she improve her business? This we would say to her, for the things we shall suggest *shall* improve the material things for her, but by improving the material things for her, it will also improve material things for God's children. We would suggest to this soul, work with the development of the vitamins that may be preserved in canisters for many years. There are many who would be in need of these. Can thy understand of which we speak?

*"Yes, Aka."*

Now, we see soul Bartholomew. We would say, do not despair, God is with thee. Do as thy have thought to do; this is right.

We would say to the wife of soul Bartholomew, walk tall. God loves thee and blesses thy thoughts.

July 15, 1970: **Thy have other questions, ask them.**

*"We have some of what we think is sage. Is this what you were referring to?"*

We have seen thy problem in this area. This is a very poor grade; therefore, we see the necessity — this thy may understand — from what grows from the root shall grow to the leaves, the stems and the flowers of such. The root is the source; therefore, in thy root is the larger quantities of what is needed. And with thy problem, we would say two ways — first, to start now. Buy thee of the commercial sage leaf. Then, for the second part of this, purchase the script [a written description] of the desert plants. The natural substances for the healing of thy bodies are in these plants. And now, we would say, before it should be too late, go into the desert and gather the fruit of the cactus, all that thy may find. Then ask again, and we shall tell you of their uses. Can thy understand this?

*"Yes, Aka. The one we are to purchase, is that the sage, what is called sage tea, or is it the sage seasoning that we should buy."*

**Nay, the sage tea.**

*"Would it be to our advantage to plant the seeds of the sage that we have?"*

**It would be better to order seed and plant it.**

*"All right."*

Therefore, you will have a better quality of what thy seek. But remember, there are very many of this plant which grows close to thee. Thy have yet to recognize it. First, take of thy script that thy may recognize what thy seek.

*"All right."*

July 20, 1970: **Now thy have other questions, ask.**

*"Aka, [R   ] is very concerned about the drugs that she took. She wants to know if they harmed her body?"*

Now we would say to [R   ] this. Listen to both, of thy life reading and of thy physical reading, and by doing of such thy will know how to bring two into one, and by bringing the two into one, then they shall have the spirit, the soul and the body, and all will be in accord.

We would say one other to this soul. Think thee not of thyself, but of others, and by doing this, thy soul shall grow and become one. Do unto others as thy would have them do unto you. Love thy brothers and love thy sisters and forgive those who have offended thee. If thy can do this, and cast all this aside, then thy have taken the first step toward God, our Father. And our Father shall come into thee in such a way, and dwell in thee, for all thy days upon this plane, and thy riches shall become seventy-thousand fold and seventy thousand again. We know thy do not understand of which we speak. But thy soon will.

July 20, 1970: **Now thy have other questions, answer** [ask].
*"At this time can you give some information on* [4-20-70-001]*'s general health?"*

Yes, yes, we have soul Andrew, body and soul and spirit. We see here, yes, if this soul at this time would think upon the word, Aka, and our Father, tonight, and for three nights, then help he needs at this time shall be given. At this time ask for another reading and we shall give [the] same. This is all on soul Andrew at this time.

July 20, 1970: **You have other questions, ask.**
*"You told us to obtain an ultraviolet light; we obtained an infrared. Will that work in its place?"*

**Nay.**
*"All right."*

But, the use of the infrared and the ultraviolet together would give thee a more complete and faster form of obtaining the things that thy desire at this time. We repeat a warning — do not mix these chemicals together. Thy have asked, "What could this be?" Then we would say to thee, as thy would call it, the root of the Night-blooming Cereus, contains the strongest natural antibiotic known or grown on thy earth at this time. Can thy understand of which we speak?
*"Yes."*

Second, as thy would call them, the saguaro blossom, these shall contain the same, as thy would call, a headache powder, or form of pain relief, used in a nominal form. Also, they are a very good natural food supplement. The contents of these in their natural form are a very good blood and circulatory system builder. They are very high in certain vitamins that thy need at this time, and shall need in the future. Thy must understand, by the year of 1998 all shall be in accord. Can thy understand of which we speak? Nay, but thy soon shall.

Therefore, we have told thee, together — of the flat-leaf fruit, the fruit of this with the root of the sage or the tea of the sage, which would be of the same — these should be used in dissolving of what thy call small tumors. These same tumors, with what thy are calling at this time — there are natural substances in these which could cure, as thy would call it, thy sinus problems. Can thy understand of which we speak?

*"Yes."*

July 20, 1970: **Then ask thy other questions.**

*"[7-15-70-001] has requested help. At this time can you give us some guidelines for her?"*

**At this time soul Ray grows very weak. We would suggest that the reading be taken for soul [7-15-70-001] at the next reading. It would also be suggested at this time, right at this time, for her respiratory system, the reduction of the amount of tobacco at this time that have same, through intake. Can thy understand of which we speak?**

*"Yes."*

**Now, we would also suggest at this time, as she would call them her "Triple X," the taking of these for her would be very good.**

**But, we also find here that this soul should change her drinking water immediately. The usage at this time for her of the sauna, as thy would call it, bath, as we have suggested, would be very, very good for the cleansing and purification of this body at this time, in the extracting of poisons from same.**

**In the next reading that we should give, full instructions for [the] same shall be given, and the building of such, in the locations of the groups, should start as soon as possible. There are certain poisons in thy system that the natural form of extraction cannot carry at these times. Also, we find one other problem here, and this thy should know of the location in which this group, here, is at this time. Due to the large amounts of mineral substances in the earth, and of the different types of [the] same, the drinking water that comes from this earth affects the nervous system in such a way that the man-animal [has], as thy would call it, temporary insanity for periods of a time. Can thy understand of which we speak?**

*"Yes, Aka."*

**Therefore, we would give further information on this subject at a different time.**

**You have one other question; we shall answer it before we go.**
[Editor's note: Aka waits for 20 seconds.]

**Then, it is time to awaken soul Ray from his slumber.**

July 25, 1970: **Now, at this time, we have here the body, the soul, and the spirit of soul [7-1-70-003]. First, of a physical nature, we would** say — we would say certain suggestions which have been given before have not been complied with. These suggestions should, at the earliest convenience of this soul, be complied with. Also, at this time, rest.

Now, we have a new problem here. Yes. This problem is what thy would call of a mastoid infection. We would suggest at this time that she consult a physician and the necessary medication for this shall come forth.

July 25, 1970: **Now thy have other questions.**

**And, again, we would say to soul Bartholomew's wife, we have answered your question [as we] did the same time we did thy sister's.**

**Now, again for soul [6-6-70-002] — the words of wisdom that thy seek are with thee. And this we would say, if thy can find peace in the house thy dwell, then the material things that thy seek are already there. But we would say one other. This we do usually not, but this time we do. The reason for this — you and your husband and your children, God has given free choice. Therefore, we would suggest a path only, the choice shall be yours. If thy would seek the mountains, yes, then do of these things. First, bring your husband and yourself into one, and your children into the same house. Second, bring all of thy worldly goods into one bundle, and then as thy walk to the market to trade them, thy shall have what thy need.**

**Now, thy ask, "Why can not I get my husband into this house at this time?" Remember, our Father has many mansions, and He loves His children in each mansion the same. And He sheds tears for [these] [His] children the same. But remember, a divided house cannot stand; therefore, we shall help thee in bringing this house into one. This thy must do. For three days and three nights think of us. Think of us early in the morning and think of us again before thy slumber, and we should come to thee. And by coming to thee that [that?] would open the door of thy household, therefore, we should enter. For we would say in this way, for each bridegroom there must be a bride. Can thy understand of which we speak?**

*"Yes."*

**And now we would say — yes — we see this problem. Yes. And for this one we would answer in this way. If thy should do the things that are necessary in thy mind at this time, there should be no problem of thy livelihood. Can thy understand this?**

*"Yes."* [A woman answers.]

**Nay.**

*"Yes."* [A man answers.]

**Nay, then we would say in this way, each of you in thought, this thought would mean something to them. Take it to your hearts and study it.**

July 25, 1970: **Then, we would answer to the old soul of** [5-15-70-001]. **Yes. We see no problem at this time. You shall have one in the future, but not at this time. But we would have one other suggestion for this soul. If thy would open the door, as we have said before, then think of our Father first, and then the word, Aka. Then we may come to thee in thy slumber tonight. Then come back and let us speak with you again.**

July 25, 1970: **Now, soul** [4-6-70-001] **would ask a question. But first, we would speak to this soul. Study, soul John, of yourself in the time before. Therefore, your problems would be less, and the understanding of yourself would be easier, for what has happened to you before is happening again. Can you understand of this?**
"*Yes.*"
**Then ask. Ask of this question.**
"[4-6-70-003] *asks* [4-6-70-001's] *question. 'As Aka has spoken before — as in our eyes, as we see it, it may not be a sin in the eyes of God — what sin in accordance to the Ten Commandments; how may we be forgiven if we sin in accordance to our Ten Commandments?'*"
**If thy sin in accordance with the commandments, first, we would say to you of this. The commandments were written by God upon stone with fire. Therefore, we would say in this way, once thy have knowledge that thy have sinned, that in itself is the ending of a karma. If thy have sinned, by knowing of this and by admitting it to thyself, and forgiving thyself, but learning from [the] same and going on to face whatever is in front of you in life, that is forgiveness in itself.**
**But remember, our Father loves His children. Our Father loves His children more than themselves. And all our Father really asks, the one commandment, love thy God greater than thyself, for God loves you greater than Himself. Can thy understand this?**
"*Yes, Aka.*"
**Then, soul** [4-6-70-001], **we would say to you, be careful in your speech. Your mind at this time is stronger than thy realize. We have given to you the power to walk upon water because of your faith. Your hands and thy mind may heal, but they may also destroy this healing. So remember, touch only with love each creature, even to the smallest of this earth. And as thy touch them, both with thy hands and thy lips, and with thy speech, then healing and love of our Father shall be known to thee. Can thy understand of this?**
"*Yes, Aka.*"
**Remember, my son, our Father loves thee with all His heart and soul. And for our Father, [work] is a great deal of love, more than your whole world has ever known.**

July 25, 1970: "[4-6-70-003] *asks* [4-6-70-001's] *question. 'As Aka has spoken before — as in our eyes, as we see it, it may not be a sin in the eyes of God — what sin in accordance to the Ten Commandments; how may we be forgiven if we sin in accordance to our Ten Commandments?'"*

If thy sin in accordance with the commandments, first, we would say to you of this. The commandments were written by God upon stone with fire. Therefore, we would say in this way, once thy have knowledge that thy have sinned, that in itself is the ending of a karma. If thy have sinned, by knowing of this and by admitting it to thyself, and forgiving thyself, but learning from [the] same and going on to face whatever is in front of you in life, that is forgiveness in itself.

But remember, our Father loves His children. Our Father loves His children more than themselves. And all our Father really asks, the one commandment, love thy God greater than thyself, for God loves you greater than Himself. Can thy understand this?

*"Yes, Aka."*

Now is the time to waken soul Ray from his slumber.


July 29, 1970: Therefore, now we see [in] the mind of soul Andrew [4-20-70-001] a question. We have told you before the problem that thy have created. We advised you at that time against taking certain steps. The one thy seek is the same one. Therefore, we should say no more.


July 29, 1970: Now, we have here the body, the soul and the spirit of soul [4-3-70-002]. This, thy must understand, in thy reading; because of the karmic action involved here with soul Ray, certain information we cannot give. Therefore, proportions of your reading cannot be given.

Therefore, the beginning we may not give. This plane must be omitted.

Your next entry was in the time of Atlantis.

From Atlantis, this is all the information on Atlantis we may give you, other than your next entry was in Egypt. This is all on this entry we may give you.

Your next entry is in a land known as, at this time, as Indonesia. At this time, again we may not give this information.

Your next entry again was what is now known, was in the city of Bethlehem. This information cannot be given you.

We can tell you of another entry, this entry was during the early voyages of what is known as the Americas, continent. And again, this information we cannot give.

We would tell thee only that thy have been chosen at this time for a task. But thy must remember thy marriage vows, and every proportion of these marriage vows. They were given to you differently for a purpose. They were given to you that thy might walk tall by thy husband. Thy must help him in completion of his mission upon this earth. He shall be used, and you shall be used, as our instrument.

If thy do not walk, as thy would say, backward, but walk forward with this man, then thy blessings from our Father and yours, who in your heart you know better than you think you do — remember this, thy have always loved our Father.

If thy will study these readings and do not misinterpret the words, this is the task we give you, which will be harder than for most. For your reward in some ways shall be bigger than most. For your task shall be a hard task, for many shall come and many shall ask. But we would tell you this much. These words, and the one who asked our Father, and the ones we are preparing a way for, is, as thy would call it, Jesus Christ — and we bestow upon thee this mighty task. We know that at times thy heart shall grow heavy from it, but thy love thy Father and He loves thee. This shall be all at this time on soul [4-3-70-002].

[Editor's note: After a long pause the tape recorder may have been turned off, then on again, for there is a loud click. Perhaps a question was not recorded.]

Ask them, for soul Ray grows weak.

*"Aka, at this, at this time — do we have time — soul [T] asks for the life reading on her son, [J]."*

Not at this time, at another reading. We would suggest at this time thy awaken soul Ray from his slumber.

July 25, 1970: **Now — now, you have many questions, ask of these questions. Permission has been given and they shall be answered.**

**First, we would say to soul [6-6-70-002] of thy question.**

**And this we would say to thee. It is not permitted for information to be given about one soul to another. But in this case, permission has been given, for the permission of the other soul involved in this situation has been given from the same. Therefore, we would say to you in this way — in the life before, the one you speak of was not a mother as in this lifetime. In the life before, as thy would call it, both mother and daughter were rivals. Therefore, their karma upon this earth, at this time and at this plane, would be as such. Can thy understand of which we speak? Other information on this subject can be given, should either of these souls ask.**

August 3, 1970: **Now, you have many questions, ask these questions.**

*"Aka, at this time we have a request for a health reading on [8-3-70-001]. Is it possible to get one on him at this time?"*

**One moment, permission must be given.**

**Yes, we see here, all is in accord; therefore, we find the body, the soul, and the spirit of [8-3-70-001]. Therefore, we should say to this soul — one moment, additional information must be obtained.**

**Yes, yes.**

**We should suggest permission for a life and a health reading be**

given at this time. We see here without both, one by itself could not fully serve in the way that is needed.

Therefore, we find that permission both from the soul and from our Father, have been given. Therefore, first, we find many problems here — old injury, first. Some of these problems, this soul through meditation, and the meditation of thy group[s], these could be helped, for permission has been given for this help — but only if in his meditation he should think of us that we may enter.

We find here a problem, in your, in a language that thy may understand, we find an [ambroious]-type cyst growth of the left pelvic. Yes. This was caused in a fall as a child from riding horseback.

We also find here — yes — a circulatory problem of the blood. We would suggest first, that this soul, in the taking of a blood tonic, such as, uh, "S.S.S," yes, this would do at this time. Also, we find fatty tissue in the blood area; this is not good. We would suggest, therefore, a change of diet. This fatty tissue is clogging the third valvulatory* area of the heart; this could be very dangerous. Therefore, we would suggest for this soul the eating of more, as thy would call it, vegetation, vegetable — okra, as thy would call it, squash, more radish, more of salad-type vegetation. Yes. Any of these would be good — also more exercise, but not of the stringent type; we see an overly, too much exercise at this time could cause complete failure of this area. Yes. We would also suggest massaging of the heart area. This could be done, starting at two-minute intervals a day; [it is] suggested early in the morning. Do not do this in the evening; therefore, at that time the heart is very taxed. This could cause, as thy would call it, heart failure. If this subject at this time could purchase, oh, there are many good vibrators, as thy would call them, on the market; vibrating for two-minute intervals in the area that is just beneath the heart, this would relieve the pressure here. Then, after this has been done for a 20-day period, it would be suggested, then, at that time, another reading be taken. And, if feasible, at that time the type of baths that we have suggested, sauna-type baths, this would do away with a lot of the extra, as thy would call them, too many white corpuscles of the blood area, overly attacking.

This, you must understand, we also find here one other problem, a problem which this soul in the settling of himself, the searching for his own soul. We would say to you in this way, no matter where thy would go, thy take thyself. Thy might find thyself anywhere, if thy should sit still long enough and look into thyself. We cannot at this time give a full life reading, for permission from this soul has not been given, only for the partial reading.

We should also find here an injury to the head area. We should suggest at this time that, that the type of medication that this soul needs, he himself could not obtain; therefore, we would suggest that he sees a good medical doctor for attendance therefore.

We see that this soul has at this time [been] taking certain astringents of the type medication [for, or] — therefore, we would suggest the continuing of these.

We see here that this soul has at times problems in remembering the taking of these, too; this is not good. We would tell this soul, it would be, you would be creating a new karma for yourself by neglecting your body — therefore, by entering our world, as thy would call [it] — therefore, then rebirth, with more lessons than thy have to learn now at this time then thy had before. We find here a psychological block in this area; therefore, certain information that is required from this soul should be asked in, in a private reading.

Now we look — yes — we find arthritic-type tissue growing. You must understand, and this it will soon be learned by your own medical doctors, this is caused by a virus, not by the things at this time that are thought of the same. As the virus attacks, not of the tissue, but of the inner tissue of the bone area, at this time you have no known medication for this area; therefore, we would suggest the eating of the Night-blooming Cereus in the quantities of two inch cubes per day for this subject would greatly help this subject.

Now, we find other old lacerations of the body.

For the present time we would suggest that another reading be given within a 20-day period on this subject, if consent is given. This is all at this time on this soul.

Editor's note: Valvular – of or relating to a *valve* or *valves*, especially of the heart. Valvular heart disease is characterized by damage to or a defect in one of the four heart valves: the mitral, aortic, tricuspid or pulmonary.

August 3, 1970: **Now we also see, as thy would know it, [8-3-70-002], soul [8-3-70-002].**

Yes, we have the body, the soul, and the spirit here. We see permission has been given; therefore, a reading shall be given. The records show, first, of your karma and your desire to overcome this karma. Then, at this time we would tell thee, if thy would drink of this wine, study it, study all phases of this wine, and in thy meditation if thy would ask permission that we may enter, help shall be given to this soul. But remember, if help is given and thy step backward, then thy shall become what is known as a lost soul. So before entering in the area that thy desire, think first of where you have been; therefore, we shall tell you from where you shall go.

Now, we see here in this soul, pulled ligament area in the third vertebrae. We find osteopathic treatment desired here.

We also find a problem here that could be corrected quite simply by dieting. This soul desires to carry more weight than the body structure at this time will handle. We should suggest more of the raw beef, more of the raw vegetations. We do not, when we speak of raw, mean, not cooked, but not overly cooked.

Now, we also see here that if this soul constructs, at this time, a bar approximately six inches above his reach, that he may for periods of five minutes per day, as thy would call it, hang from this bar, therefore, stretching this area out. You must remember, this area is permanently damaged. Through thought concentration thy may rebuild a good part of this area, but this area has been destroyed in such a manner that complete recovery is not feasible at this time.

First, take of the first of the reading, and then of the last.

This is all on this soul at this time. Another reading shall be given at his request.

August 3, 1970: *"Aka, [D    ] asks that a health reading be given or he has permission from a [JCM]. Could you give a health reading on this man at this time?"*

We would suggest that this soul place his self in a better position, that we may give this reading. At this time, he is not at the location you have given. We do not find this soul at this location. Also we would suggest that this soul be brought more in accord, that this reading shall be given.

August 10, 1970: Now, for the wife of soul Bartholomew, your time to smell the flowers is now. Your time to let others smell your flowers is now.

And we have said before to both of thee, look backward from which thy came, so thy would know from where thy are going. This time is now. There is great work for both of you. There is great work for [thy. their] children.

Now, thy ask, "Shall we survive? Should we survive this famine?" And we would say unto thee, yes — if thy stand tall in God's light, thy shall survive, all things. But for thy sake and for the sake of thy family, and for the sake of many souls where thy dwell, do not step backward at this time, for the half time[s] shall be no more.

August 10, 1970: Now, for the wife of soul Bartholomew, your time to smell the flowers is now. Your time to let others smell your flowers is now.

And we have said before to both of thee, look backward from which thy came, so thy would know from where thy are going. This time is now. There is great work for both of you. There is great work for [thy. their] children.

Now, thy ask, "Shall we survive? Should we survive this famine?" And we would say unto thee, yes — if thy stand tall in God's light, thy shall survive, all things. But for thy sake and for the sake of thy family, and for the sake of many souls where thy dwell, do not step backward at this time, for the half time[s] shall be no more.

August 10, 1970: **Now, we see, for the father of soul Andrew —
yes, we see this problem at this time, yes — we would say, this soul should
see through his work. We should also see that he should come here, that
both a life and physical reading should be given, that help in this area
may be given. Therefore, we might at this time say this, permission from
our Father has been given, but not from the soul. This is all on this soul at
this time.**

August 10, 1970: **Now, we find a soul within thy group who would
ask for healing. Yes, we see this. If thy would think upon us for three
nights. Before thy slumber, think first of God, and then the word, Aka,
and ask that permission may be given that we enter — and we shall, if
this is desired in the soul — and the healing that thy need shall come into
thee.**

**Now, we see one other problem here, in this soul. We would say,
answer you, in this way. You have the answer within yourself. There is a
course that thy might take. If, in handling this other soul, in which you
refer, to, if thy would think upon this soul only in kindliness, there would
be no problem.**

August 10, 1970: **Now, we find for the other soul. Both of these
souls would know of themselves.**

**At this time, our time is growing short, for soul Ray become tired;
therefore, we become weak. We should suggest for both of these souls,
first, before this information is fully given, if thy would study of these
works. And then, in six days — nay, nay, nay, one moment.**

**Yes, yes, yes, Father, we see this, yes, Father.**

**Then we should say in this way, our Father has asked that better
words be used. Our Father says to this soul to think of that time in your
half time, in the time of the separation when thy walked in His light. If
thy could think of this, our Father shall let us enter. But remember, thy
children shall grow old after thee, and thy children's children shall grow
old after thee. Dying, as thy would call it, is only part of life. Can thy
understand of which we speak?**

*"No."*

**Nay, then in three days come back. In these three days, use them
for meditation. In three days, all thy questions that have not been
answered in the course of these three days, we should answer for thee.
Can thy understand of this?**

*"Yes."*

August 21, 1970: *"Aka, we know that you have made certain
adjustments on soul Ray. But what can be done to ease the pressure on soul*

*Ray's overwork? Is there anything we could do to, even the pace?"*

These things he must regulate himself. He knows his own condition. He knows in his own mind the strain that is being put on his physical body by overworking. If thy could remind him.

We often remind him. But you must realize that soul Ray in awakening state is a very stubborn person, almost to the point, at times, of stupidity. Therefore, it would be suggested that you remind him frequently. The necessary adjustments have been made, but remember our Father, and us, may only do and only restore, but we cannot restore those things that he should destroy.

Can thy understand of which we speak?

*"Yes, Aka, I think we can."*

August 21, 1970: *"We have this evening, Aka, requests for several various health readings. We would like a reading on [8-21-70-O01], a health reading.*

*"Ah, have you any suggestions as to how we might conduct these different readings, health readings and life readings, as to time element and soul Ray's condition as to being tired, overtaxed? There are many requests for health readings and life readings which we haven't been able to get into our readings because of this."*

We would suggest at this time that all of the health readings that thy have requested, we would suggest that at every third day, a health reading should be taken. Do not request a health and a life reading at the same time. These do overtax.

There are times when we must give in proportion to both; therefore, it would be suggested and would save a great deal of your time, and ours, that when requests are made for both health and life readings that they be given at the same time — in other words, permission from the soul be given. Therefore we, at that time, would be free to give the necessary information.

August 21, 1970: Now we see other questions, and these thy must ask.

*"Aka, [6-9-70-001] has had some very bad nose bleeds. And [(4-3-70-002) (or 6-9-70-001?)] would like very much to know if, at this time, she could have a health reading or if she could have some explanation as to what she can do about them or what is causing them. Can you give us any information at this time?"*

Yes, we have the soul, the spirit and the body of soul [6-9-70-001]. One moment — yes — at this point we would suggest the giving of Lydia E. Pinkham in the adult dosage. Also, we would suggest here that calcium is lacking in the diet. This should be added to the diet. Also we find that more salt should be added to the diet, a lack of salt in the diet. Yes. It should also be suggested that the purchasing of a good, natural daily vitamin, and be given once per day. There are many good ones on the market. Therefore, we see a child that shall soon [spring] the first steps of early womanhood. Prepare her soul and mind for this time.

We also find here a problem of the feet area, of a rash in this area. This is not as thy think it. This is a virus. With the proper dieting these things may be corrected — but as we have told thee before, taking of the greasewood, boiling of this, of the leaf of the greasewood, boiling it to the point of boil, letting it cool, doing this three times — it shall form a jelly-like form — therefore, adding, as thy would call it, baking soda. When this application, after this application has been placed on, then placing towels over this area, as hot as the child may stand it — then taking olive oil and briskly rubbing in to this area — then using the ultraviolet light to treat this area, not over, oh, five minutes per day of the light. Over usage of this could be dangerous.

Yes, we see this. We also see at this time — yes — problem of the [lymphro] area. Yes, we would suggest massaging this area in a downward position — this could be done at home — massaging this area in a downward position; then by firmly placing both hands on the child's neck as the child lays flat on its back, stretching the neck area very gently; this could relieve the pressure in this area, therefore, secreting the necessary chemicals that would do away with this entirely.

Yes, we see this. We also find here, [mortiporeses? More psoriasis, more type-oresis? ornithorhynchus? ornithosis?]-type growth in the [flambrous? flatus? flabbiest? flexuous?] area. Yes, we find that this area, the drinking of the sage tea, and with the other treatment prescribed at this time, should take care of the medical needs of this child, at this time. We would suggest that another reading be taken in the near future.

We also would suggest that a life reading be given on this soul.

This is all, at this time, on soul [6-9-70-001].

August 21, 1970: Now, we would suggest that for soul [6-21-70-001], her problem is very simple, she is pregnant. Therefore, we would suggest at this time that the taking of Lydia E. Pinkham, also we find the area low in calcium. We also find a problem of the back area, in the [limbrone? limber? lumbar?] area, which should be corrected. This should be done a little at a time. We would suggest that she see a good chiropractor and these pressures be relieved. We also see a pressure here in the upper neck area; this is caused from, as thy would call them, pinched nerves, [nervous] system. If work was done in both of these areas we would see a great improvement.

Therefore, we could also see in this soul — yes — bring thyself closer to thy Father. Bring thyself closer to thy God. Speak to Him as thy would speak to thyself that He may understand of which you speak. Remember, if thy walk through thy plane in life with thy God, thy Father, all things are possible. And we feel that, at this time, when thy speak to thy Father, ask Him that we may enter and that we may give the healing that is necessary in thy body, and soul and spirit. Can thy understand of which we speak?

Nay.

*"I think so."*

Not fully. Thy shall, in time.

We would say to this soul, let others smell thy flowers, let others see the goodness in thy heart. Do not be afraid of this goodness.

This is all on this soul at this time.

August 21, 1970: **Thy have one other reading which is important, and then thy shall waken soul Ray from his slumber.**

*"We have had —"*

We find this before us, the body the soul, as thy would know her, [8-21-70-002]; therefore, we find — yes — your problem is from an old laceration. In this area, the upper shoulder and down through, causing pain down through the finger tips — yes — taking hot castor oil, rubbing it into this area very briskly — then applying the same castor oil into a cloth pack and wrapping this area, then taking, as thy would call it, a heating element, and placing it over this area, and leaving it overnight, this would greatly relieve these pains.

We find a[n] other problem in this soul. We find a growth. We have spoke[n] before of this growth.

Now, at this time, and we say — not of another time, but of this time, now — all members of this group shall pray. Pray each of you in your own way. If thy prayers are strong and if thy may walk on the water with us, then we should heal of this woman at this time.

Now pray of thee. [There were two minutes of silent prayers.]

Now thy should waken soul Ray from his slumber.

August 24, 1970: *"Aka, [4-3-70-002] asks if the pain in her solar plexus from over lifting is something that she needs to consult a physician for?"*

Yes, yes, we have the body, the soul, and the spirit of [4-3-70-002]; therefore, the necessary information shall be given. [4-3-70-002] **first should consult a physician.** We find pleurisy and the necessary prescribing of certain antibiotics at this time. Yes, we find congestion in the lower lung area, inflammation between the tissue.

Yes. We also find on [4-3-70-002] at this time that certain chiropractic treatment should be done as soon as possible. This we have suggested before, which was not complied with. This would greatly relieve this area also.

Also we have suggested that this soul, for the taking of a good blood tonic, "S.S.S." would do. We would also suggest that this soul go back to the taking of good natural vitamins, taking this very regularly, daily.

We find also that the saunic baths we have suggested before —
yes, this should be done — at this time, that as soon as possible the
constructing by your group of the saunic bath, that all of thy group and
the many others of this area, that these could be used at this time.

We also find here that the drinking of the sage tea would help
improve the sinus area. We find that the — as we have said before,
certain growths caused by certain bacteria pumped into the drinking
water in this area has caused nervous disorder. By the drinking of the
sage tea, this might neutralize this area. It is also suggested for the
neutralizing of the acid in thy water.

We also suggest that in thy bath water that a, the bath water used
for the vagina area be changed, that this area be bathed in a different
way. I think at this time the soul has in mind a different type of bathing
for this area. This would be good. This would greatly improve. We find
infection of this area due to the bathing at the present time.

This is all on [4-3-70-002] at this time.


August 24, 1970: *"Aka, [8-10-70-003] asks, what should he do about
his interests in mining in light of the urgency of other things?"*

We would suggest that, very strongly, retain thy interest in a
silent manner. Retain it only to the point of keeping the present claims
that thy possess. But as thy would store wheat for another day, store this
also. The time shall come when you shall need of this, but the time at this
time, do your other work first.

We find in this soul, thy are thinking of, as you would say, a
mosaic. This has also entered upon thy wife's mind. Then, we would say,
think of the Almighty; think of the records that are kept forever and
ever; and, think of the coming of the Messiah. If you may put in thy
minds a picture, this would bring all in accord with God.

We see in this soul the love for his wife and children, and his
desire to express this love. Be not afraid, for the love that thy have now
shall come tenfold, for they are climbing upon our ladder. Thy shall walk
upon the water with us, and as thy walk, thy family shall walk with thee.
Thy wife shall walk tall, as she has done before.

We would say to her, think thee of Ruth, and thy would know of
which we speak.

And now, we also see in thy minds a fear for thy children. As we
have said before, if thy would construct the saunic-type baths, this would
take care of the problem. At this time, the chiropractic treatment is only
a temporary thing.

We have a problem of arthritis here. We would suggest that the
taking of the sage root; we would suggest the taking of the flat-leafed
cactus — boiling these two substances to a boil, barely to a boil — letting
it cool, and drinking of this, this would greatly help this area. Now we

would also suggest that the eating of the Night-blooming Citros [Cereus], from the root of the same, quarter-by-quarter inch daily, also would greatly help this area. This might be done by all in thy family for a short period of time. We would give a further reading on these subjects at another time.

Now we look into the heart, and the soul, and the spirit, and the body of this soul's wife. And as we have said before, think thee of Ruth, and thy would know of thyself. Think thee of the love thy have had for our Savior, and think thee of the time of thy walking by the Sea of Gallea once before. As we have said before that the healing, both in thy children, and in you, shall come; have faith. Walk on the water with us, and thy faith shall blossom as thy have never seen a rose blossom before.

God loves thee, and God heals thee, and thy healing shall come now. [Editor's note: there is about a 25-second pause as the healing is given.]

August 24, 1970 [in Philosophy]: **Ask thy other questions.**

*"Aka, what, if anything, can I do to help my sister's situation, without upsetting her whole household?"*

Thy sister shall know the things to do.

Continue thy work, as thy have done it before, Peter. Think thee of healing, both in the mind, and the soul, and in the spirit, and in the body, and these things shall come, and they shall be made unto you a new gateway. And through this gateway shall have three sides, and the towers upon this gateway shall have of three sides, and the boats thy shall sail in shall have three sides, and the ground that thy walk on shall have three sides, and there shall be the answer into thy prayer. Think thee upon this, and we shall come to thee tonight.

And then, think thee again for three days. And then, return unto us that we may speak to thee again.

*"Thank you, Aka."*

But remember, think of thy Father who loves thee. Thy are walking the path in which thy are attended, and thy attendants shall be many.

August 24, 1970: **Thy have one other question, ask of it.**

*"Aka, the question that I have here is a, the continuation; I know you have given a small portion of [8-3-70-001]. But before he left, he consented to a health reading. Do you have time for that this evening?"*

We have given [8-3-70-001] his health reading.

*"Excuse me, Aka. I meant a life reading."*

His life reading shall come at another time. There shall be — yes, ask again and this shall be granted, for permission has been given for this.

Now, our time grows short. Soul Ray grows very tired, and we shall grow weak. But before we go, we would remind thee that now is the time of the Cherub, or as thy would call it, the cherubim.

Now, awaken soul Ray from his slumber.

August 29, 1970: *"At this time, Aka, can you answer* [7-18-70-002]*'s question?"*

Yes, we may answer your question. But you ask now as a child, for you know the answer within yourself. Walk tall, as thy have done before, and if thy still do not understand, ask again, and we shall answer thee.

Augusts 29, 1970: Then we would say to this soul, if thy could build this monument, and in your heart this monument must be of a material thing and this is the only way thy know of worshipping your Father, then do so, but do it in the way that others should not suffer, for much blood was shed in your building of your last temple. Why, then, should it be shed in the building of your temple in yourself again? Lift thyself above this. God does not expect you to shed one teardrop more than you are capable. But He should expect you to shed each teardrop that you may be able to shed. Now, remember, our Father loves you; more love than you have ever known in all of your lifetimes together, our Father has gave unto you.

There are other things we should mention, but we do not find these things are necessary at this time, for this soul knows of which we speak. And we should say unto this soul, 'if thy eye offend thee, cast it aside;' and thy shall know of the eye we speak of. But remember, should thy grow a rose in thy garden, and the smell of the bud of the rose is sweet, save the seed and plant it again. If thy fruit that thy should plant shall multiply and be sweet to thy taste, then plant this fruit again and watch it grow; and take the meat of the seed of the same, and watch this fruit grow, for this thy shall use for meat. Can thy understand of which we speak?

*"Yes."* [the person answers.]

Not fully, but thy shall within time. If thy shall take some of our fruit, think upon our name for three nights and think of God, your Father, that we may enter, the help that thy need shall come into you. But remember, you must open the door first.

Now is the time to awaken soul Ray from his slumber.

August 31, 1970: You have other questions, ask.

*"Aka, we have many questions tonight. At this time* [4-6-70-003] *is quite concerned about a very dear little friend. Is there anything that can be done?"*

First, for this friend, we should give the help that is needed.

First, change thy diet, change it for this friend. Take of the fresh vegetables, chopping them and then grinding them — take okra, take of the radish, take of the corn, take of the spinach. Then we would suggest taking of a blood tonic known as S.S.S., grinding this finely, mixing it, then taking of fresh liver, cooking it very slowly. With this, you must remember, the one you speak of has what is known as tick fever.

Now, we would suggest one other. Take of the Night-blooming Citros [Cereus], grinding this within the food. Take of the sage tea, preferably of the root of the sage, grinding this within the food.

And third, remember, if you should have the faith to walk on the water with us, and if you should talk to thy Father and it should mean something to you, you have but to ask. But have faith in yourself, and by having faith and believing that your prayers shall be answered, then your prayer *shall* be answered.

September 5, 1970 (evening): **This is all on this soul at his time. Thy have other questions, ask.**

*"Thank you, Aka. [9-1-72-002] of Globe is in Tucson tonight at the home of his mother. He has asked for a health reading, particularly because of the severe pain he has been experiencing. He wonders if you could tell him cause and possible treatment?"*

**Yes, we see thy need. One moment please. We should say unto thee, this is a traveling soul.**

**Yes, yes — yes, now that is better. Yes, yes.**

**We have before us the body, the spirit, and therefore, the soul of the same. Yes, we find this problem, and therefore, the healing that is needed shall be given.**

**We would suggest that this soul go unto the sauna baths. This should be done at least once daily for a four-week period. We find this soul should go unto either a good osteopathic or chiropractic doctor; with the corrections, therefore, that could be given [it] would greatly relieve the pain, therefore, within the same.**

**We see further — yes we see this. We should answer in this manner, that the soul in question has but little faith. Therefore, we should say unto this one, thy have come unto, before us to ask for healing, and we should say unto you these words. Have the faith of a mustard seed and it should grow and move the mountains that thy desire to be moved. Build unto our Father a temple and the temple shall be built within thyself. We see great emotional problems — yes — here, upheavals within the mind, doubts within the mind, doubts of yourself and your fellow man. Do unto the things which we have suggested and then ask for other information and it shall be given upon your request.**

September 10, 1970: **You have many questions, ask.**

*"Aka, I have a question from soul Bartholomew. He is very concerned, his physical health as to the relationship of his continuous gagging. Could you give him any helpful information at this time? It seems to*

*be quite a worry on his mind."*

Yes, we find this problem. The help that is necessary in the healing of the same shall be sent. We would suggest, first, that his problem basically is a sinus problem that, we would suggest the saunic baths at this time would greatly improve this area. We would also suggest in this way. Remember, a little tobacco as thy would call it, or of the weed as thy should say, is good for the body, cannot harm the body, but too much can harm the body. And remember, we should take care of the necessary repairs in thy physical bodies of the disciples of this work, but beware. Do not push this body too far, for we cannot create, for we are not God, we are only the messengers of God. Can thy understand of which we speak?

*"Yes, Aka."*

Then the healing at this time shall be given unto this soul. And at this time, if thy group should pause for prayer for all healing in thy group. [Editor's note: Aka paused for 25 seconds for people to pray.]

September 10, 1970: Now thy have other questions, ask of these.

*"Another question, Aka, in reference to soul Bartholomew's wife, which he's greatly concerned with...."*

We see this problem.

Yes.

We would suggest the taking of the Night-blooming Citros [Cereus]. We would also suggest that her basic problem is [in], of the nervous system, therefore, an eruption, as thy would've known, of the basic nervous interval known as the kasados [caudate or sciatic?].Therefore, we would suggest osteopathic treatment in the lower proportion of the back area. We would also suggest, there is other work necessary at this time of the upper back area. We also find that, in this soul, that if thy would change of the music thy listen to; remember, light and sound may effect your physical health. We would suggest for this soul, for 15 minutes each day, of meditation. But drink of the smoothing music, that which would satisfy thy soul, and meditate. This would greatly relieve this area.

We see the passing, therefore, of congested blood of this area. This, in itself, could bring on complications; therefore, we would suggest a good gynecologist. But we see at this time this should not be practical; therefore, we would suggest in the vagina area an acid form of douche, as thy would know it, washing of this area. This, in itself, we would also suggest in this washing, the proportions of the Night-blooming Citros [Cereus] liquid extracted from the same, be placed and used in the washing of this area. Can thy understand of which we speak?

*"Yes, Aka."*

We have one other problem in this soul. Yes. We see, as she would call them, head spasms. We would also suggest that, in seeking out a chiropractor, that certain adjustments be done on the sinus and the lybro [lympho?] gland area. These can be done quite simply by the shifting of the skull area, but be very certain in doing this that this comes about in a very gentle way — very slowly done. The music would do the same as this adjustment, but not as fast.

This is all on this soul at this time.

September 14, 1970: **Aka is here.**
*"Aka, is Ray safe?"*
**Soul Ray stands with God.**

Now, for soul Andrew and the wife of soul Andrew, we see thy need, but remember, we may not interfere with the free choice of any soul. Therefore, of thy problem, we should say, remember, thy are the parents of the child, and therefore, are responsible for the teaching of the child. And even though the child shall be, in itself, a free soul, it was given of its own free choice unto you for teaching, that not only the child could overcome its karma, or sin, but that you also might overcome your karmas and your sins.

Remember, on your earth souls shall have karmas, and groups shall have karmas, and therefore, to be born and born again into the same group, as thy would know it. Therefore, we should tell you, the son was of not a son of before; the son was a brother of the same. We know thy cannot understand fully of what we speak.

Then we should say it in a different way. As thy walk upon your plane and upon your earth, walk it in a way that thy would climb your Father's ladder, and in climbing this ladder, climb it in such a way that others may walk before you. Think not always of yourselves. If thy could do this in the teaching of the child — remember, each person on this earth shall reach his Father in a different way. No two souls upon your earth are identical; no two spirits upon your earth are identical, and no two mortal bodies upon your earth are identical. Each body must be fed its own fruit; each soul must be fed its own fruit. And above all, if the body and the soul are fed the proper fruit, then the spirit shall grow, and therefore, the immortal body shall climb your ladder as three.

September 14, 1970: *"All right. [9-5-70-002] asks about her karmic lessons that she should learn in this lifetime."*

We should say of your karmic lessons that you should learn of this lifetime — and in asking we see permission from this soul was given for partials of a life reading and partials of a medical reading, as thy would know it.

Therefore, we should say unto this soul, first, you have neglected your body before, therefore [positing] as you would call them, karmic lessons, or sin. You must remember that the overindulgence of anything that shall harm your body, or your soul, or your spirit, is sin. Therefore, first we would suggest, consult thy local physician, and in his examination, we should tell thee, we find a problem of the prostrate — or in your case, growth, growth of the membrane area known as the [muliebris, muliebridian] testicle. [Editor's note: another name for ovary.]

We find this problem. We also find this soul of great nervous pressure. We would suggest that after consulting your physician and taking the necessary steps to overcome your medical problem, this, in itself, shall be the end of a karma.

Now, of your nervous, remember, if you should trespass upon others, then this that thy have done shall be done into yourself, either upon this lifetime or the next. Therefore, drink a little of this wine we offer you.

Do not become radical in this work. For those who would become radical remember, they can no longer see the need of others, only the need for themselves. Therefore, they are no longer serving a useful purpose, for they are dominating their power upon others. This we do not want. In loving others, in building upon what is already there, in loving others enough to give them a gift from yourself, as one soul would give a gift to another — but remember, in giving this gift, give it in the same way to another that you would give it, a gift to your Father — if you should overcome your last karma, we should say, speak to your Father as you would into thyself, and speak to the ones thy love of the things that dwell in thyself.

This is all on this soul at the present time.

September 14, 1970: *"All right. Thank you.* [9-5-70-004] *has requested a health reading, mainly to find out why her legs are so large and is there is anything she can do for this?"*

Yes, we see the problem. This problem, in itself, is a problem of the circulatory system; an over-enlargement of the blood vessels, as thy would know them, which are servicing the lower limbs, are enlarged. Now, we also find a thyroid problem here, directed — also this problem is built upon infection of the kidney area, liver's — we would suggest, first, absolutely no alcoholic beverages of any type. Second, find a substitute for the salt; salt to your bladder is poison, therefore, feeding these other areas. Now we would suggest the saunic baths. This would help in the reducing of the size of these vessels, as throwing the circulatory system back into its proper scope, as thy would know it.

We also find a problem here of the mastoid. This would be very simple to correct by going to a good, as thy would know it, dentist. This also would help relieve the poison going into your system because of a bad denture problem.

This is all on this soul at this time.

September 14, 1970: *"All right. Again,* [9-14-70-003] *asks for a health and life reading. Would you like for him to read these before it's given?"*

**We would suggest thy go on to thy other questions at this time.**

September 14, 1970 [in Life Readings]: *"All right. I'm not sure of the pronunciation of this name, Aka. It is [9-10-70-005] and he asks for a health reading, a life reading if necessary."*

**The problem here, first, reduce thy imagination. The things that thy would imagine in thy mind are not necessarily so. Meditate. In your meditation, you shall seek the healing that you need. In your imagination, you are creating problems that are not there, but remember, your mind is a very powerful instrument. If you, in your mind, should think yourself sick, then your mind shall make your body sick, and the body shall decay and die.**

**Now, on this soul, thy ask for a life reading. Then, we should tell thee. You have asked from curiosity, and only in curiosity. But we shall tell you of your life in this fashion.**

**Yes, we see this.**

**This soul was born, in the first entry, in the time before Atlantis. And in your wandering in this time, thy have lost thy way.**

**Therefore, we find the next entry in servitude in the time of Atlantis. Now, in your servitude, we find thy work shall be directed for those not of the God of One; therefore, our Father, because of your ignorance, shall forgive this sin.**

**Now, we see this soul, not again until the first century after the birth of Christ. We see this soul born in that part that is known at this time as [Eutilia], later to be known as a proportion of what is now known as France. Now, at this time, we see your search. Upon this lifetime, you are a warrior, a hunter. At first, we see this has come about for the need of food, but later, we see this comes about for the lust of killing.**

**Now, we see this entry again not until, in the land known as Spain, again until 1632 A.C. This time you are born as the duke of a royal family of Louis.**

**Yes, we see this.**

**We see your father is Francisos, Don Francisos. We see many Jewish people at this time. We see your problem again. At first, the persecution of these people is something you do not like, something you feel you must do because of your father. But again, we see your liking, as you would say, this work.**

**Now we see this soul not again until the 17th century. Yes, we see this soul at 1717 — your choice, for your years are not from a light you have learned, but from a light you have seen backward.**

**Now, we see this soul again in Massachusetts as you journey in your teachings this time, and your teachings shall be the word of Christ. Sometimes your teachings are true, sometimes your teachings are false,**

for instead of the words that were written, you are using your own in their place.

Now, we see this soul again upon this plane, and we should tell this soul, you are walking backwards. Your next step shall be to lose your spirit. Turn toward your Father's light. Talk to your Father as you would talk to yourself, and love Him, and He shall give you the help that you need at this time. And in talking to your Father, if you would speak that we may enter, we would give the help from our Father, for remember, all thy must do is ask, and upon asking, pray for guidance.

This is all on this soul at this time.

September 14, 1970: **You have one other question. This is not a question that is written. We see this question that, as thy would know her, this soul, [7-1-70-003], we see this soul as the wife of Matthew, and she asked, "Why should Matthew not come to hear of this work?" Matthew shall come in his own time, in his own way, for Matthew is learning, and as he learns he shall give unto others. But remember our promise unto you, and our promise was a promise of our Father, and all things unto which He has promised shall come, as thy would know it, in this life plane.**

**Now soul Ray weakens and grows tired. Waken him.**

**But remember, now is the time of the Cherub.**

September 18, 1970: *"At this time, Aka, we'll continue our experiment release readings. We have a question, a very concerning question by* [9-18-70-001]*, concerning her daughter, M___ A___...in Globe, Arizona. She asks, 'My daughter is missing and I want to know if she is safe?'"*

We should say unto this soul, the giving of information upon another soul without the permission of this soul we cannot do. But if you should wait of a moment, permission must be given from our Father.

Our Father should speak of these words — the one thy should speak upon is safe.

But remember, in your world, you have created many things. And most of these things you have falsely created. The use of drugs is not a safe thing. You do not come closer to our Father with the use of your drugs. Nay, instead you open the door to Lucifer that he may enter and show you the wonders that he may perform. If a drug should be used in a correct manner into which it was originally created, this, in itself, would be of a good thing. But when it is used for the abuse of the body, [and] remember, our Lord created this body, and He should grow angry at those who would abuse it. But even in this form, He leaves the punishment unto yourselves.

If you could think of the beginning of what we have said, and place the ending before the beginning, you shall have the your answer to the place your daughter shall be found.

September 18, 1970: *"Aka, we have another request, experiment release, for a life reading on S___ M___ S_____. The address is...California. Can you give a reading at this time?"*

Yes, we should give both of a health and a life reading.

We see of your problem, but before we give your full life reading, we should say unto you, give of yourself unto others. This should be the first step. We see your love for mankind, and we see your love upon this earth plane and your sorrow. Understand, there are times when we would like to interfere. We should send you of the help you should need, but even this help may only enter through yourself. Without this — we should say at this time, this reading shall be continued at another time; soul Ray becomes weary. Therefore, awaken him from his slumber.

September 21, 1970: **But we do have another message for soul [6-9-70-004]. As you have walked once before in the light of teaching, let this light surround you and become part of you, and let it shine from you in such a way that others may receive this light. If your light should grow dim and, as you would call it, need rekindling, then come forth, and we shall give such help as needed. But remember, there is no place upon your earth which our Father cannot touch of His choosing. All you must do is open of the door, and through the horn of plenty, all things shall come into the soul, the body, and the spirit.**

September 21, 1970: **Ask your next question.**

*"We have another experimental release form here on [9-21-70-002, San Diego, California] who asks, first a question, 'How will I find peace of mind and tranquility?' He also asks for a health reading."*

Yes, we find this problem. First we would give of the health reading, for this is very essential. Our first suggestion would be that this soul immediately change its drinking water. Buy of the purified water.

We also find — we also find here an old lesion of the kidney area. Yes.

This problem was created as a child, in the experimentation of the body when the expansion of the bladder area was done, there was misuse here. For the child had a wetting problem, and the parents, in conjunction, to correct this, used force in such a way that the bladder area was overly expanded. Therefore, we see a very definite problem here in the prostate. We would suggest that this area be thoroughly flushed, using of the sage tea and some proportions, as you would know, as ginger. We would also suggest that if this problem is not corrected with this usage very soon, that tests be made in this area for, as you would know them, cancer-type growths. This should not be neglected.

We also find the problem here — yes — many old lesions — yes, yes — very definite problem in the back area. These problems could quite simply be taken care of by very simply going to a good osteopathic doctor or chiropractic doctor. X-rays taken of this back area would expose the necessary repairs to be made. We also find in this soul that the use of meditation would greatly help this soul. Prayer within your group, prayer[s] should be held within your group for this soul.

Now we feel your other question. We would say, drink a little of our wine. In its works you may find the answers you need. With meditation and giving of yourself unto others, your peace of mind shall be as one.

But remember, you still have another question unto which you did not ask. Fear not of our answers, for we are here only to prepare the way for a greater Prophet. Therefore, we would answer your question, for we see its need. You are faced with certain financial problems at this time. These you have created unto yourself by not being truthful with yourself and others. We would say unto you, be truthful with yourself. And remember, we are here to help; if you would open your door, first by thinking of God in your meditation, and then of the word, Aka [Atka]; we would enter and give you the help you need.

This is all on this soul at this time.

September 21, 1970: **Ask your other question.**
*"Aka, soul John asks, he would like to know why he has been having such bad headaches after each meeting we have here?"*

If you would take the time after the meetings for meditation that our messages may come through, open both your mind and your heart unto this work, for remember, soul John, we have chosen you for mighty work. There is much knowledge that must pass between God and yourself. We see your need for relief at this time, and we should take away this pain. The pain we have left there has been a reminder of the pain you have seen before, but remember, soul John, this pain you saw before was shed for the love of mankind.

This is all.

September 21, 1970: **You have other questions; ask of these.**
*"Yes, Aka. We have here a request for a health reading from [9-21-70-001.] Can you give us a health reading at this time?"*

One moment, please. We do not find this soul you mention. We feel that you have made a mistake in pronunciation of the name. Therefore, it would be necessary that you would obtain additional information, that this reading may be given.

September 25, 1970: **Now, we would say unto Paul, God is with thee; fear not. Remember, we have given you the healing of the body, and this healing shall come unto you and your family, and let not man with his foolish thoughts put God's work asunder.**

September 28, 1970: **Ask your other question.**

*"Aka, at this time are you able to give a health reading on soul P___?"*

Yes, this health reading shall be given. One moment, please. Yes, we have the body, the soul and the spirit and the immortal body of soul P___.

Yes, we find the need for, first, for corrective, a different corrective lens. We might suggest, in this case, that eye exercise be used. If this was used over a period of two-months' time, this problem would greatly improve — casting the eyesight as high in one area as it may see, and as low in another area as it may see, as far to the right and as far to the left as it may see, then returning the sight into a central point into the center.

We also find at this time that this soul should use sage tea. We shall make the corrections needed in this soul in the physical body. These corrections shall be made and the healing shall come about. But there are certain precautions that the body in itself should take.

Remember, soul P___, all thy must do is ask in our Father's name, the name of the Messiah, and the help thy require shall always be there.

Now, we see a problem and we shall make the adjustment, therefore, within. We should ask thee of one small chore, that for of three nights thy should ask [of] our Father for the healing. Permission has been given and this healing shall come about. This healing shall be for all of thy children, upon your request, for you are wife of soul Peter.

Now, we would suggest to soul Peter, we have given unto thee the healing power. Have thy so little faith that thy would not use it unto thy wife? Remember, say unto thy wife, "In my Father's name, thy shall be healed." And this shall be done unto her.

But remember, soul P___, you are dear to our Father. You have been dear to Him many times before. And we should leave this word in thy mind, thy was Helen once before. But not think of thee of the time of Christ, think of thee in the time of Isaiah.

This is all on this subject at this time. A further reading shall be taken in three days.


September 28, 1970: **Ask thy other question.**

*"Aka, soul J___ would also like a health reading at this time."*

We see her problem. And we shall repeat again this message to soul Andrew. Have thy so little faith that thy cannot believe in thy own healing power? You are becoming of five, and therefore, this power has been given unto you. We would suggest, in this case, that when soul Ray has awoken, that you consult him of this healing.

Now is the time to awaken soul Ray from his slumber.


October 5, 1970: Now, we would say unto soul Luke, for the one who should need of the healing, give unto this soul. Your Father gives you these words. "LOVE, IN EVEN THE SMALLEST THING UPON THIS EARTH, IS A MIGHTY TOOL."

Ask your other questions.

October 5, 1970: **Ask your other questions.**
*"Aka, the wife of soul Thomas would like to know if her daughter is safe?"*

As we have said before unto this soul, your daughter is safe.

Now, at this time, we would ask unto your group to give, each in his own way, into prayer for this soul. Pray for healing in all ways. [Editor's note: There is a long pause while they pray.]

And now, we would say unto this soul, we shall send the help that is needed to guide this one. But remember, even our Father will not interfere with the free choice of a soul. Therefore, we shall give what help we can. But, we would say, this soul shall return soon, and she shall no longer be a child, for she shall be a woman in all ways. Therefore, as thy should talk unto this soul, talk as one woman unto another, and remember that all things are not of sin, that the natural desires of the body God placed unto you, that thy should multiply and be fruitful. Therefore, therefore, what would be sin in your eyes would not be sin in our Father's eyes.

Remember also, there is one commandment in which your Father would ask above all others, that thy would worship no other God but He, that thy should love your God as much as He loves you, and that thy should treat the smallest thing upon your earth the same as thy self should be treated upon your earth plane.

And remember also, our Father has many mansions. And remember, our Father loves all of His children in His many worlds, for that unto which ye should create can never be greater than the Creator. In your own way, you think you have created this body that moves around the soul, but remember, this soul came unto you in the beginning of its own free choice. It shall return unto you again of its own free choice.

October 9, 1970: **Ask your other questions.**
*"Aka, at this time, can you give a continuation on soul P\_\_'s health reading?"*

We should say unto thee again, soul Peter, at this time — one moment. Our Father should give the healing at this time that is needed, both mentally and physically. We would suggest that soul P\_\_, at this time, the taking of Lydia E. Pinkham. Also, we would suggest that, within six weeks, if the problem at hand is not completely settled, then the other help shall be. But remember, our Father gives unto thee complete healing. Our Father cannot give unto thee what thy would not accept. If thy would believe this in thy mind, our Father would give it, complete healing. And before three nights shall pass, thy shall dream as thy were before and the light of our Father shall [shine] upon thee, and thy shall taste of the Lamb's blood.

This is all on this soul at this time.

October 9, 1970: *"Aka, at this time we have another experimental release on one we have brought up before, much to my error in pronunciation of the name. We would like to try again for a health reading on a [9-5-70-007]. Can you give us any information on him at this time?"*

Yes, we see the body, the soul and the spirit; we also see [their] need. Therefore, permission has been given.

We find, first, on this soul, cancerous-type growth on the facial area. We also find this growth shall inline deeply into the vocal cord area. We would suggest that this soul seek a good physician.

We find healing could be suggested within thy group, if each one, in their own way, should give of a prayer for this soul. [Editor's note: There is a 50-second pause.]

Now, we should also say, remember, in thy request thy cannot ask and we are not given permission to give information from one soul unto another. This reading was given only by permission from our Father, for this soul did not sign, as thy would know it, of the release form.

Now soul Ray becomes very weak, and therefore, we would suggest that thy should waken him. But remember, before we go, now is the time of the Cherub.

October 12, 1970: Then we would say unto thee, soul Luke, we have seen thy need, and given thee thy help in thy time of need. And we send this message into thee once again. Our Father loves thee and blesses thee, and there shall be great work unto thee. And the healing that thy have asked for shall be given.

And for those in the valley below the sea [Editor's note: Soul Luke at that time lived in Yuma, Arizona, in the Imperial Valley, where the Yuma study group was. Aka is interrupted when something falls over and the dog yelps] — and for those in the valley below the sea, we would say unto thee, come into thee.

Now we would suggest that thy should waken soul Ray from his slumber.

October 23, 1970 [in Philosophy]: Therefore, ask thy other question.
*"Aka, could you give us any thought or information as to the purpose of the organ pipe cactus, medicinally. Medicinally is the organ pipe cactus?"*

Yes, medically, as what thy know it, or internally, this cactus, as thy would know it, the pulp known from the roots is a good, as thy would know it, once dried and made into powder, and then by taking of the Night-blooming Citros [Cereus] dried and made into powder, then by taking of the flat cactus, as thy would know it, the pulp of the same, dried and made into powder, this placed upon an open wound would greatly, could be greatly used in the healing of the same.

There are other uses of this same plant. The blossom [removed] from the same can be dried and used in small quantities for what thy know of, for treatment of heart diseases. But at this time you have many other good drugs for the same.

Therefore, the use of this, make of experiments of the same, storing for the time that shall be lean. Take of all this knowledge; store it for the time that shall be lean. There are other information; your time, this same pulp may be used in the healing of radiation burns, mixed, as thy would know it, with the greasewood; therefore, displacing a virus known in your land as [cacturus], or, as you would say, cancerous.

October 23, 1970: **Ask your other questions.**
*"Aka, soul Judas asks if there is any information you can give him to help understand the personal events that are happening to him at this time?"*
Yes, soul Judas, we see thy need. Then we say unto thee that no man may trespass upon thee. Blessed are those who should follow the Lamb. For blessed are they who shall take the Sword of the Lord in his hand in vengeance of the Lord. [See *The Revelation*, chapter 19.]

There are times thy should change in thyself; there are times that others should change. As the man known as Jesus said before, "If thy are offended and struck upon one cheek, turn the other." But he did not mean to let this person continue to defile thee. Can thy understand of which we speak?
*"Partially."*
Then we say unto thee, if thy had two calves and both were fat and ready for slaughter, and one calf thy would give unto the Lord and one calf thy would give unto man, the Lord does not mean that thy should slaughter this calf and lay it to waste upon [   ] its altar. The Lord means, sell this calf and do good with it in God's name, and therefore, you have given unto the Lord. Now, soul Judas, can thy understand of us?
*"Yes, Aka."*

November 2, 1970: *"All right. At this time can you give us the continuation for [10-23-70-001]?"*
Yes, we have the body, the soul, the spirit, and the immortal body; therefore, permission has been granted and this reading shall be given. We realize our message unto thee was quite puzzling, but the light that thy shall see and have seen shall be thy guiding light. This is unto which thy have asked for, and we have given you this.

Now, remember, [10-23-70-001], each soul in their prayers shall ask for different things upon your earth. Those, our Father shall never have deaf ears, for He hears all things. For those who ask, they are given the help they need and the guidance they need. You shall soon meet one who shall need help, and you shall give this help as freely as it has been given unto thee.

We find thy have certain physical problems. Now, we should say unto thee, these physical problems are partially in thy mind. But then again, we would suggest, first, you have the problem of irritated skin, or acne, as thy would call it. Then, take thee of the greasewood, and take thee, as you would know it, of the substance known as soda, first cleansing thy skin with the substance known as olive oil, then applying these two substances made moist with the olive oil upon your skin. This corrective need shall be brought about.

We also find here that the blood, of [an] impurity here. We find of the lower count of the white corpuscles than should be; therefore, if thy would see thy medical doctor and have the tests run that would show of the same, we find this problem could be corrected quite simply.

We also find that this soul is bothered with what is known as migraine headaches. We would suggest to this soul that chocolate, as thy would know of it, is a poison unto thy system. Do not eat of this substance.

This is all of this soul at this time. A life reading, as has been suggested, shall come in a future date.

*"Thank you, Aka."*

November 9, 1970: **Ask thy other questions.**
*"Aka, have you any suggestions as to what we might be able to do in relationship to soul Ray's health and his weariness over the past months? We've been falling behind on our readings. Have you any suggestions on how we can catch up on this backlog of readings we have that we haven't been able to get to? We are beginning to get more readings than we are being able to take care of. Can you give us anything on this?"*

First, for soul Ray's physical health, we have said before that only our Father may create. We shall do much to help his physical body, but all that we may do, he may tear asunder. But we find that this soul has received our message.

First, for rest, remember, rest of the mind is necessary also. Now, we find that certain chemicals in his body shall need sleeping [feeding]. We would suggest that an additional vitamin substance be given unto this soul for a period of 90 days. We find that of this vitamin, more, as you would know it, of vitamin C, more, as you would know it, of vitamin D. We also find, more sodium of iodine compound. We find the lacking of calcium. We find, more of the natural salt. We find this soul should have more, as you know it, of the salad foods, fresh. We find this soul should need more, as you would know it, of the sea food. This should be placed in his diet at least once a week. But above all others, we would suggest that at least three times each day he should have rest. We would suggest that this soul should not perform physical labors for more than two hours at a time. If he should perform two hours of physical labor, then, of your time, have him rest for 30 minutes.

Of your other question, we have placed the necessary information in soul Ray's mind. We would suggest for all your readings that one reading a week be set aside for only backlogging of your readings. But of all readings that are brought forth, these readings, before they are suggested to be given, should be studied by the entirety of your group, therefore, giving judgment of the same before these readings should be asked for. This would greatly eliminate foolish questions. We would tell thee in this way. If, in your prayer, you should ask God a question, then bring these same questions and place them into readings. Those who would ask in this way will receive what they have asked for.

November 9, 1970: **You have other questions. Ask of these questions.**

*"Aka, we have a request for a health and life reading from soul Judas, from [8-31-70-001]. Can you give us a health and life reading on [8-31-70-001] this evening?"*

We would suggest before this reading is given that she should take one of your experimental forms and fill this out. At that time, both of the health and life reading shall be given.

But we would say unto this soul this message. If the river of two streams should run, one at your front door and one at your back door, and one would head east and the other west, and one should give of thee pure water and one should be polluted, which of these would thy drink? And if in thy mind thy knew that thy could travel of both rivers, and the one that would travel east would bring of thee into polluted land, but the one of the polluted water that would travel into the west would bring thee into a pure land, think thee then of which thy would travel. Think thee then, and then ask again.

November 9, 1970: **Ask of thy other question.**

*"Aka, [11-2-70-001] asks, "What can we do, if possible, anything to help [11-9-760-001]?"*

We say unto thee, ask thee of God.

And we say unto all of thee, pray thee unto God at this time, each in his own way, and we shall give the help that is needed in our way. [Editor's note: There is a long pause.]

November 13, 1970: **You have other questions, ask.**

*"Yes, Aka, I [4-6-70-002] have a question this evening. I would like to see, or hear, if you could give me any information on the person I saw quite some time ago in my dream of levitation in the picture. This person has been with me quite often this past week in my thoughts as well as my physical self. I feel quite good about this, yet I would like to know if there is any information you can give me on this at this time?"*

This is a member of our council which has been sent unto you to advise you in your daily life. Heed his words, for he speaks with wisdom.

November 13, 1970: **Now, we would say unto soul [4-3-70-003], we see thy need; thy thought has been received. We shall give thy help that thy ask, and blessings and healing from our Father shall come too with thee. God bless thee, and mercy unto those who would offend thee.**

November 13, 1970: **And now, we say unto soul [8-10-70-003], we have seen of thy plight, and the necessary steps have been taken that the help that thy should need shall walk by thy side. Do not fear this one, for this one comes from God, our Father.**

November 13, 1970: **And we say unto [8-10-70-002], speak of thy Father.**

November 13, 1970: **And remember, soul [4-6-70-002], our Lord blesses thee. Walk thee and take the advice of the one sent unto thee.**

November 13, 1970: **And now we have this message for soul [7-3-70-001], we see thy need, and we say unto thee that again if thy would in thy meditation think upon our Father, and the help needed shall be sent for guidance into thee. And into [7-3-70-001]'s wife [6-9-70-002], we see thy doubt. Then we say unto thee, we give thee this message, that had Lot's wife listened, she would not have been cast from the face of the earth.** [See *Genesis* 19:12-26.]

November 13, 1970: **And now, for the wife of soul Ray, fear not. Remember, the ones who would protect him do not sleep. And the ones who would protect you do not sleep.**
**Now, we would say unto thee, awaken soul Ray from his slumber.**

November 16, 1970: *"Good evening, Aka. Does Ray stand with God?"*
**Soul Ray stands with God.**
*"Thank you, Aka."*
**And now, we see thy need, soul [6-9-70-004]. And we would say of thy question, we have given unto thee, unto thy soul, [11-16-70-001], an entry; there was no entry unto this body before.**
**Therefore, we should give at this time a health reading upon this new soul.**
**Yes.**
**We should say upon this soul, the body is not, as you would know it, perfect. We should send the help that is needed into this soul.**
**First, thy should give into this soul large quantities of natural vitamins. Give unto this soul an adult dosage of vitamin D. We should also suggest that large quantities in the adult dosage of calcium be given unto this soul.**

You must understand that your job in the corrective work ahead shall be in the redirection of the brain cells. First, we should acquaint thee with the brain cells. In the [dormular, dormant?] area, no entry would accept this type of damage which has come at birth; therefore, correction had to be made into this area. Correction now has been made. You shall also find slight damage into what is known as the brainstem area. With patience, this problem should heal itself. You will find that the child, therefore, shall need corrective lenses, for the child shall have double vision, and has this now. As soon as can be found practical, if this was taken care of this would reduce the dizziness and loss of equilibrium into this soul.

We would also suggest [that] the taking of the Night-blooming Citros [Cereus]. This should be done by first drying this and grinding it into a powdery substance, therefore, mixed unto the soul's meals. We would suggest that a 2-by-2-inch square's be used daily. This should be done for at least six-month's time.

We should also suggest that as the retraining of this child commences, the child shall be very dominant, wanting his way continuously. In some things this is good, but in others this is very bad. Therefore, we would suggest that certain rules [to] his daily life be set forth and these rules carried out steadfast. A discipline at this time is a must. Without discipline, this child shall lose the repairs we have done at this point. Teaching at this time of all things should come about. The language barrier should be broken as soon as possible. If these works are done in their proper coordinance, you should find that the advancement shall soon come forth unto four, and then five.

We should say that this child shall become a very psychic, as you would know them, person upon your plane, capable, at an early age, as you would think, performing miracles. This child should have constant teachings of God. Without these, he should forget his way, and the power set forth there should destroy him.

And now we should say unto thee, think thee of God, your Father. Think of His ever-loving, of His ever-forgiving. Think thee of our Father and the tears He should shed for your — Our Father loves thee. He should prepare a way for thy grief.

November 16, 1970: **Ask thy other question.**
*"Aka, [11-16-70-004] has a question this evening. She asks, 'Will our financial picture improve shortly?'"*
Nay. Thy financial picture can only improve. We would answer you in this way. If thy have but one donkey, and load this beast of burden too heavy, thy should kill of the beast.
**Ask thy other question.**
*"Aka, last Friday during the reading — "*
**One moment, please.**
**Yes, Father. Yes. Yes, Father. Yes.**

Then we would say unto this soul, your financial, material burden shall change as thy heart should change. And it should come unto thee as unto raindrops. But we would say unto thee, return thee into thy church. Worship thy Father. Remember, unto all things who would speak unto our Father, without profanity, who in his thought and soul should seek our Father, our Father should give unto [he] thy blessings. Forgive thee those who should trespass upon thee.

November 20, 1970: **Thy have other questions, ask.**
*"Aka, this evening we have various questions. Soul Paul has questions this evening that he would like to ask in relation to a friend of his; a W\_\_\_\_ S\_\_\_\_ has asked if he will find what he is seeking, or should he redirect himself?"*

We should say unto this soul, in your own words, redirect thyself, but not in completion. Use meditation to seek thy soul. And as you find your soul, so shall your soul find its spirit. We should say unto thee, turn thy eyes toward to heavens, turn thy heart toward the heavens. But remember of this, God did not make rules unto worship unto Himself. He asks that thy love thy God, that thy love thy fellow man.

November 20, 1970: **Ask thy other question.**
*"Aka, soul E\_\_\_\_ C\_\_\_\_ has a question this evening. 'Is a move nearby feasible and reasonable?'"*

We should say unto this soul, at this time it should not either be feasible or reasonable, for your costs in moving would be more. We would say unto you, if thy continue to sell of what thy have — now is the time to stand fast. Look into thy resources as they are. Take of thy debts. First, we would say unto you, as you would call them, your hospital and doctor, pay these as you can. There is funds available to you to pay these. You are, as thy would know it, disabled. Also, if it was in your mind to use this, there are Federal, of your Government, funds available for the same. Of your other bills, go unto your debtors and plead your case. Reduce your bills. But worry not of the time, as you would know it, of Christmas. Your children shall receive the blessings of God. Open your hearts, and as raindrops, your hearts shall runneth over. At a future time, living facilities will be made available unto you. At this time, then make your move, but do not sell of thy home, retain this as seed. Can thy understand of which we speak?
*"Yes."*

November 20, 1970: **Then ask thy other questions.**
*"Aka, soul M\_\_\_\_ has a question of personal concern this evening. She asks, or is concerned about her son J\_\_\_\_'s reading and his ability to grasp his reading problem. Can you give her any information on this, or any advisement as to helping him, if he needs it?"*

We see no problem here. You have made this child lazy. Therefore, retrain his mind. You have at your disposal the use of hypnosis. Use unto this. After this has been done, ask again. Remember, those who would look after your family do not sleep.

November 20, 1970: **Ask your other questions.**
*"This evening, Aka, soul J__ has a question, questions in a series of three. Number one, 'What is causing the pain in my side and what can I do?' Number two, 'Can or will you tell me what has happened to Tippy?' Number three, 'Was Mike's dream about the lights to instruct him?'"*

**Of your pain in your side, we find — yes — strained tissue. We find strain of the mind from worry. Both of these, from the worry of the same, should cause thy pain. Then we would suggest, before thy sleep tonight, think thee of God and think thee of the word, Aka, that we might enter and cause healing into thy body.**

**Of thy other question, of Tippy, this we should say unto thee. Do thy doubt God's words? We find your concern here. One moment, please.**

**This question must be asked at a different time.**

**Of your third question, we should say unto thee, there are things of the mind which are of the mind. There are things of heaven which are of heaven. And there are those things of earth which are of earth. And in thy mind, thy already have the answer of your third question.**

**Of your fourth question, we would say unto thee, as the bride should take unto the groom, so should the groom take unto the bride, for both vows are of the same. And as doubt grows and the seed of doubt, for we have said before that even the seed of the onion, as small as it may seem, should act as yeast and coveth thy mind either with the works of God or the works of Lucifer. There is no way that you can control the thoughts of your husband. Therefore, worry not of his thoughts, but of your own. Can you understand of which we speak?**

*"I think so, Aka."*

November 27, 1970: **We see now one in need and we should answer this question. Your daughter, the gift of healing has been given, and she shall be well again. Can you understand of which we speak?**

[She whispers.]

**Then we should say unto you, remember, as Lot's wife looked backward, do not yourself.**

December 4, 1970: **Aka is here.**

*"Good evening, Aka. Does soul Ray stand with God?"* [Peter, who was conducting the evening's session, asks.]

**Soul Ray stands with God.**

*"Thank you, Aka."*

**You have many questions, ask.**

*"Yes, Aka. This evening you have a question from soul John [4-6-70-*

*001]. Soul John asks if there is any way you can help him in determining what is causing his severe dizzy spells which have come about in the past weeks?"*

Yes, we have the body, the soul, the spirit, and the immortal body. Yes, we see thy need.

First, we would say unto this soul, you have a concussion from an old injury.

Yes, we see this.

We find that during the time of this injury lesions in the muscles that control the eye; therefore, we would suggest, first, as you would say this word, an eye doctor should be consulted. Therefore, a corrective lens should help at this time. We should also say, with exercise of the eyes, first, by casting the eyes to the right as far as possible, then to the left as far as possible, then upward as far as possible, then downward as far as possible. We should suggest during these exercises that you should find a point at each, upward and downward, into which to concentrate upon. Find a point to your left and to your right to concentrate upon. We would suggest this soul should have more rest.

We would suggest a changing of the diet. We would suggest more of what is known as raw vegetation. We should also suggest that a good natural vitamin, or vitamin substance, be taken.

We find also a problem of the kidneys. We find inflammation there. Therefore, we suggest the drinking of the sage tea. We would suggest placing in this tea of ginger; also we would suggest placing in this tea of lemon. If it is found that for the taste buds you may sweeten this tea, but not with of the white sugar. Sweeten this tea with, as you would know it, the juice of the bee. Therefore, this should be taken at least once a day and preferably twice a day.

We also find a problem at this time of the thyroid, of the overactive thyroid. There are many good compounds. We would suggest that by taking — for you have not prepared, and therefore, the natural substance is not available to you at this time — then we would suggest there are many good natural food stores. You should go into these; find — mixing of the calcium, mixing of the blossom taken from the Night-blooming Citros [Cereus], taking from the blossoms of the saguaros. If these are not available then we would suggest, consult your physician.

We would also suggest by use of meditation your problem may be overcome.

This is all on this soul at this time. A reading should be taken within a two-week period.

December 4, 1970: **Ask thy other question.**

*"Aka, [4-6-70-003] has another question. It relates to a question we asked earlier. She asks, 'Is Tippy dead?'"*

We have said before, this is all on this soul at this time.

December 4, 1970: **Ask your other question.**

*"[11-2-70-00 ]this evening, Aka, has a question. It is very important to her, and would like an answer if she may receive one. She asks, 'Will my mother's health be restored to her and her sufferings be relieved?'"*

**We find we shall answer your question. Her suffering shall be relieved quite shortly.**

December 4, 1970: **Ask your other question.**

*"This evening, Aka, have you a message for soul Peter [4-6-70-002]?"*

**We should answer your question in this way. There shall be the times of doubt and frustration. As you walk upon the earth you shall see this in many souls. But once before you were asked this question, if you should have the faith to walk upon the water with us? Why do you doubt thyself? Give healing where it is needed.**

December 4, 1970: **And now we should answer one other question, unto the one who feels sorrow at this time. Our Father sees thy need, and He should prepare the way. The light of our Father shall be seen unto this one, and their parting shall be with grace and beauty. For our Father sees thy love.**

**Now is the time to awaken soul Ray from his slumber.**

December 7, 1970: **You have many questions. Ask.**

*"Aka, [12-7-70-001] has asked for a health reading. At this time can you give this?"*

**We see thy need. One moment, please.**

**We have body, soul, the spirit, and the immortal body. We see her need. Therefore, the help that she seeks we should give unto this soul.**

**We see of her present problem. We find, that as a child of eight-years old, she was hurt while climbing stairs. We find old lesions in what we would know as the [limbro] or neck area. We do not see the traction, in this case, could improve this area; we find that through either osteopathic or chiropractic treatment. The bones — as you would know them of the upper neck area — were dislodged. We find, that due to the cold weather, that arthritis, in this area. We would suggest, first, that necessary work be done in this area for correction of the same. We find that saunic baths be taken. Therefore, we would suggest [that] in the area known as Apache Junction, these baths and the necessary chiropractic treatment could be secured at this time. We also find, that due to the secretion of the nerves of this area, as you would know it, a poisonous — we find the kidney area, an inflammation of the same.**

**We find inflammation of the right kidney, inflammation of the liver area. Therefore, we find from, as you would know it, bad diet, the fatty tissue in this area, that the necessary function of the testicle [ovary] of the same, interference. We also find fatty tissue around the heart area.**

This in itself is not good. We would suggest at this time [cough] — we would suggest at this time that a very strict diet of beef, [and] no pork — of no fat in the beef, that the beef be boiled before eating — a vegetarian-type diet. We also find a good natural vitamin be taken.

We also find injury of bruise of the left hip joint area. We would suggest that the taking of an adult dose of calcium.

We would suggest, we find of the multiple [meridian, uridium?]-type growths]. Yes, we see this. We would suggest changing of the drinking water. We would suggest the taking of the sage tea. We would suggest the taking of the Night-blooming Cereus in quantities of quarter-by-quarter cubes daily for a period of two weeks.

We also find, of the lower back area, chiropractic treatment needed. We find in both feet that due faulty, of the wearing, as you would know them, shoes, we would suggest that of this, that supports be worn. This would greatly improve both of the posture and of the holding of the vertebrae[s] into place.

We find multiple breaks of the upper limb of the circulatory system. These would be greatly improved with the saunic-type baths of the same.

We also find of this soul, and we should say [on, and] it, for improvement of the same, if in your daily life, speak unto God as you would speak unto yourself. Do this in private, and remember of these words, our Father, and yours, should shed many tears for this soul. For what you have been before, you shall be again.

December 7, 1970: **Ask your other questions**.
"Aka, S____ I___ has asked the question, what is causing the trouble that he is having?"
We would say unto this soul that from a boy to a man there are many changes taking place in your body. At this time, you have the body in many proportions of a man, yet the physical development of the same has not taken place. Then we would say unto this soul, after you have worked and performed your duties, take of the warm olive oil, saturate your whole body in the same. Therefore, you shall not have this problem again. We find that this soul should go to a chiropractor for adjustment of the upper back area. We find of the brain-stem area, pinched nerves. This problem and the treatment of the same with warm olive oil should correct this problem from occurring in the future.

Of your other problem, we should say unto this soul, remember, did not Christ change water into wine?

Ask your other question.

December 7, 1970: "Aka, at this time, can you give a continuation on the reading for [11-9-70-002]?"
We should suggest, from the overtaxing of soul Ray, that this

question be asked at a different time.

*"All right."*

We should suggest at this time that you should awaken soul Ray from his slumber.

December 11, 1970: **Then we say unto the one known as soul Judas, in the very bottom of the pits of Simon there was love and compassion, even though the cuts upon their body burned of salt, for they looked up into the heavens and saw our Father and knew then that man, no man, could destroy another man's soul or spirit, or immortal body. And weep not for the wife of Lot. And this we should promise unto thee. We lift thyself from this pit. And go to the river and bathe thyself in the blood of the Lamb, and thy shall become as five. And go out into your world and give there healing and give there love, for from your body we shall have taken your sin upon us. Can thy understand of which we speak?**

*"Yes."*

**Then bless thee, my son.**

December 11, 1970: **Now you have other questions, ask of these.**

*"Yes, Aka. [8-24-70-001] would like to know if you can give her any information as to making her feel better?"*

**We should say unto thee these words. For healing we have given thee. But remember, this healing comes from our Father, and with one single finger did He not cast Lucifer from the heavens? Doubt not of His power for healing. For, if it should be of a bolt of lightening that thy should witness, this we should give, if necessary. Thy body shall become whole again, my daughter, for God loves this soul.**

December 11, 1970: **Then we say unto you, soul John, be patient. In your daily life project love and understanding. Do not be harsh with your fellow man. Give of him the blood that dripped from your Master. Give it freely. For did we not promise thee eternal life?**

December 11, 1970: **And now we say these words unto soul Luke, we see thy need. And God, our Father, shall be with thee in thy travels and give healing unto those of thy need. But remember, give of thee the blessings of our Lord and bring into thy flock all of thy sheep. Do not be, as you would know it, impatient with man, for he is but man. He shall stand and fall upon the way. Bend and pick him up, and wash his feet as you have done before. Remember, soul Luke, of the time into which I have washed yours and you have washed mine? Remember from the beginning of all time. Do not slide backward, soul Luke. You have come so far. Walk again with us. There are many who need thy teachings.**

December 18, 1970: **Thy have questions. Ask of these.**

*"Yes, Aka. Aka, we have a question this evening that I think particularly concerns the entire group. I know we've asked before, but can anything else be done to improve soul Ray's health? Over the past week he's gone through quite a lot of discomfort. Can you give us anything one that?"*

As we have said before that the mental change and the mental powers — do not think that soul Ray cannot become angry, for we know he can, and his anguish with others not to use the power given unto him wrongly at times may seem to destroy him. But with each battle within himself, he shall become stronger in spirit and soul. Can you understand of which we say?

*"Yes, Aka, I think we can."*

We would say unto you these words, from time to time he shall grow weary and tired, and shall need rest. He should know of these times, for in these times we shall let him rest.

December 18, 1970: **Ask your other question.**

*"Aka, soul [4-3-70-002] has a question this evening. Can you advise her as to the situation that exists with her mother in Yuma, as so far as helping her?"*

We see the need of soul Luke. We should say unto thee, give of this need. Give of the help that is needed. But remember also, give thy family of thy need also.

December 18, 1970: **Thy have other questions, ask.**

*"Aka, [11-16-70-004] has a question this evening that is quite important to her and her family. She asks, 'Would a visit to the coast to see my mother be a necessity during the next two weeks?'"*

We cannot see this as a necessity at this time. Prepare thyself for a later time.

December 28, 1970: **Aka is here.**

*"Does Ray stand with God?"*

**Soul Ray stands with God.**

*"Thank you."*

And now we see thy needs, soul Luke. And of the thirteen, thy shall receive healing which has been granted from our Father, healing both of thy body, thy soul, thy spirit. If thy should make of the sign, of the same, known in the days of Arcan of the sign of healing unto all, that we may enter — for as we see thy body, thy soul, and thy spirit, and the immortal body, passing through the sign of Arcan [Arkan].

Then take thee of the fruit bared from the root of the Night-blooming Citros [Cereus]. It shall be necessary that the eating of quarter-inch cubes be done.

[Editor's note: This person had inflamed, cracked and bleeding hands.]

The hand area should remain dry. We should suggest that this dryness be done by the heating of warm stones, and towels be placed upon the same, and these towels be placed upon the wounds. We should suggest the taking of the substance known as soda that this may draw the poison and absorb the same. We should suggest the eating of more citrus-type fruit in thy daily meal.

In thy mind thought thy have thought this is from chemicals of the use of the labor. This comes from unbalanced diet.

Remember, soul Luke, only our Father may create. And as you are the servant of our Father, so are we.

Though you walked with us before, you chose rebirth to be on this earth upon this plane that thy love of labor should shine upon the earth in the preparation of the preparing of the way of the coming of the Messiah. We have seen thy work. We have seen thy soul. And we should give thee a gift again of the sight and of the hearing. From this day forward, you may hear our passing and the others of both sides, for thy shall be given the gift of raising the veil, for we feel that this gift may be entrusted in thy hands.

We would suggest that the towels should be saturated first in castor oil, placing of the same upon the hot stones. Do not place this upon the hands themselves, levitating into such a manner that the heat only from these towels may reach the hands. Continue using the substance of medication thy are using at this time. But do not be foolish, soul Luke. Take of the gift that is offered, for it is given with love, and love, of beyond all things, is the teaching of our Father.

Thy ask, at this time should thy daughter, soul [4-3-70-002], journey with thee into the valley below the sea [Yuma, Arizona]? This we see, and this we should recommend. All things should go well. Do not return to work, of thy labor, before thy moon has struck again in fullness, for this shall be part of our healing. Of the financial things, these needs shall be taken care of, and as we have said before, the financial things that are needed in your lives shall be provided as raindrops, a little at a time. But, as the one known as Jesus Christ who broke bread and fed many, these teardrops shall feed many. Can you understand of which we say?

*"Yes, I understand you."* [She answers.]

Then we say unto you, soul Luke, give of thy love unto others. Protect thy veil unto which we leave this day with thee.

December 28, 1970: **Thy have many other questions, ask.**
*"Aka, we have been asked this evening to get a life and/or health reading on 12-28-70-001."*
**This reading has been given. We see no change at this time.**

December 28, 1970: *"Then, Aka, we ask for a life and/or health reading on [11-9-70-002]."*
**We have the body, the soul, and the spirit of soul [11-9-70-002];**

therefore, permission has been given for a health reading upon the same. We find, of this soul, hardening of the arteries. We find, of this soul, tumor of the left eye. We find, of this soul, circulatory problem. We find, of this soul, problem of the lymph gland of the uteria [ureter] area and should suggest the saunic-type baths be given of this soul for the same.

We find in the near future, unless certain preparations are made — one moment.

We would suggest that upon this soul no information be given at this time, for in the Book that is written, soon this form shall change.

# 1971 Health Readings

January 15, 1971: **Ask thy other questions.**
*"Aka, this evening [11-2-70-001] is quite concerned about his wife,
[C_____]'s health. Could you give her a health reading at this time?"*

We see thy need. We shall enter, and therefore, give thy healing.
By the time that thy should reach home thy healing will have come about.
This soul must take much liquids into its diet, and rest, for five days. Eat
of the Night-blooming Citros [Cereus] in quarter-by-quarter-inch cubes
once daily, using of a salt substance in a gargling manner four times
daily.

But worry not upon thy mother, for we have seen thy need and
shall take care of this.

January 15, 1971: **Ask thy other questions.**
*"Aka, this evening D__ asks a silent question."*
We see thy need, and we should answer thy question in this way.
Soon thy shall be called into a different land. Thy shall travel in a means
that thy are not used to. Do not fear, for no harm will come unto thee.
Thy mother will need thee, for she shall become greatly upset from this
need, for in her shall be a house divided.

We can see thy fully do not understand of which we speak, but
since thy ask thy question in silence, we must answer thy question in the
same way. But soon thy shall know of our meaning. Fear not, for we shall
travel with thee. But guard against the serpent, for one shall use you
against another. Stand on neutral ground.

Ask thy other question.

January 15, 1971: *"She [D____] also asks if you can give her any
information as to what caused the reappearance of the growth on [M_____]'s
foot?"*

Thy have ceased to do the things we have suggested. Do them
again, and this shall be no longer.

January 22, 1971. **Thy have other questions, ask.**
*"Aka, this evening I have a question of soul Ruth. She would like to
know if there is anything more she can do to comfort Great-grandmother
T_____, as there is a breakdown and lack of communications since their not*

*being able to speak because of her recent illness. Can you give her anything at all on this?"*

Part of her question we have just answered. We would say unto you, we see thy need; but remember, to where this soul goes is so much more beautiful now, with the message she shall take with her, than where she has been before. Then release her with love; pray that she has seen the light, for all you are holding now is the shell. The soul has departed.

January 22, 1971: **You have other questions, ask.**
*"Aka, this evening we have no questions other than pertaining to our experimental release forms."*

We see a question, and we should answer. Are you, soul John, you above all other — we have told you of the growths that may form in the body. We have told you. Then we should say in this way, to take and make of the sage tea, placing of a two-inch cubicle into the warmth of the hot tea of the Night-blooming Citros [Cereus]. This must be done unto three days. But remember, we may only enter to give healing for those who would seek it.

Soul Ray now grows very tired, and we grow weak.
Then think ye of the sign of the ankh that we may enter.

February 19, 1971: **You have many questions, ask of these.**
*"Aka, this evening we have questions. [4-6-70-003] asks this question. 'Has my mother given permission for receiving help with her leg?'"*

We find permission has not been given. We should say unto thee, we have shown, through you and through soul Ray, the power of healing. If, in thyself, the knowledge still does not gather within itself, then come to soul Ray and bid his help in your meditation. Only in this fashion may this be done. But meditate upon permission before the healing.

Ask you other question. One moment, please.

We should say unto thee, if thy are to learn the lessons that are to be taught unto thee, come in truth. In the practice and the study, as thy would know, of hypnosis, use only of truth. Only in this way may help from us be given. Can thy understand of which we speak?

*"Yes."* [She answers.]

February 20, 1971: *"Aka, we have a soul in need this evening. Soul [9-25-70-001] asks a question. She asks if you can give her any information at all on the health problem she is expressing at this time?"*

We see thy need. We shall take care of this problem. Bear with us for three days, and the fruit shall bear forth upon the earth and thy needs shall be no more.

April 16, 1971: **You have many questions, ask.**

*"Yes, Aka. Ray has asked about the great amount of illness recently in this area [Globe, Arizona], and he is wondering if it is connected with biological testing, and if so, who is doing the testing, and what should he do about it?"*

At the present time we can see no testing. None has been done since our word was given into a pact. But you must remember, the seed that is planted into the ground shall grow and bear fruit; the bird, as the wind, should catch it and carry it to the four corners of your earth. For those of the plant life who should bud their last upon this earth, in this last season their venom is much like a serpent — as you would know it, the pollen that goes into the air.

Then, we should say unto thee, we have told thee of the sage tea; we have told thee of the Night-blooming Citros [Cereus]. Take of these together, and prepare a portion, and [that] each portion should contain one-quarter cube of the Night-blooming Citros [Cereus]. This must be taken fresh from the plant. If not, most of the antibiotic you shall lose. Take also one, of your measurements, known as a [teaspoon] of honey, but it must come from this same region. This should be done twice daily. We shall give and add to this from time to time.

Remember, as individual choice was given, so was the individual chemical, of each individual. Can thy understand of which we speak?

*"Yes, Aka. But I do not understand if you are saying that we cannot freeze the Night-blooming Cereus?"*

This cannot be done without damage and loss.

*"Thank you."*

April 16, 1971: **You have other questions, ask.**

*"Yes, Aka, [4-16-71-001] of California has asked for a health and possibly a life reading. He says he is having trouble with dizzy spells and his sight blacks out. Can you help him?"*

We should say unto this one, the one who would sign this affidavit, if thy should come unto us in truth, the help that thy would need to overcome thy problems would be no more.

But we should say to the one whose writing appears upon your affidavit, thy have many problems, and for this one we shall give a health reading. First, for the good of the health, learn the difference of the truth.

We see scar tissue which is inflamed. This could be taken care of quite simply by the use of banana oil upon the wound.

The dizziness thy speak of is caused from spraying of chemicals. It, and the heavy pollution of your area, is causing growths in the sinus cavities. Therefore, it would be our suggestion that this soul move to a better climate. This must be done at a higher climate. We would suggest that anywhere from the altitude of 3,500 feet; this should not be done over 7,000 feet.

We find also that the heart has been overworked from a lack of oxygen. We find that the brain tissue and the lower [lymphoma] area, also damage occurring there. At the present time, for immediate relief, obtain oxygen mask and the usage of the same. This should be done as frequently as possible. It would be suggested that this type of apparatus be carried with this person at all times.

And for thy spiritual need, come and let us speak unto thee. Open thy door that we may enter and bring the word of our Father into thy heart and soul.

We find other health problems also.

We should suggest that corrective lenses of a different type be used.

We would suggest the sauna baths for the better stimulation of the circulatory system be used. We find uremic poisoning. We would suggest that no alcoholic beverages of any type be taken. We would suggest that in thy diet that less of the salt be used, even as a precaution at this time; there are many good substitutes upon the market. We also see that from the liver and kidney area this poison has flushed through many of the organs of the body, therefore, causing abscess in what thy would know as the long intestine.

We would also suggest that the soap, as thy would know it, that thy are using at the present time is harmful to thy skin; change this.

Should further reading be asked for, this shall be given.

Remember, come unto us into truth and thy shall be received. But remember also, thy are one of our Father's children, and our Father loves thee, and gives thee blessings.

April 16, 1971: **Ask thy other question.**
*"Aka, this evening, [4-16-70-004]...Kentucky, has asked for a health reading. She has not defined her problem."*

Yes, we see thy need. Then we should say unto this soul, bless thee.

First, of this soul, you are at this time starting through menopause. It would be suggested that thy consult your physician.

We may also find in this soul that the eating of the Jerusalem artichoke, for this soul is a borderline diabetic.

We also find thyroid, a very low count. This could be corrected in thy diet, but for thy own peace of mind, it would be better to consult thy physician.

We would suggest, for the lower proportion of your body, of the vaginal area, that washing be done with less acidy solutions. There are many other good product. At the present time, the substance in use is causing scar tissue in this area, and if not corrected, shall soon turn into an abscess.

Of the left arm, upper proportion, we find there old lesions. We would suggest in this case that hot castor-oil packs be placed upon the body. This should be done in repeated succession for 12 hours. You shall find that you shall no longer have the pain.

We find also arthritis. We would suggest that the eating of the Night-blooming Citros [Cereus]; we would suggest that the drinking of the sage tea. We would suggest that much more green vegetation be eaten by this soul.

We would suggest that for the circulatory system and the flushing of the same that saunic-type baths be taken. Before this is done, in this case, eat nothing for 24 hours before the baths. After the bath, eat very sparingly of fruits and vegetables, but no meat. This being done from two to three days prior to the bath, this would flush a great deal of the poison from thy system.

We should also suggest, and we should say unto thee these words, if thy should speak to our Father, do so in a private place. And as thy words, they should mean something to you, therefore, they would mean something to our Father.

We see thy other worries of thy mind, and we should say unto thee, fear not, for all shall mature in God's light. And as once before, remember, my daughters, that that was covered shall be uncovered. Where no light shone, light shall shine again. Fear not our presence in thee, for we shall come to thee with healing.

This is all on this subject at this time.

April 16, 1971: **Ask thy other questions.**
*"Aka, I have an unsigned reading tonight on* [4-16-71-003]. *She is requesting a health reading; it is a health-reading request."*

We would suggest that this reading form be completed in full, but we should say unto these words. Fear not, my daughter, for we, with our Father's permission, and from the prayers of our instrument, shall dwell within thy house and coveth thy needs. Have faith. Our Father loves thee. And as once before, a child shall be born.

April 17, 1971: *"Good morning, Aka. Is Ray with God?"*
**Soul Ray stands with God.**
**You have many questions, ask.**
*"Aka,* [4-17-71-001] *has asked for help, and she has not written specifically what her circumstances are. Can you give us any information for her at this time?"*

Yes, we see thy need. Therefore, we would say to thee —

Yes, that is better. Yes, we have the body, the   soul, the spirit — yes, we see thy need. Therefore, we would say to thee, as the seed is planted, if the seed is planted in purity, then it should grow old and strong, But then the seed is planted of impurity; therefore, through our instrument and his prayers work has been and shall be done.

Then we would say unto thee, give of your prayers to our Father. Open thy door that we may enter, and the ones who have bore your cross before shall bear it again.

At the present time, with the help that shall be given and has been given, the child is whole. You must have more vegetation in thy diet. This is important. At least once each day thy should have of the beef; the rawer that you can eat it, the better it shall be for you. You should eat of those things that should build blood and purify it.

And now, we should say unto these words. Go unto our instrument that he may give healing. Believe in God, our Father, and the healing shall come about.

Thy have many questions upon thy mind. These we shall answer in dream form, for we shall come into thee in thy dreams and transfer thoughts.

Discontinue eating any chocolate at all. Discontinue eating anything that contains vinegar. Drink of the sage tea, morning and evening. Sweeten this tea with natural honey from thy region.

At the present time, we would not suggest a journey back to the valley below the sea [Editor's note: Yuma, Arizona, in the Imperial Valley].

New life and vigor shall come within thy self.

We should also suggest that a salt substitute be used at this time. We see that thy are a slight diabetic. This could be corrected by the eating of Jerusalem artichoke. It would not be as suggested, that any other type insulin be used. Soon the cactus fruit shall be in abundance. On the next reading we shall go further and give instructions upon the same.

Can you understand of which we have spoken?

*"Yes."* [4-17-71-001] answers.

This is all on this subject at this time.


April 17, 1971: Yes, we see thy need, and thy concern. If these plants of the Night-blooming Citros [Cereus] were dried, and later, as the blossom forms on the *mesquita* [mesquite], grind these into a fine powder and add two equal amounts. At the present time, in a dried form, using the ultraviolet light for drying, then eating, it would gain the same purpose and could be kept over longer periods of time. Once these are dried, placing them in a pyramid-type container, they could be not only kept for months, but for many thousands of years. Can thy understand of which we speak?

*"Yes, Aka."*

Then, one moment. Yes — it has been suggested that the ultraviolet light could be used in a pyramid for drying. Can thy understand of which we speak?

*"Yes. Are the dimensions for the pyramid that we have correct?"*
**This is so.**

**April 17, 1971: Now, at this time, it has also been suggested that the defining between the sonic and the sauna. You must understand that sometimes our words shall sound as riddles, therefore, because of the difference in our planes. If thy can not understand, you must but ask. The saunic-type baths are baths of the sauna taken in smoothing music. Can thy understand?**
*"Yes, Aka."*

**April 17, 1971: Thy have other questions, ask.**
*"We have a [4-16-70-003] who asked for a health reading last night and we now have a signed release form...."*
**Yes, we see thy need. You have had corrective lenses. If thy should use these, but then again, they should be corrected again. We find that the dizziness thy suffer from is partially due from this. We would suggest that in thy diet, that no vinegar or chocolate or spinach be eaten at the present time in thy diet. We would suggest, for the purification of the body, that at the present time sage tea be drunken twice daily.**

**Of thy meditation, all is in accord. Should there be a change, you shall be told. Continue thy prayers and thy meditation unto our Father.**

**We would suggest that four ounces of a good grape wine be dranken daily, preferably before thy rest at night.**

**We would also suggest at the present time, do not lift any object over ten pounds. Be careful in thy bending. Thy exercises would come more readily in walking.**

**Continue serving thy husband. These simple tasks shall be good for the body and soul.**

**And remember, my daughter, our Lord, our Father, loves thee.**

**Remember also, for what thy should give, thy should receive. If thy give of love, thy child and thyself shall receive of this love.**

**And remember also, our Father has many mansions.**

**And as our Father has said, "WHAT HAS BEEN BEFORE SHALL BE AGAIN, FOR WHERE THERE IS NO LIGHT, LIGHT SHALL SHINE AGAIN; WHAT HAS BEEN COVERED SHALL BE UNCOVERED, AND THUS, THE HEARTS OF MAN SHALL BEGIN TO CHANGE."**

**This is all on this subject at this time.**

**April 17, 1971: Now, we suggest that thy should waken soul Ray from his slumber. But before we go, we shall give healing into thy group.**

**And we say these words unto soul Ruth, walk proud, my daughter, for our Father loves thee. And remember our vow unto thee — for thy children shall be fruitful, and whole.**

April 23, 1971: **You have many questions, ask.**
*"Aka, soul Ruth asks for a health reading."*

**Yes, we see thy need, soul Ruth. And we shall say unto thee again these words, for we have made a vow. And as Abraham made a vow, he must have one greater than himself, then any vows unto which we make, permission first must be given. And unto thy descendants and their descendants, we have promised health, without interference with their free will. We can give no more. For the Holy Spirit shall dwell within thee, and God's hand shall reach and touch thee.**

**We see thy concern, but as our promise has been made, no harm shall come within thee. New life and vigor shall dwell within thy body. For as your body is made of man and as all things upon your earth come from one source, from one power, remember this, soul Ruth, for you may destroy nothing, only change its form, for nothing ever dies upon your earth. The form is changed and regenerated into new life again.**

**For thy family and thyself, we should suggest at this time that good natural vitamins be taken with the continuation of the sage tea. Continue, of thy family, these things.**

**We have found that once before you have passed beyond the veil and returned again. This was done, even then, that thy would do the bidding of our Lord. We see that thy tasks shall grow even more as a burden, but remember, it is a burden of love, for if a place should be made ready upon your earth for the coming of the Messiah, then many hands shall be needed and many minds. For have we not said before, all that is covered shall be lighted again, and not one stone upon your earth shall not be turned, for our Lord's hand is again upon thy earth.**

**Can thy understand of which we speak?**
*"I think so."*[She answers.]

**You shall now experience a chemical change in thy body. Fear not, for knowledge that thy never have possessed before shall be there and made ready at thy disposal. For we have not called thy soul Ruth in vain, but only with the blessings of God, our Father. For remember, for those who shall know where they have been, they shall know where they are going. Give blessings each day, soul Ruth.**

April 23, 1971: **You have other questions, ask.**
*"Aka, [4-6-70-003] asks, 'Can you tell me what to do about the problem with [4-23-71-001]'s feet?' And she also asks, 'Is the diet soul Andrew is on okay, or should it be changed?'"*

**We shall say unto these words, first of the child. Go, now, as the sage shall soon be blooming and the greasewood blooms. Take of this and take of the Night-blooming Citros [Cereus]. Warm them and let them dry. Let the sun evaporate the water form. Then add soda unto this. Then take the white of the egg and moisten it, and place a compress upon the**

foot area. Do this gently, with gentle words and love, and healing shall come about.

April 23, 1971: **Of soul Andrew, we should say these words; there is at this time a dragon close to thy door. Fear this not, for thy walk in the path of our Father. But remember, our Father has given unto thee free choice.**

**We say unto thee, add more fish into thy diet, both of the ocean and of the fresh water. Take from thy diet the salt.**

**Can thy understand of which we speak?**

*"Should he use a salt substitute?"* [She [4-6-70-003] asks.]

**This would be good.**

**We would say also, of the headaches, drink more of the sage tea. We would say unto these words, that that comes from the root [and] the blossom of the same. That that comes from the sky to pollute and foul thy earth, remember, if man continues in the pollution of his world — the Allen Belt around your earth was provided as a filter unto thy earth to destruct pollution — do not overdo this or man shall become in danger.**

**Can thy understand of which we speak?**

*"Possibly, not fully, but I shall try."* [[4-6-70-003] answers.]

**Nay, not fully, but thy shall.**

April 23, 1971: **Thy have other questions, ask.**

*"[4-23-71-002] has asked for a health reading."*

**Yes, we see thy need. For remember these words. As a woman you have entered into this plane, and as a woman, you are of now. Then we would say unto you, thy are passing through the change of life. There are many good medications; therefore, we would suggest the seeing of a good gynecologist. Thy worry of the dizziness thy have experienced and in this fainting-type spells thy have had. This is all part of the same.**

**And thy worry of thy spiritual development. There is one provided for this also.**

**We would suggest that in the evening before thy departed for slumber, the drinking of six ounces of wine daily, of the grape. This should never de done in excess. This shall provide for the building of the blood that is needed in thy system. It shall also provide the necessary elements that thy may sleep in the evening.**

**We find other problems, and since a life reading has not been asked for, these cannot be given at this time.**

**We would say unto thee, those things that come from the heart shall come from the soul of the same.**

**Of your marital problems, we say unto you, all of these things shall come of past. Give blessings unto those around thee. Give kindness and love. And those things that thy should give, thy shall have unto thyself.**

Of the chest problem that thy have experienced of the lungular area, this is all part and should be treated as part of the same. You must understand, with the pollution of your area certain things must be done to extract the same from your system. Therefore, we would suggest that the taking of the Night-blooming Cereus with the drinking three times daily of the sage tea, if the [following] is done, then come back and further reading shall be given on this subject with permission from the same.

The other questions in thy mind, we should say unto thee, for as a man bears sons and gives them love, so should a woman. Let not, no man take these things from you. Can thy understand of which we speak?

"*No.*" [She says.]

Then tonight, as thy sleep, open thy door. But remember these words, no house may stand divided.

April 23, 1971: **Thy have other questions, ask.**

"*Aka,* [11-16-70-004] *asks, 'Is my hip ailment truly a virus infection, or is it caused by something else?'*"

We see thy hip, as thy would call it. We have the body, the soul, and the spirit; therefore, we should say unto these words.

We should tell thee of this. As we have said before, you are developing arthritis, and this in itself is a virus. Therefore, we would suggest the eating of the Night-blooming Cereus, the taking of the saunic-type baths, both of the water and the sound.

We would also suggest unto thee, the over consumption into the body of any foreign subject is harmful to the body; therefore, we should say unto thee, thy consumption of tobacco weed has grown out of proportion with the natural chemicals of thy body. If this consumption should decrease, thy body chemicals could take over and cause healing.

Remember of these things; we are not permitted to change thy will, for this gift was given by God, our Father. Can thy understand of which we speak?

"*Yes, Aka.*" [She answers.]

We would suggest in thy diet the eating of fish. We would suggest in thy diet the eating of more raw-type vegetables. If this could be done with less meat in thy diet, if this could be done, thy body chemicals should change readily, and thy body could complete the healing. We would suggest that this diet be followed for a two-week period. At that time, another reading should be asked for. We find that of drinking of the purple sage leaf, making a compress of this area, should help greatly in the healing. Can thy understand of which we speak?

"*Yes.*" [She answers.]

May 2, 1971: **Thy have other questions, ask.**

*"Yes, [5-2-71-002] has asked, 'Is the smoking of marijuana harmful to the physical, mental or spiritual self? Would using bring about a bad karma?'"*

Your karma shall be thyself. Of this physical nature, the use in excess of any [neurological, septic?] type of drugs would show great damage to the penal [pineal] area of the body, and permanent damage, therefore, over a prolonged period of time would come about. Therefore, it would be our suggestion that overindulgence in any manner would not be wise.

Can thy understand of which we speak?

Nay, not fully.

Then we should say unto thee, man and the man-animal is the most curious of all species. Therefore, if the need to experiment is greater than the margin of safety within thyself, do so.

May 2, 1971: **Thy have other questions, ask.**

*"Yes, Aka. [5-2-71-003] asks, should he and his wife continue with their work with the Bell, Book and Candle [bookstore], or would it be more useful to go into another area?"*

In the near future, thy business shall flourish tenfold; therefore, your usage and your service to your fellow man could be greater. Remember, drink [our words].

Can thy understand of which we speak?

*"Yes, Aka." [He answers.]*

May 2, 1971: **Thy have many questions; ask of these.**

*"Aka, this evening we have questions on experimental release forms. We have a request here for a health and life reading on [4-30-71-001]. Can you possibly give us anything on that this evening?"*

First, we should say unto these words, we have before us the body, the soul, and the spirit, and therefore, we have the immortal body; therefore, all is in accord. Permission has been granted that the information given; therefore, we should say unto this soul, remember of these words, that the over-consumption or the over-endurance of any substance is harmful to the higher health.

We find in this soul a thyroid problem. This problem could be corrected with the eating of Jerusalem artichoke, with the complete change in diet. We should suggest that, for this soul, that the eating of no pork or fatty tissue, that the eating of more of the vegetable substance. We should also suggest that a mild form of salt be used in its purest form, and very little of this.

We would suggest that this soul go, as you would call it in your time, of the banana fruit, that the breakfast meal consist of 8 ounces of milk and three large bananas; that the lunch should consist of only of green vegetables, any variety in their rawest form. This we would suggest.

Yes.

For thy evening meal, once a week we would suggest of the salt fish, that that comes from the salten waters. For once each week we would suggest of the fresh water fish. For once each week we would suggest of the liver of the beef. For once each week we would suggest well-cured beef of any variety or form thereon.

Take from thy diet the starchy foods; eat not of the potato, eat no more than one slice, no more than one-inch thick, of bread at each meal. Eat vegetation, either cooked or raw, at each meal. Use any good vinegar and oil for salad dressing, as you would know it. Use either of your yogurt or cottage cheese once daily. We would also suggest the taking of good natural vitamins daily.

We find that this soul has a scalp problem. Therefore, we would suggest that the white of the egg, mixed with vinegar, be rubbed into the scalp; afterwards, rinsing the scalp with clear, pure water, and therefore, placing hot olive oil packs upon the scalp. This would not only help in a better growth, we find that for the circulatory system of your scalp, this would increase.

We also find that as a small child, from a fall from your wagon, we find a laceration of the right, upper thigh leg; therefore, we would suggest for a period of three days, one hour per day, hot olive oil packs be placed upon this area. This must be done daily for three days. Afterwards, we would suggest that over the same area, the use of banana oil over the same area, repeated for two weeks.

We find other physical problems. We would suggest that through meditation — this should be done twice daily, putting thyself in accordance with God, our Father — if thy should think upon your meditation of the words of Aka, that we may enter, we should help thee in thy work.

At the present time we should not give all of your life reading, but we should say unto thee these words. In thy meditation thy shall know of whence thy have come, and therefore, thy should know of which thy should go.

Give blessings unto the Lord, our Father, and yours, and remember these words. Our Father giveth and our Father should taketh away. If thy go into the house to give blessings, and these blessings are not received, then take thy blessings and go unto another house.

If thy should ask again at a different time, we should give thy life reading.

May 2, 1971: **You have other questions, ask.**

*"Yes, Aka. We have a question this evening of S____ H_____. She is quite concerned about her husband, B___, and son-in-law, D__ L. K_____ of Phoenix. Is there anything she can do to help them?"*

We see thy need, and therefore, we should answer thy question in this manner. Give of kindness and love and understanding, for both of these souls thy have mentioned need much of this, for they have so little to give of themselves. Remember, in giving, thy shall receive.

Remember also that we can do nothing without our Father's permission. Therefore, there is certain information of these two souls our Father has forbid [forbade] us in giving unto thee.

But we shall give thee this. Our Father shall give thee blessings and heal thee, for thy body shall become whole again, thy spirit shall become whole again, and laughter shall return into thy life.

Can thy understand of which we speak?

*"Yes, I do."* [She answers.]

May 2, 1971: **Thy have other questions; ask of these.**

*"Yes, Aka, we have another question this evening of* [4-30-71-004]. *He asks this question. 'I have periodically had sinus attacks over the left eye, sometimes light, occasionally severe. May I be told the cause of the problem, and a possible remedy for it?'"*

Yes, we see thy need. Then we should say unto thee these words. Take of the sea water, boiling it and making a vapor of the same; breathing of this would relieve thy sinus instantly. Taking of the red sage, or as you would know it, of the purple sage, making of this a tea, placing the honey that comes from thy location in this, no more than two tablespoons. Taking also of the red sage and making a compress of this, placing it above the four sinus areas, placing this, very warm; at this time placing hot, warm towels over this area. This should be done for 30 minutes each day for five days, and thy cause shall vanish.

May 2, 1971: **Thy have other questions; ask of this.**

*"Aka, we have a question this evening of* [4-30-71-004], *the following series of questions. One, 'What is the state of health of* [5-7-71-005]? *Is there any medical advice?'"*

We should say unto these words, we are not allowed to give information, and therefore, of another soul. Should this soul desire this information and should it ask of the same, information shall be given. We should say only of this word, for we see thy need. Give prayer for his deliverance into our Father, that he may see our Father's light.

May 2, 1971: **Thy have other questions; ask.**

*"In the relation to the above question, Aka, we also have, 'What is the state of heath of* [4-30-71-004]? *Have you any medical advice?'"*

We see thy need; therefore, we should say of these words. If thy should use of the diet — one moment, please.

Yes. Yes, Father.

Then we should say unto these words. Fear not, for healing shall be given unto this soul, for our Father has seen thy need and heard thy prayers.

May 2, 1971: **Thy have other questions, ask.**

*"Number three question of* [4-30-71-004], *Aka. She asks this question, 'Is Lobsang Rampa, the author of* The Third Eye, *and others, what he claims to be, and are his writings true?'"*

We should say unto thee these words. Since thy try to guide thy life by this counsel, we should say that they are not all in truth, but partially.

Thy have before thee the scripture[s] of our God, our Father. In thy search for thy mystic world, thy shall find all [the] knowledge and truth within these scriptures. But therefore, we should say unto thee, even of the scripture has been altered by man. Therefore, truth shall be within thyself. If thy life should be in truth, then truth shall be set before thee.

For only in the psychic world can a true psychic, as thy would know them, they may only function complete and wholly within truth. Should they stray from their paths, then they see in themselves and should give of these words. And should this happen they are not giving a full truth. There are those, you must remember, who should tell a lie, and in their lie they should believe of this themselves. They have formed a new karma.

But remember also, if there is a stone to be cast, cast this first stone at thyself, and then walk thee in thy light of our Father, which is within truth.

Of your psychic world, we have many prophets, and many truths. We give blessings from our Father unto these. But to the false prophets of your earth, the blessings shall not come from our Father, but from Lucifer.

May 2, 1971: **Thy have other questions. ask.**

*"Aka, we have another question carried over from a previous reading. From* [5-27-71-005] *we have this question. She has deep concern for her husband, his health, retirement and other change. Can you give her anything on that this evening?"*

We should say of these words, thy husband's retirement shall come and thy shall live within fulfillment. Give of this man your love and your tenderness and your guidance. Listen to his counsel, for it shall be wise. Guide him toward our Father, that he may carry on.

We should say unto thee, thy should make a trip soon. We should suggest that thy should not do this. In the area that thy should travel should be dangerous unto thyself and thy descendants. For we have given the warnings before, for now is the time of the Cherub, for the Sword of our Father has struck thy Earth, and soon again, very soon, your Earth shall be struck again.

May 2, 1971: **Soul Ray grows very weary, and therefore, we would** suggest that thy should awaken him from his slumber.

But before our departure, we should ask that there is one close to thy hearts, of the small child, who should need blessings and healing, and each in his own way should pray to our Father. This is our suggestion. [Editor's note: Four minutes of silence follow.]

And now we would suggest that thy should awaken soul Ray from his slumber.

May 14, 1971: **Ask thy other questions.**

"[4-17-71-001] *would like to know if the pain in her side is due to pregnancy or to some other reason?"*

Yes, we see the body, the soul, the spirit and the immortal body; yes, we have these before us now.

We find a small nonmalignant-type growth on the ovary. We find other thyroid- [fibroid?]-type growths of the womb. As we have said before, go unto a good gynecologist, and therefore, treatments shall be given of the same. We find — yes, we see this, yes — at the present time the child is growing, is growing very strong and healthy within thy womb. But heed our words; we have told thee before of the things [thee] must do. Do these things that the child must grow.

Of thy other child, go back to the beginning and do these things, that that child may grow also. For both is important, for they are the seed of your future. And remember also, our Father has endowed into thee thy need of teaching into thy children.

We see also of the [malatoid] area — yes, we see this — a slight infection at the present time. This could be cleared up quite simply by seeing thy local physician, in use of a mild antibiotic.

We see also thy need — yes — of a complexion problem. Therefore, we would say unto thee, take thee of the soda, take thee of the olive oil, take thee of the white of an egg, each in equal parts, therefore, making a potion. This should be left on thy face for 30 minutes of thy time; afterwards rinsing with very clean, clear water. At the present time washing is a necessity. Do not use of the strong soap. We find also that thy are allergic to certain sprays that thy use. We would suggest at the present time the discontinuing of the same.

We see another problem, but at the present time., we would not suggest that this be treated until the others we have suggested have been treated first.

We see much work needed in the upper and lower backular area, preferably in the third and fourth vertebrae of the backular area. Therefore, we would suggest a good osteopathic doctor. We would not suggest, at the present time, that the use of a chiropractic doctor, for the one who should treat thee would need much more knowledge. Can thy understand of which we say?

Yes, we see this. Yes.

Then we would say on your other question, have patience and believe in our Father, and those things in which thy should desire should manifest, and therefore, become reality into thy heart and soul. Fear not, for as before, the children that thy should bear shall walk in mighty footsteps.

May 14, 1971: **Thy have other questions, ask.**
*"Aka, A_____ asks if there is anything that she can do to improve her hearing more?"*
**Yes, we see thy need. Therefore, in the mastoid area we find slight bone damage of the sound track.**
**Yes, we see this.**
**There is permanent damage into this area; therefore, one moment. Yes.**
**Before three days have passed of your time, your hearing shall improve, for God's hands have reached and touched thee, and blessings shall come within thee, and thy body shall become whole again. Can thy understand of which we speak?**
**Nay not fully.**
*"Yes"*
**Thy soon will.**

May 14, 1971: **Thy have other questions, ask.**
*"Aka, we have a [4-16-71-001] that has asked for —"*
**We see this.**
*"a health reading."*
**At the present time soul Ray now wearies and grows tired. Therefore, we should say unto thee these words.**
**For in thy [house], soul E_____, we shall enter into thy soul, into thy spirit, and into thy mind, and shall cleanse the path of righteousness. But remember, it is better, far better in the eyes of our Father, to be thyself. Pretend not to be of another. Accept thyself, for you are the one our Father loves, and there can be no other, other than thyself.**
**Awaken soul Ray from his slumber.**

May 21, 1971: **Thy have many questions, ask.**
*"Aka, I have a request for a health reading on J___ R_____ who lives at...Globe... and he has had respiratory problems and joint problems and other problems, and he asks for help."*
**Yes, we see this need. First, we should say of his joint problems, change of the drinking water, for still thy water is not pure and good. There are many good carbon-type filters available now that would do an adequate, to prepare the water into a safer form.**
**Second, we should say, of the sonic-type baths, prepare these, that in thy soul and body and of the spiritual world, thy hearts may be lifted.**
**Third, the eating of one-quarter by one-quarter of the citrus fruit daily should greatly increase this.**

Fourth, the taking of good natural vitamins, this should be done, we should say, three times daily.

We find that the circulatory system has been impaired; therefore, if this soul could take what is known as S.S.S., this is a good blood tonic. But remember these words. Even though thy should feel better at once, continue with this; do not stop.

We find that corrective lenses are in need here.

We would also suggesting that bathing, and [more] promptly, of the ear sections, should be needed.

We find also a very bad condition of the scalp area. We would suggest for this that the taking of hot olive-oil packs once daily, this should be done for 10 minutes, placing the olive oil in the hair, into the scalp and rubbing very vigorously; then, with hot towels for moisture, these being placed upon the scalp, left there to cool, and then repeat it again.

We find also that a change of diet — we would suggest that the eating of three bananas in the morning and the drinking of one glass of milk would greatly help. For the luncheon meal, eating only of the raw vegetables. Your last meal we should leave to thy own discretion.

We also find in this soul, of the kidney and liver area, inflammation of this area. This is due to the over consumption of alcoholic beverages. Therefore, we should suggest before — one moment, please.

Yes. Yes.

Yes, we also find a blockage in the [carros trap][tract?]; this is the main lateral area that should extend from the [clean]valve into the[outer]valve of thy body which would extract thy normal wastage. We would suggest that the drinking of sage tea twice daily, sweetened only with natural honey from the locale; if this is not available, then we would suggest that a good sage honey would do in its place.

We also find a problem of the footing area, as thy would call them, corns or calluses. If thy should take of hot castor oil packs, placing this on this area each evening for a period of two weeks, these should leave thy body.

We also find of domestic problems which has caused highly nervous system. We should answer your problem in this manner. If the hen should sit upon an egg, and even after the egg has cast away its shell and become a young chick, this hen still desires to sit on the egg, this is itself is not good. For remember, there is a time for all things, and now is your time for patience. Show love and kindness. Show your need for love from your mate; show your need and the need shall come back a hundredfold, even with small gifts. Yes — this would be good.

May 21, 1971: **Thy have other questions, ask.**

*"Aka, I have a number of health readings that have been asked for, and other questions. C_____ C___ would like a life or health reading, and [4-16-71-001] needs a health reading."*

We should say of soul [4-16-71-001], yes, we see thy need. We should say in this manner, first, of your constant pain, as thy would know it, in your head, this is caused from blockage of the circulatory system and also from blockage of the sinus system. Therefore, in the locale that thy should dwell, we should answer your problem in this manner. Take of the sea water, boiling it and placing a cloth completely over this, constructing, as thy would know, a tent above it; do this for 20 minutes daily, eating of the [jacinta, yosinta?] plant; this grows in your area. This is from one thy would know as the eucalyptus plant, placing the leaves of the same in water. We should also tell thee that saunic baths should be needed.

We find also denture work is needed, that pressure, therefore, in the upper area is giving great pain; therefore, we should suggest that this matter be taken care of. We also find the need here for a good osteopathic doctor — yes — a great deal of work. We find problems all over this one's body.

Yes.

Our time is too short at this time to describe in detail the necessary work. Go unto this doctor, and as progress is made other readings shall be given.

We find the need of more rest, of more open meditation.

We also find a problem of the mastoid area. We would suggest, in your case, that, as thy would know it, consulting a good eye, ears, nose doctor. This problem could be corrected quite simply with the cleaning of this area and packing of the same.

May 21, 1971: **You have other questions, ask.**
*"Yes, Aka. A while back, we had a release form on J_____ B_____; you said it was a forgery and that the one who had written it, you gave a health reading on. Was that T_____ B_____? And if not, can you at this time give a health or life reading on her?"*

Soul Ray is very tired; therefore, the time should be needed for healing into the same. Therefore, give him time and then awaken him from his slumber. The reading that thy ask for shall be given at another time.
*"All right."*

And now we shall give the healing that is needed into our instrument.

Awaken soul Ray....

May 28, 1971: **Thy have other questions, ask.**
*"Aka, [4-16-71-001of A_____, California] requests a health reading. He has been suffering from dizzy spells for about seven years."*

Yes, we see this need, but we have given this reading. Therefore, ask thy other questions.

June 4, 1971: **We find other questions in thy minds.**

And unto soul Paul we should answer his question. Of thy prayer for thy friend, healing shall be granted. For thy have remembered in thy asking in thy Father's name, and thy Father should walk beside thee, and give His blessings into thee.

June 5, 1971: **Thy have many questions, ask.**
*"Aka, [2-19-71-001] asks, 'Will you please give me help to obtain my correct weight and keep it there?' Also, she says, 'Thank you,' for helping her hearing."*

Yes, we see this. Yes, we see thy need. Then we should say to thee, of the morning eat not but of the fruit, drinking, as thy would know it, one glass of milk. For thy lunch eat not but of the green vegetable in the raw form. Of thy evening meal, taking one ounce of olive oil before the meal, and then thy can eat as thy heart desires. This should be done daily. If done in this manner thy weight shall be stabilized, and therefore, with our help, you should have no problems in this sort.

June 5, 1971: **Ask thy other questions.**
*"Aka, [6-5-71-001, Globe] asks for a health reading."*

Yes, we see thy need. Then we should say unto thee, as thy are a woman who should pass through menopause, then we should suggest in this manner — that the taking of the Lydia E. Pinkham — but we should also suggest in your case that thy should consult thy local doctor and that help through hormones should be given. We should also suggest that through daily meditation, would greatly help in this area.

We also find sinus growths; therefore, we would suggest for this the drinking of the sage tea. This should be sweetened, if preferable, with the local honey. If this cannot be had at this time, then we should suggest placing a little ginger, and the use of sage honey.

We also find a scalp problem. For this we should suggest, one moment, please — yes, we find this. We would suggest, therefore, if thy should take of the hot olive oil, rubbing very vigorously into the scalp area, afterwards washing thy hair with a good shampoo, after this, rinsing thy hair with one ounce per gallon of vinegar water, this would greatly help in this area.

We find thy have other denture problems. This could be readily corrected with a visit to thy local dentist.

We find that as a small child, an injury to the kidney area and lacerations of the same, of the left kidney area. Therefore, we would suggest — first, do not at any time take into thy body any alcoholic substances — third [second], less of the medication thy are now on; this is affecting this area — third, taking of hot castor-oil packs upon this area, as hot as the skin should allow. This should be done in intervals of two hours. It should be repeated for three days.

We find many problems of the back area and upper neck area. Therefore, either with a visit to thy local chiropractor or an osteopathic doctor corrections could and should be made. Manipulation of the scalp or skull area could relieve this tremendously, especially your headaches. In the lower back area, as thy would know it, in the base of the spinal area, because of old injuries here, we would suggest that by constructing a bar approximately 3 inches above thy reach, stretching this area daily. This will not cure this injury, but would relieve much of the pain from the same.

We find that thy have a problem of the feet area.

Yes.

We find that with corrective shoes this could be relieved. Do not at any time wear shoes that belonged to someone else. Because of this thy bones have curved. With corrective shoes in this area this could be eliminated.

We find infection of the vagina area.

Yes.

We would suggest in this case, one moment — yes — the washing of this area twice daily would help. But also, a good antibiotic prescribed by thy local physician would also improve this greatly.

We also find scar tissue below the breast area, and frequent pains from the same. We would

suggest, with the use of warm banana oil on this area would lighten, and therefore, dissolve this area.

Yes.

Thy have other questions, ask.

*"Yes, Aka. I have questions for health readings from thee other people."*

One moment.

Yes, yes.

In this case we should suggest that a follow-up reading be given in two-week periods.

Yes — this is all on this soul.


June 5, 1971: **Ask thy other question.**

*"Aka, [6-05-71-002] asks for a reading on his health because he has been having headaches."*

Yes, we see thy need. Therefore, if work was done on the back area, upper back area, and manipulations of the skull area, these would be greatly relieved. We also find that stronger vitamins and mineral substances should be used.

Yes. Yes, we find this.

We should also suggest for the circulatory system saunic baths be taken at least once a week. We also find a slight infection of the mastoid area; this is caused through the sinus glands and from the area, therefore, in which thy are residing now. Therefore, we would suggest that for thy entire family, we find certain minerals in thy present drinking water that are not — therefore, we would suggest that this water be filtered through carbon-type filters.

Yes, we see this.

The drinking of the sage tea twice daily, this must be done as a ritual, and continued until a time that we should tell unto thee to make changes.

This is all on this soul at this time. Therefore, we would also suggest that a follow-up reading be given in a two-week period.

June 5, 1971: **Thy have other questions, ask.**

*"Aka, [9-5-70-002, California] has asked for a health reading because he has had dizzy spells for about the past seven years. Do you have anything, any help that you can give him at this time?"*

Yes, we should say unto this soul — first, we would suggest that the drinking of no alcoholic beverage of any kind. We should also suggest that the use of no chocolate of any type. Third, we would suggest that a change of altitude. We also find in this subject, as thy would know it, a low blood sugar; therefore, we would suggest that through the use of vitamin substances this could be corrected. We also find that in thy daily, day-to-day duties, if thy would carry, as thy would know it, candy bars, using this at different intervals.

Yes.

We also find — yes, we see thy need, yes — we would suggest unto this soul that the mental strain that thy are now under is greater than thy body was built to sustain. Through the mind and the mental torment of the mind — yes, we see thy problem — if this was relieved in this manner, taking not from thy work, taking thy time to relax, taking time for laughter, taking time for sleep, taking time for the duties thy should perform into our God, our Lord, our Father, regulating thy life in such a manner that thy have no radicalism, we find that with this thy whole health, thy whole body structure would increase.

We would also suggest for thy circulatory system saunic baths be taken, twice weekly.

We would suggest also unto this subject —yes, yes — the changing of thy diet. Do not miss meals. Eat at least four meals daily. Eat them promptly; eat them on time. We would suggest of thy morning meal, let it consist of some fruit, fresh fruit. Let it also consist of milk. In your case we would suggest the use of goat's milk. This, in itself, would help neutralize and take away part of thy problem. We also would suggest that before thy slumber in the evening the use of a small amount of hops be placed within the milk and sweetened, therefore, with honey. This would greatly help thy slumber.

If this problem continues, we would suggest a further health reading within a three-week period.

**Yes.**

June 5, 1971: **Thy have other questions, ask.**

*"Aka, are the seeds of the acacia plant, the plant that has a round, yellow blossom that grows by my home in the canyon, are these seeds medicinal, and if so, should they be used?"*

**We would not suggest that these be used. They have domestic purposes. But for the present time, we would suggest that thy do not use them.**

June 5, 1971: **Ask thy other question.**

*"I have no other question, Aka."*

**Then we should say, of thy last question in soul Ruth's mind, we have promised thee that thine and thy descendants should have of good health. And thy ask, then why should we give a medical reading upon thy son? This is not to take away as our Father has promised unto thee, but only to insure that no outside infections may enter this body.**

**Can thy understand of which we speak?**

*"I don't know."* [She answers.]

**We see this. Then in thy slumber upon this night, so shall we enter.**

**Awaken soul Ray from his slumber.**

June 11, 1971: **Then we say unto thee, for the children thy have asked help for, then we say, bring them to us. For our Lord, our Father, has given permission, for He has heard into thee thy prayer. And healing shall come into these that thy should ask. Can thy understand of which we speak?**

*"Do you mean that you wish to give a health reading on these, or do you mean that you wish to have the children brought here?"*

**We say unto thee, bring of them in spirit, for healing has been answered into thy prayer. Can thy understand of which we speak?**

*"Yes, Aka."*

June 11, 1971: **Thy have other questions, ask.**

*"Aka, [6-11-71-001] in Globe, asks, 'What is wrong with my left ear, and can anything be done to regain the lost hearing?'"*

**We say unto this one, for three nights thy should think of the words of our Father, and think thee of the name of Aka, that we may enter, and therefore, give blessings into thee. Thy hearing shall improve. Can thy understand of which we speak?**

**Nay, not fully. Then we should answer thee in this manner. Sometimes in your prayers, thy would think that your Lord has forgotten**

thee, but remember, not one tear has been shed upon your earth that your Lord was not present with thee. But as the Lord has given unto thee free choice, only upon your request may we enter and change the damage thy have done into thyself. Now that thy have asked and permission has been given, healing shall come into the same.

June 11, 1971: **Ask thy other questions.**
*"Aka, [6-5-71-001], asks for an explanation of the health reading on her. She would like to know if she is pregnant, and if not, will she bear another child?"*

(Chuckle.) Yes, we see thy need. And we should say unto these words, the instructions that were given unto thee were given for a purpose. There are certain chemical changes taking place, from the spray and other environmental conditions; therefore, corrective procedures were needed. We would suggest that these corrective measures be taken. We suggest once again, that of the medication that you now take, this should not be taken in the quantity it is being taken. Therefore, take into thy heart, do unto the things that we have said unto thee, and we shall take care of this child thy soul should want. But remember, it is not in the wanting that should count, it is in the giving.

We have said before that in a two-week period another health reading should be given. If, when this time period, the measures we have suggested are done, and in their proper perfective, then we should give unto thee another health reading. We should not at this time answer your question.

June 11, 1971: **Ask thy other questions.**
*"Aka, you spoke of the two little girls to which I gave healing today, and I have a request for a health reading on each of these little girls And the first girl's name is [in Globe. 6-11-71-002A]. She says, her mother says, that she wants to know what to do to restore the health of her child."*

For the present time, we would suggest continuing as thy have at the present time. Healing shall come; this we have promised unto thee. Then we should see these children again, for as we have said before, for we can give nothing more than what our Father has given already. And as our Father is greater than any other, that that has been given should be sufficient at this time.

June 11, 1971: **Ask thy other questions.**
*"Aka, [6-11-71-003...Globe], asks — he says, 'I am concerned about my health.' His number is [6-11-71-003.]"*

Yes, we have this. We have the body, the soul, and the spirit; therefore, the information that thy should seek we should answer. Yes, that is better — there, there — one moment, please.

Yes, we see thy need. We should suggest that this question be asked at a different time.

June 11, 1971: **Thy have other questions, ask.**
*"I have other quick questions on the H_____ children, Aka. Would you like me to ask on those?"*

At the present time we would suggest that nothing be asked on these children; there is work that the Council must do. At your next reading ask these questions.

**Soul Ray grows weary. Awaken him from his slumber.**

June 18, 1971: **Thy have other questions; ask of the same.**
*"Yes, Aka....Aka, [6-18-71-003] of Yuma, age 6, his mother asks for a health or life reading on him; she is particularly concerned about the lack of affection between her and her child. Can you explain this?"*

We should say unto these words unto thee, "as thy sow so shall thy reap." But remember also, that as a soul should enter into your life plane, this soul was a brother of before, and therefore, he should treat unto thee as a brother and the love should be that of a brother more than of a wife and mother.

Give of this child of this child of this wine. But remember also, our Father has many mansions, and that He loves all His children, and each in their own way shall reach upward unto our Father. Give unto this child love and blessings. Give of this child your knowledge, but be firm, for as his star and as he was born of the same, you must realize that these do not hold of a true pattern. But there are certain tests that must be made of this child, for he shall be in the time of one of our Father. And that this time should be made of fullness for this one, let him go on, for we see unto this child.

As he was before, he shall be a dealer of the money of your time. For in his life of before he sought unto riches. Of his food supplement was of the same, and so because of this, he killed into his own body. Therefore, we would suggest that if thy should follow a strict diet for this child, making certain that he eats three meals per day. Make certain that for the morning meal let him have of this of the goat's milk, and fruit. For your luncheon, let him have of some of the meat of the beef. Add to this as many raw vegetables as possible. For thy evening meal, take forth unto the meat of the lamb, take forth unto the meat of the beef. Feed this child as many of the raw vegetables as possible. Make certain that this child should take at least three times daily a good supplemented vitamin and minerals.

These things are needed to set a pattern for this child, for remember, the sins of the parents shall dwell unto the sixth and seventh generation. So therefore, beware, for this child was given unto thee for learning and care. Teach him well. Plant the seeds of the mind. As he should grow older we see there are many times when life shall be balanced. Do not overprotect this child; this, in itself, should be wrong. Let his appetite for knowledge go into all areas. Store, as we have said before, knowledge for the time of the famine.

June 18, 1971: **Ask thy other question.**
*"Aka,* [6-18-71-007] *asks if you can tell her about her health problems?"*

**One moment. We should ask unto thee, what specific information she should desire?**
*"She's been having headaches, Aka. She wonders what is causing the headaches?"*

**Then we should say unto thee — yes, we see this — therefore, now the records are available. We have the body, the soul, the spirit, and the immortal body before us, and the records that were began in the beginning, and therefore, shall remain for all time.**

**First, we should say unto thee, as the body should build every moment that thy should live new cells, and as this building is taking place the body in itself is rapidly changing. It should make adjustments for all proportions of your health needs. That part of itself should cause thy a certain amount of what thy would call of thy headaches.**

**But to be more specific, as man should pollute the ground in which he should dwell, then man should die in a polluted land. Thy ground was polluted first by the spray. At this time, in your area, which is a mining area, the atmosphere of the same is polluted.**

**We have suggested before that the drinking of the sage tea be used and with, if possible, honey from thy present locale. If this is not available, then we should say unto thee, use of the sage honey for the same. This should be done at least twice daily. We should also suggest that, do not eat of any chocolate. We would suggest that thy reduce in amount of the sugar used in thy diet. We should suggest that the eating at this time of the avocado. We would also suggest that as thy would know of it as the safflower seed, obtain this seed, turning it into the oil form, using this in all of thy uses of cooking.**

June 18, 1971: **Thy have other questions, ask.**
*"Yes, Aka.* [6-18-71-008] *also asks for a health reading."*

**We can see into thyself. At this time, this in itself is not needed, other than a correction of the diet unto the same. Therefore, we would suggest, first, that of the safflower seed, this should be made into the oil form and be used for the cooking of all of thy food of this family. We should also suggest that of more of the raw vegetables be eaten.**

**We should also suggest that calcium be obtained and taken in the adult form. We also find the lack of iron in this subject; therefore, we would suggest that more of the same be made available in the diet.**

We also find that this soul is developing into the adult form of the human beast; therefore, we should suggest that the taking of the Lydia E. Pinkham. We should also suggest that of the "S.S.S." liquid be used.

We should also suggest that a good natural, not of the synthetic, but of the natural vitamin and mineral be taken. We find this could be used into all of thy family.

We find, as we have said before, that thy air has become polluted, that the use of the sage tea sweetened by the sage honey. We should also suggest that soon the cacti, of the saguaro cacti, should be made of the same. This could be eaten in its rawest form, and therefore, as the plant should purify that of the seed, it would greatly help as an [antitoxic] body substance.

June 18, 1971: **Thy have other questions, ask.**
*"Yes, Aka. [6-16-71-008] also asks about her health."*
Yes, we see thy need, and therefore, as we have said before, our Father should give blessings and healing into the same. And of this, we should look both into thy soul and of thy body, and the need of the same shall be fulfilled. But remember, that unto which we should build could be taken away if thy should desire, for what we have to offer is but a gift. Therefore, we should say unto thee, if thy should follow of the same reading at the present time as that that was given before, this would be good.

June 18, 1971: **Of all of these subjects, a follow-up reading should be made within three week's time, for they are growing rapidly and certain adjustments should be made.**

June 18, 1971: **Of that, unto this soul, that thy think is bad at this time, remember, our Father did give unto you at birth a gift, and unto this gift shall turn that part of your heart into gladness and happiness, for thy shall know unto the Father for all of thy days.**

We should say unto thee, [be blessed], those who should walk with his hand in that of the Father.

June 25, 1971: **Thy have other questions, ask.**
*"Yes, Aka.[2-19-71-001] asks, 'Do I have a repressed anger? Do I have it pinpointed as to cause and effect, and what can I do to express anger without damage?'"*
(Chuckle) Now thy talk as a child. We should say unto thee, thy anger is with thyself. Anger, in itself, was given unto man to release that proportion of his emotions that has built into him. Therefore, go into thyself, and let this flee from thyself.

But remember, at this time, in the time when the raindrops do not fall upon your earth and the ground becomes parched, man's tempers should flare. As thy would know it, thy should have what is known as temporary insanity. This, in itself, should cause much harm in your area at this time.

Believe in the God "of our kind." Believe in the words of the Son "of our kind." Believe in the words that we have given unto thee. If, in thy place of anger, thy must say unto thyself, thy should cast this out, for this is part of thyself that is not beneficial to the body or soul or spirit. For if thy had upon thy face a boil, would thy not use soaking lotions to remove such? Do the same with thy souls. Pick a time of day and use this for meditation. If thy could do this for 15 minutes each day, these emotions would leave thee. This is what we have said before, place thyselves in accord. Place thyself in accord with thy soul; place thy soul in accord with thy spirit; place thy spirit in accord with God. In doing such, there is no place for anger, in itself. In this manner you will approach all your problems in a sensible, logical manner. We see thy need, and we should take care of the same.

June 25, 1971: **Ask thy other question.**
*"Aka, [11-16-70-003] was supposed to request an additional health reading at this time in regards to his problem with headaches that he was having."*

Yes, we see thy need. Therefore, we should say unto thee, thy are growing again in spiritual and physical [fulfillment]. Therefore, be patient with those of the same, that we may enter and therefore, bring blessings and curing unto the body. Can thy understand of which we speak?
*"Yes."* [11-16-70-003 answers.]

June 25, 1971: **Ask thy other question.**
*"Aka, [4-6-70-003] asks, 'Can you tell me what is causing the nausea and the sore spot under my right ribs?' Also, she asks, 'What was the name you called me reading before last? Can you give me a more complete life reading?'"*

For the last shall be first; therefore, we should tell thee of the time of [Alecha]. [Alecha] was that of a maiden that stood by Mary and tended her in her time of need. Upon this time our Lord did give unto thee blessings.

And as once before, thy were handed unto thee a [child] of suckling, we give unto thee this work as a child, once again. And treat this child as the time of the Cherub. Nurse it and watch it grow into the minds of men. Thy should before thy time stand tall by thy husband, for remember unto thee thy marriage vows.

June 25, 1971: **Of thy [4-6-70-003] first question we should say unto thee.**

We see this, yes.

We would suggest that thy should go unto thy local chiropractor, having certain adjustments made in the back area. We should also suggest, that through physical strain thy have pulled ligaments into thy arm down through thy breast area which should encircle into the backular area — yes.

We find the use of hot Epsom salts, adding to this four lemons; this should be done once a day, soaking for at least 30 minutes of your time. We would also suggest that the whole body be submerged as much as possible.

We would also suggest that for your facial area — yes, we see thy need — we would suggest  the grinding of the raw beef, placing this into that area which is swollen, then doing unto this 5- minute intervals, using of the raw pulp of the potato plant, placing this into the same area. This should be done unto two days.

We find also — yes — one moment, please.

Yes — we would suggest a change in thy diet.

First, we would suggest, of thy morning meal, as many of the raw fruits that are available at this time be eaten, one piece of your bread made into the toast substance.

Of thy lunch meal, we would suggest the drinking of one ounce of safflower liquid. We would also suggest that the taking of the raw safflower and drying it into pulp; this could be used for seasoning on thy food of the evening meal. For thy luncheon meal, eat what thy is known unto thee as a curd, or in your time, one moment .

Yes, we see this, yes.

Therefore, the eating of what thy would know as cottage cheese. If possible, the eating of small quantities of yogurt; nothing else for the lunch period.

Therefore, in the evening, again drinking of the safflower oil, eating only of the meats of that that thy may boil, nothing that is fried in any of thy diet, eating as many raw vegetables as thy desire. We would not suggest any of your dressing to be placed upon this.

This is all on this subject at this time.

July 1, 1971: Now we have here soul J_____. Yes, we have here the spirit, the soul, and the body; this is good. Therefore, the information which she seeks shall be given.

The adjustments that are being made are slightly incorrect. As we have said before, the correction of the pelvic area must be done in a downward motion, then by working out to the vertebrae area. He has corrected one, but not the other. The seventh is still not right or through.

Yes, now this is better.

Still we find she has not complied with the suggestions we have given her for improving her complexion; therefore, it would be useless at this time to give any further information on this subject. If, it would be suggested that a recording be made from the tapes that they [you] now have in thy possession, and send to her, that she may follow the rest of her reading.

And we would say to her, for her other problem, there is a time for waiting and a time to act. But now is not the time to act. Wait; be patient. The things that thy seek shall come to you.

Now we see through at this time with soul J____; it would be suggested before any other readings be given on this subject, if she would place herself in a better position, it would be easier for us to give these readings.

July 1, 1971: **Now we see E_____. Yes, soul E_____, yes, we** have here her body, her spirit and her soul; yes, all is in accord here. Therefore the information that she seeks shall be given her.

You ask, "Why, since I have had most of the other elements in this removed," and we would [say], thy are still a woman. And thy chose to be this, and thy should remain such until the say that thy die. Therefore, there are other organs in thy body which need tending to. If you would do this, you will find that the problem you have at this time will vanish.

Now we also find here the problem of the upper neck area, yes. Yes, we find what you would call the neck bone area, which is known as the brain stem area; we find here pinched nerves. This could be corrected very simple by the visit to a good osteopathic doctor, should this be done. There are many good osteopathic doctors; there are a very good osteopathic hospital in the area in which you live at this time.

Then, yes, we see a deterioration here, an old lesion of the back area. We would suggest that a bar be erected which would be precisely two inches above thy reach, that thy might grasp this once a day. Do not strain yourself to do this; do it a little at a time each day. Build up at it. This will straighten the area out. It will not cure it, but it will keep it separated and functioning properly.

Yes, yes, we see the problem of the feet area. Yes, we would suggest that the eating,...of your problem mostly from not healing, you are a diabetic, therefore, the eating of Jerusalem artichoke; you will find there a natural substance that would feed thy body and take care of its needs. If thy do not care to do this, then consult thy doctor, a good medical doctor, having the necessary tests run for this, and they will probably find that at this time two grams of insulin daily by pill form will take care of the matter. Yes, but the artichoke, eating it in its natural form, either, even in the natural form or placing it in a salad, would not harm you. You will still get the necessary elements from this. [This] Would stabilize this area very,...yes, this is good,...one moment — yes, yes, yes — but at this time we would also suggest soaking of the foot in very warm water, what thy would call Epsom salts would help to extract some of the poisons from the area.

Now we find here over the body in various places arthritis. We would suggest also, for slight circulatory problem here, we would suggest that what thy would call sauna baths be taken. This would help. Go on with these very gradually; do not overdo it. Let your body regulate itself to this. If you would do this once a day, the poisons that are now in your body would be extracted from it. The heat there would help increase the circulatory system, also relieving the arthritis tremendously.

Now, we also find a problem here, in this. We would suggest a, if you would use eye exercises here, finding two objects approximately 20 feet apart, looking as far over to one side as possible to one object, and casting your vision back to that object on the other side, doing this at first five minutes per day, then, finding an object as high up as you can see, and an object as low as you may see, and casting your vision upward and downward. The whole exercise in the beginning should not exceed five minutes, two even would be sufficient. Yes, yes, if you would do this, gradually working this exercise up, trying to do it at the same time each day.

Now for your other problem, and yourself know of this problem which we shall not speak of at this time, we would say this. If thy would meditate first, one moment, please,...Yes, yes, this is much better — yes. In your meditation, do not exceed, in the beginning, over five minutes. Do it simply in the beginning. Think of God wherever you are. Do not think of Him as someone else would think of Him; think only of what He means to you. Think of Him and talk to Him of the things that mean something to you. By reciting something that someone else has thought or said, it means nothing to you; therefore, if it means nothing to you, it can mean nothing to God.

A more extensive reading on this soul can be given at a different time. Should it be asked for, it would not be necessary at any time that she journey here for this reading to be given. We may give it no matter where she is. At this time we would not give a life reading; later this can be done. Now this will be all on soul E_____ at this time.

July 2, 1971: Thy [7-02-71-001] ask again of thy physical. Then we would say unto thee, we see this; therefore, information of the same shall be given.

First, we would say unto thee — remember first, upon this plane thy have chosen to enter once again as a woman, and thy shall be as such for all of thy days upon this plane thy have entered. Remember also that the choice was thine. Therefore, we would say unto thee, first, of the constant headaches thy have suffered, these in themselves are from mental pressure.

We would suggest that thy should take a time for meditation, a time when thy can completely relax away from all of thy worldly problems. Open thy mind. Let thy psychic self come into thee. And project it outward, first, by lying upon a horizontal position, that thy should first relax all proportions of the body, then, by opening the mind as the body is completely relaxed — therefore, starting at the base of thy body, with the movement upward, that it may pass through the spinal area, coming up and projecting from the base and upward to the upper [labordial] area of the skull — therefore, placing thyself in complete healing, that the body may heal itself. If this was practiced, thy would soon find thy health would greatly improve.

We find also, of the left hip area, from old abrasions therefore.

Yes, we see this.

From a fall suffered as a small child, this area did not heal correctly, therefore, has given problems in thy walking.

Yes, we see this.

We would suggest for this, that the use, first, of a diet, changing thy diet in such a manner that of the breakfast meal thy would eat one glass of milk and one piece of brown, toasted rye bread — yes — nothing more. Thy luncheon meal, we would suggest eating of some yogurt, some of the cottage cheese — yes — as many raw vegetables as thy would desire. Of thy evening meal eat no meat that is fried, only the meat that is boiled.

Yes.

Eat okra.

Yes.

We also find in thy diet should be added to that of the Jerusalem artichoke. We find that this soul is a diabetic. We would first suggest that thy go unto thy physician for treatment of the same. Remember, there are many things we could tell thee of, but thy physicians, as that of Luke, a physician, was placed here by our Lord for a reason, and for those physicians who should follow the teachings of the same, our Lord should give unto knowledge.

We find also, of the evening meal, drinking of no more than one glass of milk at this meal. Yes.

We would suggest that before each meal the drinking of one ounce of safflower oil.

July 2, 1971: **Of thy [7-02-71-001]** other question, we should say unto thee, since this question remains in thy mind, and it is, as thy would know it, as a secret question, we should answer it in this manner. For, as in the beginning, thy Lord planted upon thy earth all fruits and [forms] of His kind, He should plant in thee of the same.

We find other problems in this soul. We would suggest at a later time a health reading and a life reading be given in accordance with the same.

July 2, 1971: **Thy have other questions, ask.**

*"Thank you, Aka. [7-2-71-002] has asked that — she says, 'Is there anything I can do to improve several bad health conditions that have existed for 18 or 20 years?' And she would also like any help you can give her regarding her current problems."*

**We see thy need.**

**Yes, we see this.**

**We should say unto thee, of the vitamin substance, in itself, is not in completion; therefore, add more of the E in that of which thy are using at the present time. We would also suggest, that in these same diets should be changed radically, or basically, if the diet is wrong, the substance into which thy are using would not greatly change that of the body chemicals. The body first must be cleansed. By cleansing the body, therefore, you cleanse the soul. And by cleansing the soul, therefore, you cleanse also of the spiritual outlook of man.**

**Of thy own private problem, we should say unto thee, beware of the dragon that comes as a friend. Do not always trust those who speak too smoothly. Can thy understand of which we speak?**

*"No."* [She answers.]

**Then we should say unto thee, do not take unto what is given to you as truth, for thy have with thee a liar.**

July 2, 1971: **Thy have other questions, ask of the same.**

*"Yes, Aka. Do you have any message for Paul in his healing efforts?"*

**We should say unto thee these words. For a short period of time, man, in this area, should be of a violent nature. Remember in thy healing, thy may heal only of those who should want this healing.**

July 3, 1971: **Aka is here.**

*"Good evening, Aka. Is Ray with God?"*

**Soul Ray stands with God.**

**Yes, we see thy need. Thy have many questions, ask.**

*"Aka, [7-3-71-001] asks for a health reading on her daughter, [7-3-71-002]. And she says, she asks for a health reading because of health problems."*

**Yes, we have the body, the soul, the spirit, and the immortal body. Yes, this is good; therefore, the information thy desire shall be given.**

**First, thy must realize that as an entry was made upon this plane, this entry was made as an act of love on the part of our Father.**

**We should say unto thee, first, of the [pinalian] [pineal?] gland, we find in this location problems.**

Yes.

Underdevelopment of this gland has reacted in such a manner as not to give off the necessary gene to fight off disease. Therefore, it should be necessary —

Yes we see this.

Therefore, it should be necessary that this soul be given adult dosage of that proportion of vitamin E. Also this soul should be given in accordance adult dosages both of calcium and of the vitamin C.

We see the use of the drug known as [gamma globulin]. This in itself is good. But you must remember that over dosage of this substance, the body will become, and build, immunity to the same. Therefore, it would be far better that the body functions be brought back into their natural form.

We would suggest also that the extraction of any type of the white sugar be taken from this diet, the usage of either honey of the local, or of the use of sage honey, in the sweetening of substance for the same.

We see thy need, and our Father has given, therefore, healing into the same. But remember also, that as a parent, your duty lies in the protection of this soul. Therefore, it would be deemed necessary that those precautions that we have given unto thee be taken.

We find also the use of the Night-blooming Cereus in cubes of one proportion of cube of your inches one-fourth, therefore used once daily.

It should also be suggested for further development of both the growing of the hair and the hardening of the fingernails, therefore, the use of [trickle] gelatin. This you should find in that substance tonic known as the tonic known as S.S.S.

We find the lack of substance of iron.

Under no circumstances feed this soul any of your substance known as chocolate. The soul, in itself, is poisoned by the same substance.

Prepare a very healthy diet. We see the need for more nourishment than usual. Then we should say unto thee, let this child eat at least six meals per day.

Can thy understand of which we speak?

*"Yes."* [She answers.]

Thy other questions, ask.

*"Yes, Aka. I would like to pause for just one moment and pick up a microphone. Would it be all right to pass around soul Ray?"*

Yes, we should wait.

*"Yes, Aka. Could you give me the dosage on the S.S.S.?"*

Yes, we see thy need. Therefore, we see of the child's dosage.

Yes, this would be good.

No more at the present time.

Yes.

July 3, 1971: **Thy have other questions, ask.**

*"Aka, [7-3-71-002] asks for a health reading on herself."*

Yes, we see thy need. First, it should be our suggestion — one moment, please; the records must be checked.

Yes, we see thy need. We have before us now the body, the soul, the spirit, and the immortal body. Yes — all is in accord.

Therefore, we should say unto thee, go unto a good gynecologist. Your problem is relatively simple. We see the large intestine.

Yes.

The intestine itself has become, as thy would know it, kinked or crimped off. It is not aligned [for] proper digestive of the same. We would also suggest that of this soul a different, as thy would know it, of the vagina and [liverkine] area, a different wash be used of the same.

We find a problem of the thyroid; therefore, certain, as thy would know it, precautionary procedures must be taken. We could give further information on this area, but this should be taken care of by the physician.

We also find — yes, we see this — of the [malatosin] area, we find, therefore — one moment, please.

Yes. Yes, yes, Father.

Then we should further define, this is of the mastoid area, of the inner ear problem. This is caused basically from infection of the inner ear, caused from sinus problems. We would suggest the drinking of the sage tea. We would further suggest changing of the present drinking water.

Yes.

Or the filtering by carbon of the same.

Yes, we also see this.

We would also suggest that this subject have corrective lenses. We find the problem —

Yes.

This could be simply done. It, in preference, would be done by thyself with exercise of the eye. This could be done in finding two objects approximately 20 feet apart, and then finding objects approximately 10 feet in height, placing both eyes, without moving the head, on the left object and then of the right, then up and then down. This should be done at first five-minute sequences a day, increasing unto 10, then gradually unto 15 minutes each day. If this were done over a four-week period this problem would take care of itself.

Yes, we see thy need.

Yes.

We would further suggest that this subject go unto what is known as a dentist. There are certain problems here which are causing intensive head problems or headaches. This is caused by the misformation of the teeth. Should these be straightened, or the teeth pulled and removed, it would allow the skull itself, the [formular] area of the skull, to come back into place.

Yes.

We also find that this subject — yes — of the back area, both of the fourth and fifth vertebrae — yes — problems here. This is causing the subject to endure unnecessary cramping during the [pinal?] period of her cycle. Therefore, if this was taken care of, she would no longer suffer this problem.

Yes. We find, also, there is a great deal of work here in the back area. We find also of pinched nerves of the upper, as thy would know it, brainstem or neckular area, that proportion which connects the brain with the spine. Therefore, we would suggest that either a good osteopathic doctor or chiropractic doctor be seen.

We would further suggest that a follow-up reading be given on this soul in two-week sequences.

This is all at this time on this soul.

July 3, 1971: **Thy have other questions, ask.**
*"Yes, Aka. [7-3-71-003], and he asks for a reading on his health problems."*

Yes, we see thy need.
Yes.
On moment.
Yes.

These records are in order; therefore, this reading shall be given. We find, therefore, body, the soul and the spirit, and the immortal body.
Yes.

Therefore, we would suggest, at the present time, soul Ray grows very weak, therefore, we would suggest that a continuation of this reading [can] be given at a different time.

Awaken soul Ray from his slumber.

July 9, 1971: *"Thank you. [7-2-71-001] has asked, Aka, that she was instructed to go to her doctor for a check for diabetes. And she says that the tests turned out negative. 'Could you please give me any further information and advice on this subject?'"*

We see thy need; therefore, we should say unto thee. Thy tests at the present time are negative, but unless certain precautions are taken at this time, thy are what is known as a borderline diabetic. If the precautionary measures that we have given unto thee are not done at this time, then thy shall be in chaos. Therefore, we may only, as we have said before, suggest unto thee. But for the good of thyself and thy family, take of these suggestions.

July 9, 1971: **Thy have other questions, ask.**

*"Aka, [7-9-71-003], and she asks, 'Am I in danger of physical violence?'"*

Nay, we cannot see this at this time. We should say unto thee these words. Go unto thy brother and forgive this brother who has offended thee, and therefore, this brother may offend thee no more. But if thy should go unto this brother, and still, thy do not make, as thy would know, of the peace, therefore, then take with thee two witnesses, and therefore, again go and try and make unto this peace. But remember, thy must forgive of this brother, therefore, that he may forgive unto thee. Can thy understand of which we speak?

Nay, not fully. Then we should say in a different way — first, of the violence that thy fear, mostly is in thy own mind, but secondly, of the anger that thy feel, this is very real. Take this anger from thy heart, for this anger can only harm thy own soul. For remember, man may harm thy body, but only you yourself may harm your soul. And by harming the soul, thy would be, in itself, harming the spirit and driving it farther away.

July 9, 1971: **Thy have other questions, ask.**
*"Aka, [11-2-70-001] asks for a health reading."*
Yes, we see thy need. And we should say unto this soul, because of thy deliverance into the Lord of thy body, thy soul, and of thy immortal body, then we should say unto thee, as has been promised before, fear not for thy mortal body, for thy Lord has much work for thee. These things that are needed within thy family shall be taken care of. As time should pass, we should give of thee the necessary knowledge to make of this [soul].

July 10, 1971: [Editor's note: This was a private reading to an individual whose family lived in Kellner Canyon, Globe, Arizona, where runoff from Pinal Peak where the U.S. Forest had sprayed Agent Orange was causing serious health problems for residents and animals.]
Yes, we see thy need. First, we should say unto thee — yes, this, as we have said before, should be safe. Most of that unto which thy would know as the spray has left, or dissipated, as thy would know. Therefore, the milk of the goat should be of purity, and the meat of the same should be of purity. Then we should say unto thee, fear not.

July 10, 1971: **Thy have other questions, ask.**
*"Yes, Aka. My mother [B____ Mc____, who is presently in California for a few days has found that she has cancer inside her and she is going in next week for an operation, and she has asked for a health reading and your guidance as to what she should do and how she can best recover from this?"*

We should say unto thee, we see thy need. Therefore, we have the body, the soul, the spirit, and the immortal body. Yes, this is fine; this is good.

Yes, we would say unto thee, we find there, of the vagina area, the [mesomorphous, metamorphosis]-type growths.

Yes.

Yes, we see thy need [sigh], and at the present time, we would say, go unto thy physician for treatment of the same. We should say, with meditation, these of the same should leave of thy body.

That thy might fully understand of this type growth, these are very much as thy would know of as a skin cancer. We should explain from which they have come. The spray of thy area has changed of the body genes. [Editor's note: Agent Orange was sprayed on Pinal Peak, Arizona, by the U.S. Forest Service for defoliation, as it was in Viet Nam.]

All matter is made of cosmic matter; should this be disturbed in any manner then growths of the same should take place in the body. The spray used, in forming of the same, should attack of the pineal glandular area; therefore, causing this glandular area to produce more of the [antivaccine]-type serum into the blood. This same [vaccine] should create of a virus, which in itself is to fight disease. But an imbalance causes growth of its own, or foreign-type malignant nature. These are variously of a parasite nature.

Therefore, we would suggest the taking of what thy would call of the seed of the mistletoe, making of the same after drying into a powder, using of thy measurements 2 grams per day of this powder, this would greatly help in the healing of the same.

Within time, the body should become whole again.

This is all upon this soul at this time. Should further information be needed, if this soul should ask of the same, information pertaining to this would be given.

Awaken soul Ray from his slumber.

July 16, 1971: **Thy have other questions, ask.**

*"Aka, [7-16-71-001] asks for a health reading. She was born May 8, 1957, in Los Angeles, California."*

Yes, we see thy need. And we should say unto this soul — one moment, please.

Yes, that is better.

Yes, we see thy need. Therefore, we have before us the body, the soul, and the spirit, and therefore, we have before us unto the immortal body.

Then we should say unto thee, first, thy diet must be changed. And we say unto thee, [eat] of one piece of toast; this toast must be cooked well done. This should be eaten with one glass of milk in the morning meal. Of thy luncheon meal, one glass of milk and not more than five bananas; nothing more. Of thy evening meal, one ounce of safflower oil before a meal; this should be done at least 30 minutes before the meal. She should not eat any of the fried meat of any kind. Do not use either of that of the butter that comes from the cow, or of, as you would know it, your imitation butters. This cannot be used. Eat as many raw vegetables as thy desire, no more than one-fourth pound of meat; none of the pork may be eaten. This meat must be boiled. It cannot be fried in any form. Take of unto the leaves of the petals of the rose. As these are dried, make unto them a powder, mixing 10 grams of this substance with one teaspoon of honey. This must be done before the evening meal and afterward. We would also suggest for the other necessary mineral[s] and vitamins lacking in this soul at the present time the usage of the substance known as Lydia E. Pinkham. We would suggest that an adult dosage of vitamin E be taken. Of the morning, before the morning meal, vitamin C should be taken. Before the morning meal vitamin B should be taken. This should be done before the morning meal and before the evening meal. This diet must be followed for a two-week period. At that time we should change certain proportions of the same.

We find that there are certain dental work that should be done in a corrective manner. We find that there are pressures from a secondary, wisdom tooths, which is putting [proportion of] pressure toward the brainal area. These should be removed.

There are other corrective measures in the backular area that should be taken care of by your local chiropractic doctor. We would also suggest for this period no loud music of any kind, only of the smoothing nature. Avoid loud noises as much as possible, and the healing into the same should come. We would also suggest that meditation be taken twice daily. Can thy understand of which we speak? Nay, not fully, but thy shall. We should also suggest that calcium be added into thy diet.

Thy have other questions, ask.

*"Yes, Aka, one other question on the same subject. They asked, 'Do you mean that the meat should be broiled or boiled?'"*

The meat should be boiled.

*"Thank you."*

July 16, 1971: Thy have other questions, ask of the same.

*"Yes, Aka, a number of times you have referred to the Night-blooming Cereus for medicinal purposes. There are, I am told, about a hundred varieties of this, and most of the varieties are available through nurserymen. Ah —."*

We should say unto thee, if thy should check into thy health food stores, thy shall find the dried variety. These have already been processed and are available in the dried variety of the same.

July 17, 1971: Thy have many questions; ask of these.

*"Yes, Aka. G____ C____ asks, 'Are occasional items, such as commercial ice cream or root beer, harmful once or twice a week?' And then she also asks about her child, L____. She says, 'L____ won't drink S.S.S. tonic because of the taste. Would the same vitamins found in children's chewable vitamins, such as Super Plenamins Juniors, be just as good? Would they also supply the necessary calcium?'"*

We should say unto thee, first, of thy first question, this is good. These things thy should give unto a child are good. But as a little wine is good for the body, so should these things be good, but not taken in excess.

Of thy second question, of the vitamin substance thy have mentioned, we should say unto these words, seek out a natural vitamin that is extracted in such a fashion that it comes out in a natural form. If the child cannot take of this — yes, we see this — then we would say unto thee, go and take of the natural vitamin form. There are many of these that are good. There are those which are of a malt flavor; these would be good, and the child should take of these.

We see this. Yes.

And of thy child, we see into this also, and we should say unto thee — we would suggest for a short period of time, do not let this child walk upstairs or downstairs by herself. Make certain that some adult is with her, for she shall fall, and this should not be good. This should be only done for one week. Her star shall be different within that period, and therefore, her chances of accident shall have passed. We see there are things thy have done up into this time, and these things are good.

We would suggest unto this child, after this one-week period has passed, let her be a child. She may bruise herself or fall at times; let her pick herself up. But she shall know that thy shall be there to help her if you are needed.

And now we should tell you of this child. For she shall grow into a lovely young lady. At the age of 17, she will at that time want to be married, but this urge shall pass. When she has reached the age of 23 she shall marry. She shall bear unto you four grandchildren, one boy and three girls. She shall use the education, as she has done before.

But we should say unto thee, this is all we may tell thee of the child's future at the present time. In her next reading we should give more of the information that is desired.

Thy have other questions, ask.

*"Yes, Aka. I have one other question on this child. How many days should the Night-blooming Cereus be given?"*

We would suggest that this should go onward unto a month of your time, and another reading should be taken again. You must realize that the body chemicals change every moment of thy life. This is all done according to God's plan. As she develops, both mentally and spiritually, forward, as new ideas are born within her, so should her body chemicals adjust to adapt to this. Therefore, changes at that time shall be made.

July 17, 1971: **Thy have other questions, ask.**

*"Thank you, Aka. G_____ C_____ was supposed to request a follow-up health reading on herself. Do you have any information for her?"*

Yes, we see thy need; therefore, we should say unto thee of these words. At the present time, we should suggest, before each meal, the drinking of warm milk. This would be preferably of the goat's milk. This should be done approximately 30 minutes before the meal. We would suggest again another follow-up reading on this soul in a two-week period of your time.

We would further suggest, with the continuations of the plans thy have in thy mind, fear not, for God, our Father, has heard thy prayers, and they shall be answered.

But remember of these words. As thy speak unto [thy] Father, speak unto Him as thy would speak unto thyself. Spend a little time each day in meditation; put thyself in accord with thy God. Do this in the morning as thy rise, and these things that thy should desire shall come into thee a little at a time, as raindrops should fall.

But as thy prayer is a sacred thing, we should answer unto thee in a secret way. These things shall come in joy for those thy have desired it for.


July 17, 1971: **Thy have other questions, ask.**

*"Aka, G_____ C_____ would like a health reading."*

Yes, we see thy need. And as before, the records are clear to us; therefore, this reading shall be given.

But first, we should say unto thee of these words. Of thy past life, thy were much as thy are today, in a different world. There are many times thy have seen, from close, to the Greek people. And this is not surprising. For as once before, thy were a student of philosophy, thy shall be again.

And of the medical reading, we should say unto these words. First, thy problem of thy feet, of the arch of thy feet, we see this. And therefore, we should say unto thee, first go unto your stores of footwear, and therefore, obtain corrective shoes unto the same. This should be done with a full-arch support. Also, we would suggest that a crepe-type-cushion instrument be used as thy soles, for in thy present work, this is not only affecting thy feet, but it should cause arthritis, much worse than the small amount that is in thy body at the present time. Therefore, we should say unto thee, go then unto the saunta baths, at least once a week. This would be good, very good for these soles — and as a family unit, go as a family unit with all of thy family.

We should also suggest that because of the unusual noises of thy work, some of these noises could be detrimental to thy health and thy nervous system. We would suggest no walking of thy daily leisure time.

We should also suggest that no alcoholic beverages of any type be taken for at least 30 days. We should suggest a diet of the same because of inflammation — one moment; these words must be placed in thy language.

Yes. Yes, we see this now.

Then we should say unto these words. Because of inflammation of the kidney areas, we should give of this area a short rest. This also should be done in the diet. We would suggest that more of the raw vegetables, the eating of the greens of the same — this would be good. We would suggest this be done at least once daily. Thy have at this time available of the melon plants, [forss], one moment — yes, your word of cantaloupe. It was spoken different before — yes. Of the cantaloupe, it would be good; this would be very good for thy system. The rest of thy meals could be taken much in the same fashion as thy are presently taking them.

Yes, we see this. Yes.

We would also suggest, after thy have left thy work, take a time then for meditation, placing thyself in accord with God. Thy shall find thy shall be able, therefore, to leave a little of your worries at work with thee.

Yes, we see this.

We find also that as a small child you quarreled with thy brother. Thy did injure unto the same and cause lesions unto the left kidney area. We find, as a child also — yes.

First, we should say unto the first. If thy should take of both above the right and left kidney, hot as thy may stand this, using of thy castor oil — yes, this would be good — making a compress of the same; doing this in 30-minute intervals.

Yes.

If this were done for four days this matter would clear up.

And of thy second, we find an injury of the right thigh bone area. This area was, in your words, fractured. We cannot see this area mending quite properly. Therefore, we should give unto thee of thy luncheon time a little different of the diet. We should suggest the taking of calcium of the natural form. We would also suggest —

Yes, we see this.

We would also suggest that for thy lunch, one glass of, either of the cow's milk or of the goat's milk. It would be preferably, the goat's milk would be much better. This should be taken also with only of the banana, not succeeding [exceeding] six of the same.

We would also suggest on this soul —

Yes, we see this.

Both of the morning, the noon, and of the evening meals, 30 minutes before each interval should be drinken of the sage tea. It would also be suggested in the evening, because of the congestion of the same, of the sinus area, making, therefore, a steamed broth of the same, placing over thy head a tent made of a towel and breathing inward. This in itself would help to quicken the immunity to the same and break down this congestion.

There are many other small complications of the body of area. We would suggest either of a chiropractor or a doctor of osteopathic of the same, be used to straighten out the backular area, working upwardly. This would help to relieve unto the same of the nervous headaches.

This is all on this soul at the present time. Additional information should be given as it is desired.

July 23, 1971: **Thy have many questions, ask.**

*"Aka, [7-23-71-001] asks for a health reading. He says, 'I have asthma and have allergy difficulties, also eye muscle difficulties.' He asks if you can help him?"*

**Yes, we see thy need. But ask your other questions first and then this shall be given.**

*"[5-7-71-004] and he asks for a reading because of health reasons."*

**This shall be given. Ask thy other question.**

*"[7-16-71-003] has asked for a health reading."*

**We should say unto this soul, strengthen thy faith in God. Thy have been given certain instructions. Take of these. With these, thy problem shall no longer exist. But as we have said before, thy shall have of thy son.**

July 23, 1971: **Thy have now two health readings; ask for these and they shall be given.**

*"Yes, Aka. The first health reading that I had was for [7-23-71-001], and he asked about his asthma difficulty and his eye muscle difficulties."*

**Yes, we see thy need. And we should say unto this soul, we have before us both the body, the spirit, and the soul, of this immortal body.**

**Then we should say unto thee, first, of thy eye problem. This can be done quite simply. But it must be done as a ritual every day of your month and must be carried out for three months. First, finding two objects approximately 20-feet apart in a vertical line, then by finding two objects 20-feet apart in a horizontal line, first by casting of the horizontal line upward and downward, and then to the vertical of the north and the south — do this, each daily, placing thyself on a north-south axis. The help thy should need should come. Stand erect, doing this in such a manner one day that the sun should cast on the right side of the face, the next one, the left side of the face. This must be done, first, for five minutes of each day of the first week, and increased up to 45 minutes. If this is done in this manner, thy eye problem shall be no more.**

**Then we should say, of thy sinus problem. First, thy have not done as instructed unto thy family. Drink of the sage tea, placing, if**

possible, the natural, local honey — placing of the sage tea once a day and making a vapor of the same. This should be done.

Third, we should say unto thee, give of meditation. Talk unto thy Lord. Open thy mind for expansion. Do not close thy mind. But do not become impatient.

If the things we have mentioned have been done, the healing thy desire shall come into thy body, in fullness, and awareness shall come of the same.

July 23, 1971: **Thy have other questions, ask.**
*"Thank you, Aka. [5-7-71-004], and he has asked for a reading because of health reasons."*
**Yes, we see thy need.**
**Yes, we see this.**
**Then we should say unto thee — one moment.**
**First, we should say unto this soul, for the records, therefore, have been checked, and as we find of both the body, the soul, the spirit, and now, of the immortal body, permission has been given for information of the same.**

**First, we would suggest that this soul go unto a dentist. The removal of all, therefore, as thy would know it, of the wisdom teeth should be done first. This would relieve the headual and backular area and stop the secretion of poison entering in the body. There is other dental work that should be done, and done as soon as possible.**

**We also find arthritis entering, therefore, into the body. Basically, this is not of a true arthritis; this is caused by an imbalance of the pineal glandular area and the [autum] glandular area. We would say then, go thy either unto a good osteopathic or chiropractic doctor. If the manipulation of the bonal area that houses, and therefore, encloses the brainstem area, certain corrective measures, and pressure relieved from this, would, therefore, let certain of fluids return back into these glands.**

**We also find — yes, we find this — that this diet should be radically changed. First, we should say unto this soul, fish should be eaten, of the salt water variety, at least three times a week. And this should be done in such a manner that all the vitamins, therefore, are kept within the same — this, by taking of what thy would know as thy tin foil, wrapping all fish to be cooked in the same, and baked. We would suggest that there be no fried foods of any type consumed. And therefore — yes, we see this.**

**We also see his need. (Chuckle). Then we should say unto thee, as thy ask in this form, as a child, then our answer of this problem can only be answered in the same manner. Of this problem of thy sex life, this is all of thy mind. If thy would think positive in this area, thy would have no problem. But we should also say of these things unto thee. Our Father only sees sin, therefore, that is cast out of thyself into another. For our**

Father asks but two things, to love of Him unto one-tenth of that love that is given, therefore, unto you, and to love of thy brother in the same manner.

Of thy other problems, should these be asked in such a manner that they are sincere, these other things in thy mind shall be answered.

July 30, 1971: **Ask thy other question.**

*"Thank you, Aka. [4-6-70-003] asks — she says, 'You said [ 4-13-70-002] should have frequent readings for her health. Can you give one now, and also, anything on her life if necessary?' She also asks, 'Would it be good for M\_\_\_ and Andrew to continue their flying activities? Do you have any other advice for the family?'"*

We should say, first, of the first question, the health is relatively good at this time. The child shall go through certain, as thy would know it, growing pains. These are not things to worry about. But as we have said before, teach this child of the waiting, not of the sin.

Of thy second question we should say of these words, we see no danger at the immediate time.

July 30, 1971: **Ask thy other question.**

*"Aka, M\_\_\_\_ V\_\_\_\_ asks, 'Will I get the child who was offered to me this week?'"*

We do not see this; nay. But be patient, for we see children ahead. Grow nearer unto thy male that thy have chosen. Become and grow as one. Build of thy love. Be patient with others around thee, and thy wishes and thy prayers shall be heard. But remember, as has been said before, the Lord should act in mysterious ways, sometimes unbeknowing to yourself. But as your prayers have been heard, those who have suffered in the same manner into which you have, and who have conquered their karma, should be sent unto thee for guidance. Give blessings unto the Lord, your God.

July 30, 1971: **Ask thy other question.**

*"Aka, L\_\_\_\_ D\_\_\_\_\_ asks, that she would like a general health reading."*

One moment, please. Yes, we see this.

Therefore, we have before us the records.

Yes, that is better.

Now we have before us the body, the soul, the spirit, and therefore, the immortal body.

Yes, this is very good.

Therefore, that which thy request shall be given, but we should give of thee healing. But remember, we are nothing; we are not great. We may only give unto this one that that our Father permits us. Therefore, the healing that she desires shall be given. Then we would say unto this one, go then unto thy home, and for three nights we should come to thee.

Upon the third night give thanks unto the Lord for this healing, and the healing shall come in fullness.

August 6, 1971: **Thy have many questions, ask.**

*"Yes, Aka, [8-6-71-001] of Yuma says, since the age of two when she had polio she has walked with crutches. When she was 12 she had a severe attack of inflammatory rheumatism. She is now in her early 60's and she has considerable pain in her back and her knees, particularly her knees. She states that she realizes that there is no cure for the overall condition; however, what, if anything, can she do to ease the knee pain to make walking less difficult and less painful?"*

Then we would say unto this one, we have before us the records — yes, yes — therefore, we have the body, the soul, and the spirit, and therefore, the immortal body. We see thy need.

First, we would suggest, take time for meditation, first, by placing thyself in accord with thy God. Pray for forgiveness, but pray first for healing unto thy body.

Second, we would suggest the use of the [saunta] bath. This should be started in very small intervals at first — yes — no longer than five minutes at a time. This should be done each day, gradually over a two-week period increasing up to 10 minutes, over a three-week period, 15 minutes.

We see thy need also. Most of thy pain comes from that upper back area; we find in this soul the stiffening, therefore, of calcium deposits of the same. We would suggest, if thy should go unto thy chiropractor and this area be very gradually worked over — at no time should he forcibly place any of these back in their proper perspective. This treatment must be done over a very long, prolonged period. We would suggest in this case that the use of an osteopathic doctor.

We also find that bonular [bony] area of the heel, calcium deposits, therefore, of the same. These are giving pain upward into the upper lumbar area. We would suggest, therefore, that the use of the vitamin E be used, with more of this than the other vitamins and minerals, therefore, needed in the diet.

We would also suggest that during this diet thy should eat of at least three meals per day. Thy morning meal should be made up of toast and milk, no more than one glass of the same. Thy noon meal should be made up of warm, either [other] tea that thy prefer of the Orient, or therefore, of the sage [tree] of the same. Therefore, only of the green, raw vegetables of thy own choice would do. Of thy evening meal, we would suggest that thy meat be eaten as raw as possible. We would also suggest that no fried foods be used in this diet. We would suggest, therefore, that fish be taken at least once per day in small quantities. We would also suggest that one meal of each week should be made of fish only. We would also suggest the use of the evening meal, that thy would take upon this meal food supplements [low] in protein as possible.

We would suggest, therefore, that before your retiring in the evening that additional tea of the red sage be used, or in your case, the purple sage. We would also suggest, this can be obtained at your local food store, it is of the herb called of the laxative herb. This is in ingredients of several herbs. If this was used, this would put thyself on a daily program which, in itself, would help relieve in thy pain.

We should suggest, therefore, that if the program we have laid out before you at the present time cannot be followed in full that thy go unto thy local doctor, and therefore, through surgery, have the calcium removed from the heel area.

August 6, 1971: **Thy have other questions, ask.**

*"Yes, Aka,* [8-6-71-001] *wants to know about the general health and attitudes of her two children. The first child is* [8-6-71-002]. *The second child is* [8-6-71-003]. *"*

Yes, we see thy need. Therefore, we should say unto thee these words. Remember, even as a snowflake is individual, these are two separate, completely different individuals with individual needs.

Therefore, we should say unto thee these words. Their needs are completely different, both of the food for the body and the food for the mind. Remember also that as these two souls have evolved through time, they have grown and their plane has grown. Therefore, their need is no longer as husband and wife, as before. The lesson that they did not learn in the time of before is not the same lesson of now.

Their lesson of this plane is tolerance, of humility of mankind. For in them and the deeds they did do of another lifetime, that we should look ahead, and we should say, first of the girl. She should marry at the age of 18. She shall have three children; all three of these shall be girls. There shall be many trying times in her life, but she, in her search for her Lord, shall overcome these. She shall take of the education thy have given unto her and bear witness forth unto the time which shall come, for remember, as we have said, now is the time of the Lord. Give her these things. But remember, also, there is a time for laughter; there is a time for sleep; there is a time for work, and there also is a time for this. Let her drink of all wines, that she may become a full and complete person.

Then we should say of the boy — yes, we see this — and in the lad, itself, he shall grow onward into adulthood. He shall go to war, at a war that man has never seen before, and he shall go through this. He shall have the time and knowledge, therefore, to study to become a physician and heal. But his new revolutionary ideas shall bring a form of healing unto your mankind that you have not seen before. This need shall grow from this time. Therefore, let him go unto the needs of his body. They shall direct him, and those that walk with him, who was with him before, shall serve him well. Do not be in a hurry. You shall see your grandchildren from this one, but this should take time. For time heals all wounds, even yours.

For remember, we see thy need also, and therefore, we send thee blessings, and we should send unto thy house those that are needed to see thee through this time ahead.

August 6, 1971: **Thy have other questions, ask.**
*"Aka, [8-6-71-004] in Miami...asks if you have a message from her mother?"*

We are sorry, but the message that thy seek is not permitted. There are those which should come unto thee in thy slumber, and therefore, the message shall come into thyself.

Can thy understand of which we speak? Nay, then we should say in a different way these words. For in thy slumber, the message that thy should receive should come unto thee. For remember, your God and ours should carry the blessings into thy home in a strange and mysterious way unto thyself. But remember, within time, all things that belong unto thee should come back unto thee.

Thy have other problems unto which we see. And we should say unto you these words, for this thy have not asked, so therefore, it should come in a secret way in a secret answer. But as a Rose should be given without thorns, so should the love that thy wish should come unto thee.

August 13, 1971: **Thy have many questions, ask.**
*"Yes, Aka, [6-18-71-009] would like to know what causes her knee aches, and what she can do to prevent them?"*

Yes, we see thy need, and therefore, give healing into this soul. And we should come and assist thee in thy effort.

But we also see in her diet, one moment — yes, yes, yes, Father, yes, Father — yes, we see this. Then we should say unto these words, we have before us the body, the soul, the spirit and the holy body; all is in [intact], for therefore, we see the immortal body. Yes, we see this; yes, we see this.

Then we should say unto this one, as thy have give[n] forth thy soul and thy spirit into the Lord, take our hand and we should guide thee. Do not walk backward, but forward, for in the time of [men nelbs?] time of thy birth, we see this and we see thy need. As then, and as thy eyes were cast into the heavens, keep them upon the Lord, thy Father.

Take therefore these words, and dine upon them as fruit. And as thy should bear fruit unto man, take this fruit again, and feed those that thy should bear. And let thy descendants, and thy descendants' descendants should bear the same fruit, and therefore, walk always in the blessings of our Lord.

Of thy diet, we would say unto these words, eat more of the raw vegetation. Take also of the salt that should come from the sea. Once each week, dine from the fish that should come from the sea. Eat more liver. Consumption of more protein in thy diet, this could be added as the substance.

We would also suggest — yes, we see this — we should also suggest, therefore, the taking of the sauna baths, if this could be done at least of two-week intervals.

We also find in this one, both of the upper and lower backular area wherefore could be much correction. This could be done quite simply by the chiropractor. This also should relieve of the child's headaches.

If certain other work were done of the 6th and 8th vertebrae — yes — this also should relieve of that of what thy should call of thy menstrual periods. We should also suggest that the consumption of what is known as Lydia E. Pinkham be taken. We could not suggest at the present time the usage of calcium in the diet, for as the system, in itself, is not rejecting that that is fed in, we must first correct the system that it may digest all minerals and vitamins to the body.

August 13, 1971: **Ask thy other questions.**

*"Thank you, Aka. I am not sure if I understand how to meditate. I have always felt that I know how to pray, and I wonder if you could tell me the difference in prayer and meditation, or how you would have us meditate?"*

In your time of prayer, this is the time that you pick to confess all things unto your Father, and this is good.

In meditation, listen to your Father. Open your mind. Place yourself with your God, your Father, your creator. Listen to Him well, and He should talk unto thee. And as His words come into thy mind, thy whole body shall, should ring on a spiritual beam. Spend this time to listen to God.

Can thy understand of which we speak?

*"Yes, Aka."*

August 13, 1971: **Soul Ray grows weary; therefore, we should give time unto his healing, and then awaken soul Ray from his slumber.**

August 15, 1971: **Thy have other questions, ask.**

*"Yes, Aka, there is a request for a health reading on a child, [8-15-71-001]. The problem seems with the digestive system."*

**Yes.**

*"At this time can you help the parents?"*

Yes, we see thy need. Therefore, we have before us the records, and we have before us the body, the soul, the spirit, and therefore, the immortal body.

Yes, we see this.

Therefore, as the substance thy would know unto this child, change on its diet, give unto this child of the goat's milk. But do not give it to the child in a cool form; give it in its natural form. We find the lack on this soul of calcium, also the lack — we would suggest that thy should take of the mesquita wood, char it, and let this child, as thy would know, teethe upon the same.

We should also see in this child other problems. We would suggest that this child be taken unto a physician and correction should be made in the limbs at this time. The bone structure in this area has not developed as it should; therefore, should braces be used at this time, the limbs themselves could grow strong and true. Should this be neglected, this should be a problem unto the child the rest of its life.

August 15, 1971: **Thy have other questions, ask.**
*"Yes. Aka, there has been a request for a health reading on the child [8-15-71-002]."*

Yes, we see thy need. Then we should say unto these words, we find no radical problems in this child. Give this child normal, healthy food; add to the child's diet certain vitamins and minerals of a natural course. We find that if this child is left to grow and mature, this child should grow onward, and at one time, at the age of 24, should marry into one of your statesmen and be very instrumental in the changing and betterment of your laws. This is good. We find no problem here.

August 15, 1971 [in Philosophy: **Thy have other questions, ask.**
*"Yes, Aka, [8-15-71-003] of Yuma has given permission for a health reading, and would like to know, will she live to see her children grown, and also asks how many more lives does she have to live before she will be allowed to rest?"*

We should say unto these words, thy shall live to see thy children. But remember also, thy have free choice, the choice, as thy would know it, of life or death. For remember, our Father is not the God of the dead, but the living. For some there is many; for some there is none. The choice to re-enter and to repeat again is your own. The choice to decide that thy should rest by thy Father is your own.

As we have said before, in the beginning, man created death, as thy know it, in the means of learning, and therefore, purifying thy body, thy soul, and thy spirit. There is some who should lose sight of this. Upon losing of the sight of our Father, they should lose of the spirit, and therefore, become a lost soul to wander forever in nothingness.

Look upward; look within thyself and thy should see God. Look upon the ground, thy earth, and thy should see God.

Our Father, as He said in the beginning, created man and woman in "our image, of our kind;" therefore, He placed Himself within you. For thine are the most pure of creations upon the earth. Destroy this and thy should have nothing. But remember, thy can destroy nothing; thy can only change its form. For in its beginning, our Father gave man — and as we speak of man we speak also of woman — for remember, from where we come all spirits are of the same. And all is equal in the eyes of God. Only man makes this difference.

Our Father asks unto you two things, to love unto our Father one-tenth that love that He should give unto His children, to love unto thy fellow man the same as thy should love unto thyself. Do not run from thy churches, from thy faiths, for remember, "our Father has many mansions." And there is many truths.

August 15, 1971: **Thy have other questions, ask.**
*"Yes, Aka, [8-15-71-004] has asked, 'Is there any physical condition that needs attention? If so, please elaborate on the condition and seriousness.'"*
We should say unto these words, the only condition that we find, therefore, of the same — one moment, please.

Yes, we see this. Therefore, we have before us the records; we have before is the body, the soul, and therefore, the spirit and the immortal body.

Therefore, we should say unto thee these words. Should thy go either into an osteopathic doctor or a chiropractic doctor and have of the lower back area — this should not be forced. This could be done quite readily in four different visits and the correction, therefore, become as whole.

We would also suggest a different type of exercise. This could be done with the use of the eyes, in the strengthening of the same. We see in this soul is starting, if what is known as [glaustiformia, claustrophobia?] [glaucoma?]. Therefore, we would suggest that each day objects be placed approximately 30 feet apart, the eyes cast first to the left and then to the right, then objects as placed as high above the eyesight and as far below, this be done, and the eyes first upward and then downward. Increase this for a period and this problem should take care of its same.

We should also suggest that more of the vitamin B be taken into the body. We would also suggest, in thy case, the eating, if possible, of the Jerusalem artichoke. We should also suggest the changing of the diet within the same. We would suggest, for a period of three days, the eating of nothing but milk and bananas. This in itself would help to flush the system.

This is all on this subject at this time. Should it be that this is asked for, there are other things that would be added at a later date.

We also find a need within the spiritual development of this soul. But permission has not been granted; therefore, it should be given at a different time.

August 15, 1971: **Thy have other questions, ask.**
*"Yes, Aka. Are the treatments that I have been taking developing properly?"*
Yes, we see this. We should add to these treatments the treatment of the saunta [sauna] **bath. This should be done at least once every two weeks.**

August 15, 1971: **Thy have other questions, ask.**
*"At this time, Aka, I have no other written questions."*

Then we should answer the question of the one who asks. And we say unto this soul, our Lord and yours, our Father and yours, sees no sin here. Our Father brings thee blessings and love. Take from thy heart the hatred; replace it, therefore, with the same. And cast no stones. Should thy need arise to cast a stone, let us stand before thee, and cast thy first stone at us.

August 20, 1971: **Thy have many questions, ask.**
*"Yes, Aka, [8-20-71-001] asks, 'Do you have any advice for me or my husband regarding our family welfare and spiritual growth?'"*
**Yes, we see thy need.**
**Then we should say unto thee these words. If thy should go to a market and buy there a leopard to stand watch of thy household, beware of this leopard.**
**For in thy heart we see doubt. Then we should say to you in this manner. Thy would know of the things to come; then we should say unto thee, look backward into the things that has been, for thy have made thy own future.**
**[Remember…these words], if thy should kill with a sword, thy should be killed with a sword. But if thy should take a field, and therefore, plant wheat in one and barley in another, and harvest both crops and keep of the best of the crop for seed, then plant this seed again, and ferment the earth. And thy crop, therefore, should come in fulfillment. But add yeast to thy crop.**
**In thy mind thy have what thy would call a secret question. And we should answer this. For the dragon thy think that walks by thy husband does not.**
**We should say in this manner, change thy diet. Place in thy diet more of the vitamins, both B and E. Take into thy body more calcium. Eat more of the citrus fruit. Take forth for thy breakfast that that is known of the grapefruit. Take forth for thy luncheon meal as many of the raw vegetables as thy desire. Place more fish in thy diet, at least once a week, both of the fresh water and of the salt water. Eat less of the sweets that thy desire.**
**If from time to time thy should desire more information on the same subject and permission is granted, we should give thee further readings of the same.**
**Fear not for thy children, for they shall develop into normal, healthy children. Do not take them from their religious paths. Let them seek out this. But remember, as parents to your children, even though they have free will and have chosen [it] themselves, thy have chosen unto you, that thy must give discipline into the same.**

August 20, 1971: **Thy have other questions, ask.**

*"Yes, Aka, soul Ruth would like to know if anything can be done about the rash on her face and the bloody patches in her hair?"*

Yes, we see thy need. And we should give healing into thyself. But first, we should give unto thee a task to perform. And we should say unto this one, for the rash, take of the plain soda, take of the white of the egg, making a paste of the same and placing this upon thy face. Thy have other areas into which this virus infection has touched. Thy should use this in the same manner. Of thy patches of blood, we would suggest in this form. Take first of warm olive oil, placing this into thy hair, rubbing very vigorously; taking then of — yes — of the vinegar, adding [of a] tablespoon to a gallon, of your measurements, rinsing the hair thoroughly with this. Then after this has set for 20 minutes, wash the hair with a good shampoo, and then rinsing it again with clear water. We should say unto thee, this should be done at least twice a week. It would even be better if this was performed every three days.

When soul Ray should awaken, we should have placed in his mind [the need] that he should give healing into thy body. Fear not of this. And fear not the one we have placed by thy side, for remember, as thy would call it, thy guardian angel. For remember in your prayers, your Father and ours, blesses thee. And remember....

[Editor's note: This portion of the message was lost because the tape recording was inaudible due to a loud hum.]

...[We also find, therefore, infection of the same.] We would suggest the use [also] of the sage tea with [either] the Night-blooming Cereus or the blossom of the mesquite. either would do, preferably of the Night-blooming Cereus. This should be taken in quantities of quarter-inch cube over a period of two weeks. If this is not available, go unto thy physician. There are several antibiotics that could be used in the same manner.

We should say unto these words, of thy anger, remember, all things upon thy earth have been placed here for a purpose. If thy should need to cast a stone (cough), if thy should need to cast a stone, let us stand before thee, and cast thy first stone at us. But remember, all things upon thy earth in the [near] future should come out, as thy would call it, in a manner both beneficial in financial and physical needs unto thy family.

We would suggest, of thy diet, find first a good general, natural vitamin and mineral. Take of this daily, but take also of the vitamin B and C. Of thy other proportions of thy diet, at the present time, we would suggest thy add to thy diet of [the] morning of the citrus fruit, and more of the raw vegetables. This would do at the present time.

But our Lord also sees thy need. But remember, we should give unto thee healing, but our Lord cannot restore what thy desire to tear away, for in thyself, thy possess free choice. And if thy should use thy free choice to destroy that that thy build, then the permission should be taken away.

Then we should say unto thee these words; we should give healing, but we should need of thy help.

This is all on this soul at this time.

August 20, 1971: **Thy have other questions, ask.**
*"Yes, Aka. Soul Andrew asks what is causing his two health problems and what to do about them?"*

Yes, we see thy need. First, we should say unto soul Andrew, go unto thy physician, and therefore, request a urine take. [There] shall, for they should find unto the same — yes, we see this — and therefore, medicine could be prescribed that would help in this area.

We have suggested before, soul Andrew, that thy should go unto the osteopathic doctor and have certain adjustments made of the backular area. If thy should do this, thy would not need any other corrective measures. Thy would receive both relief of the kidney area and of the headaches.

We see this.

August 20, 1971: **Thy have other questions, ask.**
*"Yes, Aka. B_____ M_____ asks what would you have her do? She is unable to obtain mistletoe seeds, as you have suggested, because they do not seem to be in season at this time. Can you suggest anything that you would have her do at this time?"*

Yes, we should suggest, therefore, taking of the red sage, and therefore, taking therefore of soda, and taking therefore of hops, making, therefore, a broth of the same.

**Thy have other questions, ask.**
*"This broth is to be drunk, Aka?"*
Yes.

August 20, 1971: **Thy have other questions, ask.**
*"Yes, Aka, I have one other question. [8-20-71-002] in Yuma, Arizona, has asked for a health or life reading."*

Yes, we see thy need; therefore, we should say unto thee these words. Soul Ray grows very weary, and this should be asked at a different time. Therefore, awaken soul Ray from his slumber.

August 27, 1971: **Thy have questions, ask.**
*"Yes, Aka, [8-27-71-001], that is here tonight, asks if you can give her information on what causes her headaches and what she can do to prevent them?"*

Yes, we see thy need. Therefore, we have before us the body, the soul, the spirit, and the immortal body; therefore, all is in accord.

We find, therefore —

Yes, we see this.

We find the problem of quarrels between the mother and father, and the child, in itself, feeling rejection from the same. This has caused, as thy would know it, nervous tension within the child, and rebellious attitude of the same. Within time, this problem shall dissolve within itself. But unless this child is taught of love, of kindness, and of the teachings of our Father and of the Son — for remember, the love, and in this word thy use so lightly, matures both of the mental and the physical nature of the same. But beware, these parents, that they do not assume the karma of their child.

August 27, 1971: **Thy have other questions, ask.**

*"Yes, Aka.* [8-27-71-002] *asks, 'What advice can you give me in regard to a certain individual, very powerful, trying to rule my life?'"*

We should say unto thee these words. If thy were given a free choice, exercise this free choice. For there is no one who has the right to rule another, for as the spirit was given of love, and as the soul was given of love, and as our Father did create man and woman with love, we should say unto thee these words. For our Father has heard thy prayers. And those who have been placed in the same situation, of another time, have been sent therefore [unto] give guidance unto the same. Fear not of these, for they shall walk with thee both day and night, and they should look after thee. Be not afraid, for they should send thee messages in thy slumber. And in thy meditation they should come unto thee and give thee guidance. Thy would know of these as a "guardian angel."

But we should say unto thee at this time of these words. Give notice unto this one of the same. Thy have turned thy other cheek. Now is the time to stand forward, and should this one attempt to slap thee again, stand firm, and with the light of the Lord strike back.

**Can thy understand of which we speak?**

*"Yes."*[She answers.]

August 27, 1971: **Thy have other questions, ask.**

*"Yes, Aka, I overlooked, a little while ago, an important reading that I should have asked.* [28-08-71-001], *he was born...,and he asks for a health reading and any other advice that you can give him."*

As soul Ray grows very tired, we would suggest that this be asked at a different time. But yet, we would give of now this information. For we find inflammation of the liver. We find, therefore, of the kidney area great strain. We would suggest that this one to go unto the chiropractic doctor and certain adjustments be made of the same. But as these adjustments should be done in a prolonged period, readings should be made upon each adjustment of the same.

August 29, 1971: **Yes, we see thy need, soul E_____, and we should say unto thee these words. Beware of the dragon in thy household.**

But of thy illness we should say unto thee, continue thus with the medication thy are now taking. Stay away from all barbiturates, for they are part of your dragon. Go into the arts. There are many groups in thy city; join of these, work of these, learn of these. Go into thy university, and therefore, learn, for thy shall learn for eternity; and what thy do not learn of this plane, thy shall learn of the next and the next.

September 1, 1971: **Thy have other questions, ask.**
*"Yes, thank you, Aka. [8-28-71-001] has been to the chiropractor as you had suggested, and he has been quite ill. And do you have any other recommendations for him at this time? You have mentioned in the last reading that he had kidney trouble and, I think, liver trouble. Do you have any suggestions for him now?"*

Yes, we find this; therefore, we would suggest that the continued visits be made. We find also that an improper adjustment has been made, therefore. Therefore, he should return unto the same. This treatment should be done as we suggested before, not to force this area. This should be done, first, of the sixth and the seventh vertebrae. This should be moved outward and downward. We find, therefore, that this area should be massaged. Thy could use of the wintergreen oil, therefore, use, therefore, with that — yes, we see this — therefore, we would suggest that of the tonic used. One moment, we must see this again.

Yes, we see this; this is better.

We would suggest, therefore, that the tonic of the S.S.S. — we find, therefore, that the subject would be declined to take of the same, so therefore, we would suggest a good, natural vitamin be used, strong in the iron content. We would also suggest that the minerals of the same be used.

We also find, therefore — yes, we see this. We would suggest that four times daily that that of the red sage be used. We would also suggest that that — yes, we see this. Therefore, we would suggest — yes, yes — we would suggest that a visit be made unto the local medical doctor, and therefore, prescriptions of antibiotic of a strong nature be taken. This should be done for a period of seven days. This would greatly improve in this area.

We find other problems here. Should, as we have said before, these that have been suggested be done, follow-up readings of the health be done of the same.

You must remember of the massage. This must be done each night before retiring. If possible, it should be done of the morning also. We find that this should be done in such a position to go clear unto the lower limbiar [limb? lumbar?] **area.**

This is all on this subject at this time.

September 3, 1971: **Aka is here.**
*"Good evening, Aka. Is Ray with God?"*
**Soul Ray stands with God.**
**Yes.**
**Now all is in accord.**

September 3, 1971 [In Health and Life Readings]: **Thy have many questions, ask.**

*"Aka, [8-20-70-002] of Yuma is supposed to have a follow-up reading on health or life. Do you have anything this evening on him?"*

**We see thy need; therefore, we should say of these words. We find, therefore, into this soul — yes, that is better.**

**Yes, we have before us now the body, the soul, the spirit, and therefore, the immortal body. Yes, we see thy need. Therefore, we find into this soul the need of more of your vitamin B. This could not be taken in the regular, oral manner. We see the need, therefore, to go unto a physician, and therefore, this be given directly by the physician of the same. If this is not done — we find many other problems into the soul of the same. But all of the problems unto this soul go back unto the need of the vitamin B, and therefore, taking orally into the vitamin D.**

**We also find into this soul a radical change of the diet is needed. We should put more fish into the diet, at least twice a week. We should, therefore, place more of the green of the vegetables. We also find that, as this soul is allergic to the cystic-type foods, we would suggest that the taking of vitamin C orally would greatly help unto this soul. We find, therefore, as this soul is allergic to these of the same, we would suggest that the honey from the local locale be taken twice daily. This should be placed, therefore, in with two [microdrops] of vinegar, therefore, placed into the same, of one tablespoon of your measurements of honey.**

**We should also suggest of the taking twice daily of the sage tea, this should be done also, sweetened, therefore, with the use of the natural honey of the same locale.**

**We find the greatest problem, therefore, into the soul of itself.**

**Yes, we see this.**

**And we should say unto this soul, thy have brought forth unto this plane great karma, for the one thy have chosen for a father of this plane thy did kill in thy last lifetime, and therefore, thy are placed, both with praise and misgiving. Of the lifetime of before was in the locale thy known at this time as the land of Colorado. The man of this time, of thy father, thy were partners with in a mining claim, and therefore, thy did slay of him for the riches — later, to be slain by a gambler, therefore, that is thy mother of this plane.**

**We would suggest, therefore, that the necessary karma be lived out, and therefore, [reparation] within the same be done.**

**We should give of thee this knowledge. And remember, our Father has given unto thee free choice. Neither our Father or ourselves may interfere with this free choice. But "if thy right eye should offend thee, cast it aside." And therefore, as in karma, find thy karma, and therefore, overcome of the same. And this can be done only in forgiveness.**

And therefore, as it has been said before, "respect thy mother and father."

We can see that, at times, this is a hard task on your part. But of the same, we should say unto thee, it can only be done in pureness and in love. And give it of the same love our Father has given unto thee.

September 3, 1971: **Thy have other questions, ask.**

*"Yes, Aka, you suggested for my mother, B___ M_____, that she use mistletoe and hops and sage. And I wanted to ask if the mistletoe which Ray obtained can be used in the same proportions, of two grams a day, as the mistletoe you have spoken of previously?"*

Yes, we see thy need. Therefore, we should say unto this soul, if in the preparation of the same this could be done, made of the morning, and drank, therefore, of the evening, letting this seep into the same, therefore, it could be rewarmed at that time.

**Can thy understand of which we speak?**

*"Yes. Only the proportions are in question, Aka."*

The proportions should be done, therefore, in this manner — of two parts of the hops to one part, therefore, of the mistletoe of the same. We would suggest, as there is a difference, placing of the sage in one proportion of the same. Can thy understand of which we speak?

*"Yes, only the amount in the proportions — do you mean spoonfuls, or grams, or what quantity, Aka?"*

We should suggest one teaspoon of the mistletoe to two teaspoons, therefore, of the hops, to one teaspoon, therefore, of the sage tea. Can thy understand now of which we speak?

*"Yes, thank you, Aka."*

September 3, 1971: **Thy have other questions, ask.**

*"Aka, [8-28-71-001] was advised to request an additional reading after each adjustment by the chiropractor, and he also has been taking the medicine which you recommended. He cannot get the doctor to give him antibiotics because the doctor does not know what is wrong with him and won't prescribe for him when he does not know what he is prescribing for also."*

**There —**

*"Excuse me."*

Therefore, we should say unto the same, of the adjustment of the same. And as thy are going unto, therefore, the chiropractor, we would suggest that x-rays be made of the back and lower proportions of that of the back, and the upper proportion, therefore, of the back. We should suggest also that x-rays be made of the ribular area. Adjustments should be made in this area also. This, in itself, would give the physician, or as you would call of this, the chiropractor of the same. We would, therefore, suggest, of the antibiotic needed, take of the Night-blooming Cereus, therefore, of the same, in proportions of one-quarter-inch cube per day. If this was done for a two-week period — remember also unto this soul, the improvement will come gradual. Upon the third week of the treatment of the same, this soul should greatly improve.

September 3, 1971: **Thy have other questions, ask.**
*"Yes, Aka. We have a request for a health reading from J____ H____ of...Mesa, Arizona. He has diabetes, he believes, and his health is not good, and he asks for any advice you can give him."*

Yes, we see thy need, and therefore, we have before us the body, the soul, the spirit, and the immortal body of the same; therefore, the information that thy request shall be granted.

We find unto this soul diabetic — yes — but not of a great proportion; therefore, we would suggest the eating of the Jerusalem artichoke. This should be done twice daily. If would be preferably done before each meal.

We would also suggest, for a period of two months, the eating of no raw sugar forms should be done. If thy would eat of the fruits of nature, this could be done into the same.

We would, therefore, suggest that we find also into this soul that of the grout [gout] of the same, and therefore, we would suggest the vitamin D be increased, and therefore, vitamin C be taken. This should be taken twice daily. We find also the need into this soul of a good, natural vitamin of the same.

We would also suggest a change in the diet, therefore, of the same. For the morning meal, we would suggest one glass of milk, and therefore, of one-half of grapefruit of the same. Of the evening meal, therefore, we find — yes, we see this.

Of the evening meal, this should be done, only take away of thy salt at the present time. This could be done in its manner as it is at the present. But remember, this should be done, eating of three meals per day. We find that in this soul that quite often it has forgotten to eat because it becomes so interested in its work. If during the day the need should arise for additional food, this should be done, only of taking of the grapefruit of the same.

We also find into this soul rashes of the skin, and therefore, we should say unto this soul. Take first of the warm olive oil, placing this upon the skin; second, we would say, taking of the white of the egg, therefore, mixing of the baking soda of the same, making, as thy would know of it, a paste of the same and applying it to the areas needed.

There is other work that should be done, and therefore, we would suggest that thy should visit unto either an osteopathic doctor or a chiropractic doctor. This could be done quite simply for the treatment for the lower backular area. We find, therefore, that from a fall as a child — *yes, we see this.*

We also find that in thy childhood thy were struck in the backular area, which added, therefore, unto the injury of the same. This could be corrected, therefore, with manipulation of the same.

September 3, 1971: **Thy have other questions, ask.**
*"I have a release form which I do not have with me for the friend of J_____ H_____, Mr. C_____, who had requested information as to why he feels cold on one side. Can you help him in this?"*

Yes, we see thy need, and we should say, this shall be given in parts. Therefore, we find unto this, the soul; we find nothing more. And we should say unto this, look upward into thy Father's light, for thy shall lose the body thy possess and wander into nothingness forever.

Of thy illness, thy warmth is the lacking of the warmth of our Father.

We should leave thee with these words. Now is the time of the Cherub. Therefore, look upward unto [our] Father's light. And remember, our Father weeps for His children.

Awaken soul Ray from his slumber.

September 5, 1971: **Thy have other questions, ask.**
*"Yes, Aka. I had one, I think, brief question that had to do with a health reading. [9-5-71-001] has a rash on her foot and skin, and also a problem of swelling which she has been unable to get any help from doctors or specialists with. And I gave healing to her on it, but I wondered if you have any advice for her on it in regards to anything additional that you would like her to do?"*

Yes, we see thy need. And we should say unto these words — to take of the mistletoe, and therefore, make a powder of the same, to take of the olive oil and add to the same, this should be done that a gelatin should be made of the same — to take, therefore, of the soda and add of the same; to take, therefore, of the white of an egg, and therefore, add of the same; to take, therefore, of the sage and add of the same — if this were placed upon the feet in a [poultice] of the same before this soul should rest at night, this rash would soon leave of this soul.

September 13, 1971: **Thy have questions, ask.**
*"Yes, Aka, [9-13-71-001] has asked if she should tell her friend of the doctor that is in Germany? And is there anything that she can do to help this friend?"*

And we should say unto thee these words, for we see thy need.

First, of thy friend's illness, it is not in completeness as thy have; such information is not full. And we should also say unto these words. Should thy friend ask for the information needed, we should give of this information. But of thyself we should say, nay. Show thy friend the light of our Father. Pray unto our Father that she may accept this faith.

We also see thy need, and we should say of these words.

Yes, we see this.

We find unto this soul. Therefore, we have before us the body, the soul, and the spirit of the same, and therefore, we have before us the immortal body.

We should say unto thee, do we, therefore, have permission unto the same to give a medical reading of the same?

Yes, we see thy need, and we see that permission has been given, unto soul [9-13-71-001].

Therefore, we find unto this soul, first, of the digestive tract, we find problems here — yes. Of the lower intestine, we find [tublars], therefore, of the same. Yes, we find of this lower part of the stomachal area into the entrance of the same, abrasions, therefore, of the same. Of the short intestine, therefore, we find abrasions, therefore, of the same.

You must first understand that the subject in mind is of a highly nervous structure. Therefore, we say unto this soul, first, to combat the lesions and tublars of the same, it should take a very radical change of thy diet. Thy should eat of no fried foods. For a period of 30 days, this soul should take only the [insumption] of foods that have been boiled down into, as you would call them, or crushed, therefore, unto the same. Thy may find, as thy would know it, of the baby food, eating none of the acid-type foods of the same. If this were done for a 30-day period, this would give the same a chance to heal. We also find into the same the drinking of goat's milk. If an earnest effort, therefore, was done unto these two areas, this would greatly improve this soul's health.

We should also find that, of the hops should be taken before thy slumber; this should be taken with warm milk unto the same. In the preparation of this it should be done — bring, as thy would know it, the hops in warm milk, therefore, straining away the hops of the same. A slight bit of honey, preferably from the local locale, could be used. This could be done also of the morning, luncheon and the evening meals. This, in itself, would help to control the nervous tension of this person.

At first, this person should be inclined to sleep a great deal. Worry not about this; this should be good, for in her slumber she should heal of herself.

We should also suggest, of your morning meditation — in the morning upon awakening, take five minutes, placing thyself in complete accord with thy God. Open thy mind; listen to thy God. Reach out unto the lovely, wonderful things upon thy earth that thy Lord has placed before thee.

And we should say unto this soul, of that that has passed beyond, do you not trust thy Father? Then show Him respect unto the same. For what has passed on unto thy Father's keeping should be enough for thine eyes to see. Release of this and have gladness unto the same that new life should come. And therefore, all should be in accord with thy Father, thy God.

We find, also, that corrective lenses should be worn by this individual during all of its awakening time. This also, because of thy loss of eyesight, has brought upon nervousness into thy [system]. Worry not about thy vanity, for thy husband loves thee; is that not enough?

Then we should say unto this soul, therefore, go unto the chiropractic or osteopathic doctor; therefore, there is corrections to be made unto the same of the backular area.

We also find unto this soul abrasions upon the sides of the left toe. This is caused by not wearing correct footwear. We should, therefore, suggest the taking of hot castor oil, rubbing it very vigorously into [these] areas. This should be done each evening before thy slumber, and these callous areas shall soon remove themselves.

Yes, we see this.

We find old abrasions on the left — yes, we see this — [of] the left shoulder. This was caused as a child from a fall on a stairway — yes, we see this. We find hard scar tissue of the same. We would suggest the use of banana oil. This should be rubbed into the scar tissue at least twice daily. Of the inner abrasion on the collarbone of the same, therefore, we find lesion.

Yes, we see this.

Therefore, we would suggest the use of warm, castor-oil packs unto the same. These could be prepared quite simply by folding a cloth large enough to cover this area, taking two cloths, saturating the same with castor oil, therefore, warming each cloth. If this was done for a three-day period, we could find healing unto the same.

We also find congestion, therefore, of the right and left lungular area.

Yes, we see this.

We find this caused from a flu virus of the same; therefore, we suggest that the same castor oil packs be placed over the lungular area. We would also suggest that most of the congestion, therefore, from the same is from the sinus area. Therefore, we would suggest the taking of the sea water, making, therefore, a tent over the same as it is boiled, and breathing of the same. This should bring up and out, and drain these areas. We should, therefore, find that the drinking of the sage tea, sweetened with honey from the local locale would greatly help. But we find most irritation from the dry climate that thy dwell in. Therefore, the use of the sea water quite frequently should be needed.

We find other symptoms unto the same.

We should suggest unto this soul that frequent medical readings be given.

We also should suggest these words, for there is different type of healing, both mentally for the mind and soul, and physically for the body. Therefore, therefore, we would suggest — as we have said before, now is [not] the time of Lot; therefore, thy are allowed to look behind into thy lives. But in your case, we should say unto these words. Yesterday *was* yesterday, today is today, and tomorrow shall be tomorrow. Therefore, live unto today unto its fullest. For blessed are those who give not of a dead lamb into the Lord, but the worship of the Lamb in itself unto the Lord. And do not give Him of yesterday's meal; make it of today.

Now is the time of the Cherub.

Awaken soul Ray from his slumber.

September 16, 1971: **Aka is here.**

*"Good evening, Aka. Where is Ray?"*

**Soul Ray stands with God.**

**Yes, that is better; now all is in accord.**

September 16, 1971: **Thy have many questions, ask.**

*"Yes, Aka. [9-16-71-001], her mother is in poor health at this time — because of this will she be called on to console her?"*

**We see thy need. And for the peace of thy mind and for the peace of thy soul, we should give thee this information. Thy mother — yes, we see this.**

**One moment, please. We should need the name and location of this soul.**

*"At this time?"*

**Yes, we see this.**

*"Her name is [9-16-71-001A]; she's in Pittsburgh, Pennsylvania"*[a woman whispers.]

*"What's her last name?"*

*"[9-16-71-001A]."*

*"Could you hear her, Aka?"*

**Yes, we see thy need, and we should give healing into this one.**

**But we should say unto thee these words. Give thy blessings into thy mother, and let her know that her daughter loves her and has forgiven her. And the healing thy seek shall be granted into the same.**

**But we say unto thee these words. All souls upon your earth plane have free choice. And even though our Father should grant the healing, our Father, or us, does not and cannot interfere with free choice; so therefore, give this soul a reason for living, as you would know it. But remember, our Father is the God of the living, not of the dead. Can thy understand of which we speak?**

*"What do you mean by Father, God?"*[the woman asks.]

*"I think she will, Aka."*

September 16, 1971: **Thy have other questions, ask.**

*"Yes, Aka. C____ [C____] asks if she should consult a specialist about her foot?"*

**Yes, we see thy need, and therefore, we should say unto thee these words. Go unto the specialist, for we see — yes, we see this — the removal**

of the calcium deposits upon the same. But remember also that within this soul is that of which thy should call arthritis. Your technology at this time has yet to harness the cosmic powers of your earth. Therefore, we should say, with the knowledge that thy physicians bear at the present time, surgery should be necessary.

September 16, 1971: **Thy have other questions, ask.**

*"Yes, Aka. I have two questions this evening."* [4-3-70-002]. *"First of all, the hot olive oil treatments that you have recommended for many people, is this for restoring hair — will it help the growth of new hair, or would it be better to use the Tesla current to restore the growth of new hair?"*

Yes, we see thy need, and we should say unto thee, the use of both — first, of the hot olive oil. But remember also that as each individual has free choice, and therefore, the body chemicals of each individual are different, each person, as you would call him, or soul, should be treated accordingly. Do not take the reading for one person and try to apply it to another.

Thy have other questions, ask.

*"Yes, at this time, I am quite concerned about the rash that has appeared on my hands. Is this anything to be concerned about, and if so, what can I do to stop it?"*

Yes, we see thy need, and therefore, we should say unto thee these words. For we have before us the body, the soul, the spirit, and therefore, the immortal body of the same.

Yes, we find this.

First, of the rash in itself is caused by the plants thy would know as ragweed, into the same, has come into bloom, and therefore, the seed from the same. We find, therefore, thy are allergic to the same. Therefore, we would suggest taking — yes, we see this — we would suggest the taking of the mistletoe in one part, taking of the sage tea in two parts, adding, therefore, natural honey in the third part. This should be done three times daily. Prepare this that it may [steep] for one hour. We should also suggest — yes, we see this. In thy work we would suggest the use of gloves be worn for a short period of time. We find that in the system, at the present time, that any gold that should come in contact with the body, therefore, would cause a chemical reaction of the same. We would suggest that this of the wedding band only be worn during the day, and at any time thy are using the chemicals in thy work, it should not be worn. Can thy understand of which we speak?

*"Yes, Aka."*

Therefore, we should find further into this area — yes, we see this. We would suggest that more of the vitamin C be used at this time. We would further suggest that more of the vitamin D be used, preferably in adult quantity. We should find also that more minerals should be added into the diet, and therefore, we would suggest the eating of more of the green vegetation. It would be preferable if this vegetation came from thy own locale. But we see this is not practical at this time; therefore, we would suggest the taking of any good mineral at this time would do.

Yes, we see this.

Thy have other questions, ask.

[4-3-70-002]: *"On the tea that you told me to take — is the mixture I have at the present time, would that be sufficient?"*

This would be sufficient.

Yes, we see this.

September 24, 1971: **Thy have many questions, ask.**

*"Yes, Aka. An old friend of mine, [9-24-71-001], has failing eyesight, and I have attempted to give healing to him, a number of us prayed for him, and to restore a part of his sight so that he could see, and we have been unable to noticeably help him. And he has asked — let me step back a minute; his name is — "*

We see thy need. And we should say of these words. For as an apostle of before, we have given unto thee, thy disciple, the power of our Lord unto healing. But we could not give thee something we did not possess. For we may not interfere with the free choice, and neither can thyself.

But we should say unto this one — that thy may see more clearly, thy sight should fail, that thy may see the light of our Father, that the lesson thy have chosen to learn upon this plane may come more clearly in your later days. But fear not this passing, for it should come in great joy.

In thy mind, thy should ask us of thy son, and we should say unto thee these words. For the father shall be first before the son, and they shall be reunited in a short while. Can thy understand of which we speak?

*"Yes, Aka."*

September 24, 1971: **Then ask thy other questions.**

*"[5-7-71-002] asks, should her husband, [8-27-71-001], continue with the chiropractor for the price of $252? And also she asks, 'Why is he ill after he eats?'"*

Yes, we see thy need, and therefore, we should take the last first.

Therefore, first, we should say unto these words. We find that of what thy would call of a nervous stomach — secretion, therefore, unto the stomach area and the lining of the same.

We should say unto thee, first, take of the warm goat's milk, and therefore, add of the myrrh. This should be done 30 minutes before eating.

And of the second, we should say of the same. This, in itself, should be fulfilled, for as a man should do a day's work, and therefore, do it in honesty, we find, therefore, he should be paid for the same. He has not asked for overpayment, and you shall find that in fulfillment, shall be just rewarding unto the same.

Of these other things that enter thy mind, we should say unto this — nay, we do not see this. We do not find these things, for as they are said, they are not in truth.

As we have said before upon this soul, there should be continued follow-up readings of the same.

Ask thy other questions.

*"Yes, Aka, if I may, one question — did you say add myrrh to the goat milk?"*

Yes, we see this.

*"We would not know where to obtain this, Aka."*

We should say unto thee these words. These things may be obtained at the health food store. If they cannot be readily available, then we should say, take of two parts of the hops to one part of the mistletoe. This should not be as good, but it would do at this time.

September 24, 1971: **Ask thy other questions.**

*"Thank you, Aka, C____ asks, 'Is soul Mark in any physical difficulty or danger at this time?'"*

Nay, we do not see this.

But we should say unto soul C____ of these words. Our Father has looked into thy soul, into thy spirit, and therefore, that thy should come into the immortal spirit of our Father, we should say unto thee these words. If thy should have faith, our Father should come into thee and give thee healing, and should make a vow into thee for the remainder of thy days upon this earth. If thy should serve unto our Father, therefore, your wish shall be granted.

September 24, 1971: **Ask thy questions.**

*"[6-18-71-008] would like to know the cause of swelling in her feet and hands."*

Yes, we see this, and we should say unto the soul, take from the diet at the present time of the salt; add, therefore, unto a salt substitute of the same. Give of this child of two parts of the sage to one part of the hops. Find, therefore, of the laxative herb; add unto the same. This should be done once daily.

October 8, 1971: **Thy have other questions, ask.**

*"Yes, Aka, [10-8-71-001] is disturbed about her daughter who lives in San Diego, and she says that her daughter has mental and emotional problems and is very desperate. How can she be helped?"*

Yes, we see thy need. Therefore, we should say unto thee for the good of thy soul, we should give of this information. But thy must understand, we do not have permission to interfere with the free will of any soul.

But we should say unto thee these words. For thy daughter shuns the psychic world; thy daughter fears that man should look within and see, therefore, her karma.

But we should say unto this one, we see no sin, as thy would know it. We see the small karmas thy have brought forth. Yet we see these are minor. We find, therefore, thy would think of thy body as the temple of sin. And we say unto thee these words; we do not see this. Your Lord, God, did create thee, and give thee of all of His knowledge, of His emotions; therefore, these urges of the body are not of sin. Seek out and satisfy that of the same, but do it with love. This in itself would cure a frigid woman.

But we find physical problems unto this one. We do not have permission to give of the information that is needed. Therefore, we should say unto thee, go forth unto this daughter that permission could be given.

But we find into the soul of your same, physical problems; therefore, we should say, for we see permission has been given. We find, therefore, numerous problems of the backular area. We find, therefore, through bad use of a chiropractic doctor certain nerves in this area have been, as thy would know them, crimped off, therefore, giving pain into the same, and therefore, the nervous condition of the same. We find, therefore, this is secreting fluid into the stomachal area and of the lining of the same.

We also find that as a small child thy did take a fall. We find that as thy played thy fell over what thy would know as a saw horse, did strike of the right side of the kidney area of the same. We find, therefore, pains, both of this area and of that of the crimped nerves of the same. We would suggest, therefore, first seek out a good chiropractic or osteopathic doctor; in this case, we would suggest an osteopathic doctor. We would also suggest that of the hot olive-oil packs be placed on this area, that a [poultice] of the same be made, therefore, and applied. This would give thee immediate relief for a time, but unless the backular area has made corrections in the same, the pain should return.

At a different time we would suggest a full health reading on this, [thine] soul.

October 8, 1971: **Thy have other questions, ask.**
*"Yes, Aka, [5-7-71-002] asks, 'Why is [8-28-71-001] so ill after each meal?'"*

Yes, we find — for we have before us the body, the soul, and therefore, the spirit of the same, and therefore, the immortal body of the same. And we should say unto this one, because of the prolonged period of the uncorrected, of the backular area, we find that that proportion of the upper neckular area that has been damaged, that that should secrete the acids into the stomachal area has been cut off. This in itself would cause nausea before eating and after eating, and therefore, would cause of the backular [bowelular?] area, therefore, not proper digestion of the same. Therefore, we would suggest — yes, we see this. One moment.

We would suggest that thy go unto the valley below the sea [Editor's note: Yuma, Arizona], and therefore, give unto the physician known as Dr. Caine the information from this reading, and therefore, the necessary corrections can be given.

October 8, 1971: **Thy have other questions.**
*"Yes, Aka,* [10-8-71-003…Miami, Arizona] *and he asks for a health reading."*
We would suggest that this soul be placed in a better, proper position, for in the position we find this soul at the time, a health reading would be very unpractical. If this could be asked for at another time, the information would be given.

October 8, 1971: **Thy have other questions, ask.**
*"*[10-8-71-004] *of —.just a minute, Aka — of Buckeye, Arizona…asks for a health reading."*
This should be given at a different time.
Soul Ray grows weary; therefore, awaken soul Ray from his slumber.

October 9, 1971: **[Aka is here.]**
*"Good morning, Aka. Is Ray with God?"*
Soul Ray stands with God.
Yes, that is better; now all is in accord.
Thy have questions, ask.
*"Aka, A____ H____ sister's daughter, A__ F_____, is missing, and her sister, S____, is very disturbed about her daughter. We have asked before about this missing individual, and we wonder if you can help us with information to ease their minds?"*
Yes, we see thy need. And we shall answer thy question for the good of thy soul.
Yes, we see this.
We should say of these words, we find this soul well at this time. We find of this soul at this time of sentence [area], in the province of, Brazil? We find that — yes, we see this — we find interference, therefore, by the law officers.
Yes. Yes, we see this.
We find that, that this soul has made attempts to contact its parents. We find that these letters have been intercepted.
Yes, we see this.
We find that this soul is held in incognito.
Yes, we see this,
We find that — that should this soul be needed for the further persecution [prosecution], she shall be brought back into these United States.

But we say of this. This soul has fled of its own free will. We can not interfere with this free will.

This is all on this soul at this time.

October 29, 1971: **Thy have other questions, ask.**

*"Yes, Aka.* [8-6-71-001] *would like to ask if she should...."*

We see thy need. Therefore, we should say unto thee these words. We did not complete the physical reading upon this person, of thy husband, [7-23-71-002]. Then we should say unto thee these words. This person's biggest problem is that he is mentally deranged. His problem could be corrected. But we would say unto thee that thy are not in a position to administer healing. Therefore, we would suggest first, as thy would know it, commitment, that he may receive the proper medication for the same.

We would also suggest that thy should continue in thy present employment.

We would also suggest that thy should resubmit to the proper authorities the necessary documents of the same. We shall say unto thee, protect thy children and thyself, for if thy should not do of these things we have suggested, then we shall tell thee of the other path before thee. And we will say unto these words. As the karmic action should take place, which therefore, is not a necessity, harm shall come not only to your children, but to yourself. And remember also, your children were placed in your care. If thy do not look unto this care, then thy shall build upon thy self a new karma.

Remember also, return unto the faith of thy worship. These things have been told unto thee before. Go unto the bishops of thy church, and therefore, ask their advice. And this shall be given and the help shall be given.

Yes, we see thy need. And the Lord shall put grace upon this. For remember, the Lord, our God, did make thee "of our kind." All the emotions of your body are a natural thing, and we see no sin. Then go. And take the blessings of our Father, and take His hand that He may guide thee.

We see other problems that shall arise, but we shall take these a step at a time.

When the time comes, we shall answer your other questions.

October 29, 1971: **Thy have other questions, ask.**

*"Yes, Aka.* [10-8-71-001 of San Carlos] *has asked for a health reading."*

Yes, we have before us the body, the soul, the spirit, and therefore, the immortal body of the same. One moment, please.

Yes, yes; now we have this. Yes.

We would suggest in the future, that for all of your health readings, place these who should request of the same in a positive location. This would be better. You must understand that if the body in mind is over exercising or doing other things, it makes the readings very difficult.

Therefore, we would suggest that before this reading is given, bring her here, or find one location that we may find her. Can you understand of what we speak?

*"Yes, Aka."*

October 29, 1971: **Thy have other questions, ask.**

*"I also have a request for a health reading for* [10-29-71-002]. *I do not know if she is at home. Would you like me to delay this also?"*

**Yes, we see thy need.**

**And therefore, we should say of other things.**

November 5, 1971: *"Yes, Aka, C___ B_____, age 6...she says — her mother is asking for her; she says her daughter has a beggar's growth behind her knee. Can you help?"*

**Yes, we see the need. We would suggest at the present time that the necessary knowledge that thy desire for the removal of the same, any good physician could do this. But we should say unto thee, since this is a test of faith, then pray thee and we should assist.**

November 5, 1971: **Thy have other questions, ask.**

*"[10-8-71-001] asks for a health reading."*

**Yes, we have before us the body, the soul, the spirit, and therefore, the immortal body of the same. And we should suggest, once more, that this be done in a private reading. There is certain information that could be given, but should only be for the ears of this soul. The healing that is needed shall be granted, and therefore, healing shall come within the same. But the healing of the mind, we can only tell thee that this may come with full enlightenment of the mind of the same. Therefore, we [may] remove these things that should cause physical problems, but they should return unless the mind is treated.**

November 5, 1971: **Thy have other questions, ask.**

*"Aka,* [10-29-71-002]...*in Globe, says that she is concerned about her weight and asks for a health reading and a diet."*

**Yes, we see thy need. Therefore, we have before us the body, the soul, the spirit, and the immortal body of the same.**

**Yes, we find this; yes, all is in accord.**

**Therefore, we should suggest first, for the scalp condition of the same, the use of plain vinegar with that proportion of water used as a rinse twice a day. We would further suggest that the use of a hot olive oil treatment be used here.**

**Yes, we find this.**

**We further find in this —**

**Yes, we see this — a skin condition, yes.**

We would suggest, first, the washing of the skin with, not of soap, as thy know it, but of just pure water. We would suggest, therefore, the use of hot olive oil packs on this area. We would also suggest the use of the white of the egg, placing equal amounts of soda into the same to perform a paste, and this be placed to perform a mask.

Yes, we see this.

We would further suggest a radical change in thy diet.

For the morning heal, we would suggest the eating of one banana and one glass of milk.

For your luncheon, we would suggest the eating of any good green vegetable growths, and one glass of milk.

We would suggest in the evening meal, adapting to the same — we would suggest one meal each week of the fresh water fish; we would further suggest that one meal each week of the salt water fish. We would suggest once each week the eating of the liver of the beef. We would further suggest the eating twice a week of good beef — this should not be fried within the same; it should be broiled in its own juice. We would further suggest that before the eating of the evening meal one ounce of olive oil be taken internally.

We would further suggest that for the luncheon one ounce of olive oil be taken internally.

We should say unto thee that thy, because of your own nervous condition, should desire the intake of further food substance. We would suggest taking of either the black or the green olive, eating as much as thy desire between meals of the same, but of nothing else.

We find other physical problems within the same. We find a slight condition of the heartal [heart] area. Yes, we find this.

This is due from fatty tissue overcrowding the intestines. We would suggest, therefore, exercise be taken. We would suggest after exercise — at first, this exercise should be done for 15 minutes in the morning and in the afternoon. Do not overdo this. We would suggest that at least once a week [saunic] baths be used unto the same that the respiratory and circulatory systems can be increased.

We would further suggest — yes, yes, we see this — that the use of either a good chiropractic or osteopathic doctor at the present time be used to correct the backular [back] area.

We should also suggest that the use of a good dentist be used to correct the dentular [dental] area. We find problems in this area.

Yes.

From this area we see secretion, poison being administered into the body, which at the present time is causing infection into the [vaginular] [vagina] area.

Yes, we find this.

Of the bladder area.

Yes.

We would suggest that twice daily the use of the sage tea be used, once in the morning and once in the evening, to cleanse this area. We would further suggest that a washing be used in [the] same area. There are many washes, as thy would know it, upon the market. But do not use an acid content of the same, [before] the body would reject of the same.

Yes, this is all at this time. We would suggest that a follow-up reading be given on this soul at a different time.

November 5, 1971: **Thy have other questions, ask.**
*"Yes, Aka, [11-5-71-002]...Central Heights...has asked for a health reading because of weight."*

**We see thy need. But therefore, as soul Ray grows very tired, we would suggest that any further medical readings be given at a different time.**

November 9, 1971: **Thy have other questions, ask.**
*"Yes, Aka. V_____ W_____, a longtime friend of my family, who I asked about once before, she lives in...and she's in St. Luke's hospital in Phoenix, and she has cancer. Apparently it has turned into a runaway cancer and they are sending her home within any cure. And my question is, is there anything that we can do to help her? She has asked for help."*

**We shall say unto thee these words. At the present time, your science has not developed far enough to cure such needs. If thy should look backward into our back readings, thy shall find, of our talks unto thee, of a cosmic generator, of the chemicals that could be extracted from the sperm. But only the generator within itself could extract these. For remember, the only way unto cure this is to place the body into what you would know as that period that the sperm is incubated into life. This can only be done with a pyramid-type structure that should gather into itself cosmic magnetic rays. But even that, within itself, must be placed at the right and proper height, that the body must be placed at a precise north-south axis. Should this be done, the cure could come into reality.**

**But you must remember also, man shall develop great science; he shall go forward into the creation itself.**

**But, there are those who have chosen death that they may live again. For now, above thy earth is a gathering of the soldiers of God. This soul shall be taken there. There she shall meet many friends.** [See *The Revelation*, chapter 19.]

**We are sorry that thy should feel remorse. But do not feel this. Thy Father loves His children — and as a father should, He should take them to His breast and lift them gently from one world to another. Fear not for this one, for we shall make the passing easy.**

November 12, 1971: **[Aka is here.]**
*"Good evening, Aka. Is Ray with God?"*

Soul Ray stands with God.

Yes, we see thy need. And we should say unto thee these words.

November 12, 1971: **Unto soul [5-7-71-002] we should say unto these words; the passing shall come soon. Fear not for this one. But the karma should be relived again. Our Father has seen fit to forgive, this as thy would know, soul [7-23-71-002]. And we should send unto him in his last hours the necessary teachers that he should need to pass over. And they shall wait for him, and therefore, guide him through the threshold between the two worlds. But we should say unto thee, go unto thy heart and ask forgiveness of thyself, that thy may assist those that are needed.**

**We see thy other needs. And we should say unto thee in these words. As thy would know it, the beggar on the street should stand next to our Father, and yet give Him advice, if [it] he should enter into the kingdom of God in the right manner.**

**But you must remember also, these things that happened unto him, he has asked for them to happen. And unless he should learn the lessons that were placed before him, he must do these things again. And so should your daughter and yourself do these things again. Therefore, release this soul with your blessings. Send him to our Father with full forgiveness in your hearts.**

**Thy have other questions, ask.**

November 12, 1971: *"Aka, [11-12-71-001] is concerned about her family situation, and she asks for help, for advice."*

**Yes, we see thy need, And we should say unto thee these words. The dreams that were given unto thee for guidance thy did not fully understand. But as thy walk in the light of God, and therefore, should be a shepherd unto the Lord, then we should answer your question in this manner. If thy should take of the rooster to market, and therefore, your children should bring horses to the market, you cannot trade the chicken for a horse. But you can learn to do the work of a horse.**

**But our Lord did not mean for a man to labor in such a manner. Our Father did place upon each child his own conscience, but yet He gave them free choice. Should you love your children any less than our Father loves His? Yet our Father placed into your hands the duty to raise your children, to guide them, to place in them your own conscience, as He did place into you. Therefore, in the time of Moses it was said, "Honor thy father and mother." And in the time of the one known as Jesus it was said, honor thy father and mother as thyself. But give unto them free choice. Give them the paths to lead in righteousness.**

**We find of thy first problem, at the present time, as our Father has done, place unto this one the knowledge of yourselves. If he does not accept the same, let him stand by himself; yet he must stand with his own choice. If**

this was offered in this manner, we see that he should *stand* by himself, but yet, stand with you.

We should say to you in this manner, should this one marry and not marry unto the faith of God, then he himself should create his own karma.

Yet, we should give unto thee the knowledge and the guidance that is needed. And fear not, for as we should come into thy home, all thy must do for guidance is to open the door, that we may enter. Remember, we are not great. We are here but to prepare the way for the coming of the Messiah. We may do nothing that our Father does not allow; we may tell thee nothing that our Father does not allow, for we are the servants and the messengers of our Father.

Of thy second problem, we see this. And we should say in this manner, give unto the other the necessary knowledge for schooling. You have given the necessary knowledge of God unto this one. But remember, there is food for the mind and food for the soul. Remember also, that as Joseph did before, yet he in his own way bore his father's sin, and therefore, stood before God and made it whole again. You cannot carry the cross of this one. It must carry its own cross, in its own time. Do you understand of which we speak?

*"Yes. Yes, I understand."* [She says.]

Then, we should give unto thy hands this gift — the gift of love from the one known as Jesus Christ. For as he stood before as your savior, so should his spirit walk with thee.

November 12, 1971: **Thy have other questions, ask.**

*"Aka, H_____ DeL_____...has asked of his children and future. Do you have anything additional to say to him?"*

Yes, we see thy need. And we shall answer your question in this manner. At the present time, the help thy need is within thyself, for thy need of the healing. And we should give of this. But remember, do not overload the burro or it should become lame and not be able to carry any load at all.

Stand firm, first, as the husband of your wife. Respect her in all manners, that she should respect thee in all manners of your household. Give thanks unto your Lord. But remember, there is two things that our Father asked of His children, that they should love unto the Lord one-tenth of the love that God should give unto His children, and that they should love of their fellow man in the same manner. Can you understand of which we speak?

*"Yes, I understand."* [He answers.]

November 12, 1971: **Thy have other questions, ask.**

*"Aka, [11-12-71-003] is asking for a health reading in regards to a problem of eczema."*

Yes, we see thy need, and therefore, we should say in this manner. Discontinue the use of washing with [the] soap. Wash only with clean, fresh water. Apply the white of the egg mixed with the soda. Do this four times daily. At night, before thy should go unto slumber, apply hot castor-oil packs to this area. This should be done unto a two-week interval.

We should say unto thee, thy should change of thy diet. Add more of the protein to thy daily diet. We should tell of thee first, in your case, take twice daily one ounce of the safflower oil. For the morning meals, eating one grapefruit and one glass of milk. For thy luncheon, eat as many of the green vegetation as thy desire. For the evening meal, eat again of one grapefruit daily; thy may supplement this with as much of the citric food as thy desire. Eat twice weekly of the fish that should come from the salt. Eat once weekly that of the beef liver. Eat *no fried foods* at all. Eat once weekly of the fish that should come from the fresh water. Of your other weekly meals, thy may eat as thy please, but only of the evening meal. We should further suggest that a good supplement, general vitamin, be used. We would further suggest that vitamin C and E be taken in adult quantities daily.

We find in this soul other medical problems. We would suggest that chiropractic or osteopathic treatment be used for the upper backular [back] area.

We further should suggest — yes, we see this — that the use of eye exercise be done. This should be done in such a manner as placing objects 20 feet across. This should be done with placing objects as high above thy eyesight and as low as thy could see, looking at one and then the other. Do this for five minutes intervals daily. This would greatly improve unto this area.

We would further suggest that the use of the saunic [sauna?] baths be used to stimulate both of the respiratory system and help the circulatory system unto the same.

We find that follow-up medical readings should be given at different times, as they are asked for.

Thy have other questions, ask. One moment.

Yes, we see this.

We would suggest that a visit to your local physician, therefore, for infection to the bladder area — yes, we see this — this should be done promptly, antibiotic be given unto the same. We would suggest that the drinking twice daily of the sage tea — yes.

Yes.

This is all on this soul at this time.

November 12, 1971: **Thy have other questions, ask.**

*"Aka, [11-12-71-004] has asked me to give him healing. I wonder if you have any advice for me in regards to this?"*

As we have said before, we may not violate one soul unto another, but we shall give unto thee this knowledge. Suggest that the necessary tests be run for a diabetic. We find that this soul is a borderline diabetic of the same. The healing that thy should ask for shall be granted; give of the same.

November 16, 1971: **Thy have other questions, ask.**
*"Have you a message for E____ H____?"*
As we have said before unto this soul — yes, we see thy need. Then we should say unto thee, prepare a haven unto the children of the Lord there, that they may have a meeting of the minds. But first, open the door into thy soul that we may enter.

We shall tell thee, at the present time do not enter into the business transactions that thy have in mind, for a dragon dwells within. Within the sixth month, the financial condition that worries you at the present time shall be no longer. But remember, these things shall come as raindrops upon the desert, a little at a time. Answer the needs of thy heart. This should be done now.

November 16, 1971: **Thy have other questions, ask.**
*"Aka, do you have any advice for [4-17-71-00_] and/or the children?"*
Yes, we see thy needs. And we should say unto thee, if thy should stand tall as a woman, thy mate shall come to thee, but he should be strong of mind and clean of soul. Then, therefore, prepare thyself. We shall say unto thee in this manner, a woman who should give birth to a child has a responsibility to the child. But she should also have a responsibility to herself, and in this manner, she should have responsibility to look her best. Therefore, take the necessary steps to make thyself, on the outside as well as on the inside, a beautiful woman. Do not neglect thy looks. Remember, if thy should go unto a good tree to pick a fruit, and the fruit does not look pleasant, thy stomach shall not eat of the same.

We shall take care of the other needs of thy body. We shall give healing into the same. But remember, we are not great. We may only do these things that our Father permits us to do, for we are the servants of God, our Father, and we are here for but one purpose, to prepare the way for the coming of the Messiah. Therefore, we should ask in return, make fallow his bed.

November 16, 1971: **Thy have other questions, ask.**
*"Aka, is there anything that can be done to comfort Mrs. McN___ about the loss of [5-2-71-001]?"*
Yes, we see her need. And we shall say unto thee in these words. We do not approve of the manner in which she chose to take of her life, but remember, our Father is the God of the living, not of the dead. But she has seen her mistake. For the present time, she should need schooling and she has asked for the same.

But, she shall choose again for life, as thy would know it. Then we would say unto thee, look unto the newborn children, [for] remember, none may enter the kingdom of God who has not suckled upon his mother, and none may enter who has not entered into heaven first.

November 16, 1971: **Thy have many questions, ask.**

*"Aka,* [11-12-71-001] *is not clear on what you meant when you were talking about taking a chicken or a horse to market. And I wonder if you could clarify it for him, what were you trying to tell him when you said that one was not equal to another, but that he could learn by watching, he could learn to work as a horse?"*

We said unto these words, that the man was not meant to work as a horse. As thy should take of a chicken to the market for trade, and as thy children should own of horses, and therefore, take of the same, thy cannot carry the full burdens of thy children alone. For remember, they are souls within their selves. They have free choice. And as thy should walk and find a beggar in need and thy lift the beggar to walk again, thy cannot be a crutch. As the chicken is thyself, as the horse is thy children, thy children should not ask of either their father or mother to carry forever their burdens. Can thy understand now?

*"I understand."* [He says.]

But remember, as a good father should, our Father sheds many tears for His children. He loves them *all.* But as a good father, He must let His children fall, sometime. And sometimes He should bend and pick them up and love them unto His bosom. But He should send them out again of their own free will, for as He said in the beginning, He did create both he and she in our image, of our kind, and this cannot be done unless they learn to pick of themselves up, and choose to go on. And as they should learn of their own mistakes, then they shall be given children of their own. And their children shall make mistakes because each of these are souls, souls who have chosen to enter unto life, as you would know it, to learn lessons. They have chosen their mother and father long before their mothers and fathers are born. And some must wait patiently for this time.

There are things that thy should learn from thy children, and things that they must learn from you. This is both the beginning and the ending of a karma. For did He not promise unto thee a new heaven and a new earth?

November 16, 1971: **Thy have other questions, ask.**

*"Yes, Aka.* [11-16-71-001] *And she has asked, 'Can you advise me about my stomach problems?'"*

Yes, we see thy need. Then we should say unto thee, we have before us here, the body, the soul, the spirit, and therefore, the immortal body into the same. Yes, all is in accord.

We should say unto thee first, thy should go unto a radical change of thy diet. First, we would suggest the use of only of the milk of the goat. For the morning meal this should be taken, one glass of the goat's milk. This should be done in this manner; the egg must be poached in the milk of the same. Then by taking toast and placing the egg in warm milk of the same, this should be done for the morning meal. Before the morning meal one ounce of safflower oil should be taken internally.

Yes, we see thy need. For thy luncheon meal — yes, we see thy need — for the luncheon meal, thy may eat as many of the green vegetables as thy desire, but none of the acidy [acidic?] content. Again, take one ounce of safflower oil before the meal, and one glass of goat's milk unto the same.

For thy evening meals, [you] may do it in any manner that thy choose. Eat no fried foods at all. Eat of one each meal of the seafood, and toast. Eat one each meal of the freshwater fish with toast and milk. Eat of the beef liver, one each meal. Eat, therefore, any other substance for the proprietor of the meals in the week.

Take of a good — yes, we see this — take, therefore — yes — of a good natural vitamin; this should be done daily. Take more of the vitamin E and D into thy body. This can be done in a natural vitamin form; therefore, of vitamin C in the same manner, and therefore — yes, we see this — we would other suggest the taking of the substance known as Lydia E. Pinkham into the same.

This would be all at the present time on this soul. But we should suggest that a follow-up reading be done in two-week intervals.

November 19, 1971: **Thy have many questions, ask.**
*"Yes, Aka. Mrs. B_____'s daughter, B____ [T____ K____] has asked for advice on the behavior of her daughter. She is very concerned about her daughter's behavior."*

Yes, we see thy need, and therefore, we shall say unto this one in this manner. A child is born unto its mother and father of its own free will. But the parents of the same should give it discipline. And at the present time, this is a childish whim. Therefore, we should say unto thee, spare not the rod unto this one. But do it in a manner that this child knows the wrong it has done.

We see because of the age of this one, at the present time, it is not responsible. Yet, it remembers from the life before. As we have said before, for this, thy husband, was cruel, a cruel master unto this one in another lifetime. And these things thy must realize. But you must be firm and explain to this child that you love it.

But, also give of this child knowledge of God. We see thy have not gone into the churches of thy choice. This is needed, at the present time, for the wine that is offered into the same; this child needs to know of the love of its Father. Through this knowledge, give it of your wine, also, but do not place new wine in an old vase.

November 19, 1971: **Thy have other questions, ask.**
*"Aka, C____ [C____] wants to know if a specialist in Phoenix should read her x-rays that were taken here?"*

No, we do not see the need. The proper diagnosis shall be made here at this time.

November 19, 1971: **Thy have other questions, ask.**
*"Yes, Aka. [11-12-71-004], and because of the problem with his arm, which I discussed last time, and his other health condition, he has asked for a health reading."*

Yes, we see thy need. And therefore, we have before us the body, the soul, the spirit, and therefore, the immortal body of the same.

Yes, yes, this is good.

Yes, all is in accord. Therefore, permission has been given and the information desired shall be given.

First, we should say unto this one, there is much damage here. We find in the kidney area much damage, bladder area.

Yes.

We also find a thyroid or a thyroid secretion of the same.

Yes.

First we should — first we should say unto this one, under no, for no reason, do *not* take into thy body any type of alcoholic beverages. This is killing thy body. This comes from an old karma of before. Thy must realize that of another life, of a time of a Roman, this one did drink to forget what he saw on the cross. Yet he drinks now for the same reason. But look at the love that was given from this cross. For did he not say unto you, "Forgive them, Father, for they know what not they do." Therefore, fear not of this. For if this is not stopped at the present time, we find cell damage in the brainular [brain] area, both of the left and right lobular [lobes].

Yes, we see this.

Therefore, we should suggest, at the present time thy are taking certain antibiotics. These are too strong for your body. These should be changed and reduced in the amount. We find inflammation of the right lung area.

We find — yes, we see this — high sugar content; therefore, this soul is of a diabetic nature.

We find growths, [subformian] growths, of the [lopian] type — yes — under the surface of the skin. If these are not treated and taken care [of], they should grow on into the bonular [bone] area of the rib cage, and therefore, cause very severe damage unto the same.

We find, if this patient into itself does not reduce, take away some of the fatty tissue, give room for your own organs to move, give them room to heal into their selves — this could be done by changing your diet.

Yes, we see this.

First, we would suggest, that for thy morning meal, the eating of no more than two grapefruit. Yes — this could be followed with a little coffee or tea, using an imitation sweetener into the same, but no milk in the coffee or the tea.

[However] we would suggest that a sub-meal be eaten at approximately 10 o'clock. This could be done with a little toast and tea again.

For the luncheon, we would suggest that any combination of the green vegetable type, followed again with a glass of milk. We also find of an ulcer-type growth in the stomachal [stomach] area, of the lower tract. If this is not treated at the present time, it will start to bleed, for we find of the stomachal area — yes — a sub-form of the blood vessels — yes — which is known as a nervous stomach. Therefore, the milk used, we would suggest into the goat's milk of the same.

Of thy evening meal, we would suggest no fried foods. You may eat broiled or baked meat; eat no pork. We find that the diet toward lean meat would be better in this case. We would suggest that for one meal each week — yes — fish from the salt water should be added into this diet. For one meal each week, the liver of the beef should be used. The rest of the meals of the week can be made as thy please at the present time, eating as much of the raw vegetables as possible; eating okra either cooked or raw would be good — yes — eating as much raw carrots as thy desire.

We also find that this soul has a hearing problem; the hearing comes and goes.

Yes, we see this.

We would suggest that either from a chiropractic or osteopathic doctor — we see pinched nerve[s] in the third vertebrae — we see that the relief from the same would greatly help both the nervous system and the backular [back] area. We would further suggest of the [saunic] baths.

Yes.

This would be good.

This is all on this soul at the present time. Should further information be desired it shall be given.

November 19, 1971: **And now, we see in the mind of one, the question of a loved one which she is greatly concerned about. And we shall answer your question in this manner. Go as thy heart directs thee. Do not look backward, but look forward, for what has been before shall not be again.**

November 23, 1971: **Thy have many questions, ask.**

*"Yes, Aka, [_____] in Miami, and she asks for help in regards to a health problem of eczema."*

Yes, we see thy need, and therefore, we have before us — yes — we have before us the body, the soul, the spirit, and therefore, the immortal body. And as we have said before, place these souls who should require health readings in a location that we may find them more easily. But we shall give of this.

Yes, we see thy need. We would suggest a very radical change in the diet. For this one, The use of the safflower oil should be done three times daily in the diet, one ounce before, and preferably 30 minutes before — yes — 30 minutes before the eating of each meal.

And to this one we would suggest the eating of three regular meals daily.

For the morning meal, we would suggest — yes — the eating, preferably, of one grapefruit and a little tea, no coffee.

Yes, we see this.

For the luncheon meal, we would suggest the eating of as many green vegetables as possible. These should not be canned or cooked in any manner, but should come as they grow from the earth.

Yes, we see this.

We should suggest, that since thy body has become used to the drinking of coffee, that thy may have your coffee at 10 o'clock in the morning, but no more than two cups. We would suggest that this be done without sugar, if possible, or sweetened with the natural honey of the same.

We would suggest that in addition to thy beverage of the morning and noon meal be added one cup of sage tea, sweetened, if preferably, with the sage of the same, either in that proportion, or honey which is taken from thy own locale.

We would further suggest that for the evening meal — yes, we see this — we would suggest that no hot foods be taken into thy stomach at the present time. We would suggest the eating of as many cooked vegetables for the evening meal as possible. For this one, we would suggest taking out of thy diet any meats for the present time, for at least six weeks.

Yes.

We would further suggest that the taking of a good natural vitamin supplement — we would further suggest that the vitamins C and D, and E, be taken in accordance with the same, for we find that the body at the present time is not using that which is being brought in in the proper manner. Therefore, more should be added.

We would further suggest — yes, we see this — that at no time should any of your known detergents touch this area. We would suggest taking — yes we see this, yes — making, first, a portion [poultice?] of what thy would know of the mistletoe; this should be applied to the area, and therefore, heat be placed upon the same. This should be done for one week, and a follow-up reading be taken at this time.

This is all on this soul at the present time.

November 23, 1971: **Thy have other questions, ask.**

*"Yes, Aka, I have a request for a health reading for* [4-16-71-003]. *I have not ascertained if she is at home."*

Yes, we see thy need. And therefore, we have before us the body, the soul, the spirit, and therefore, the immortal body. Yes, all is in accord here.

Therefore, we should say unto these, this of thy soul. We have seen thy travel through time and as you would know it, energy form. And we see thy need at the present time.

As we have said before, that a child shall be born unto you, as of before. And we shall tell thee of this of thy need. But as before, thy did take Moses into thy arms and love of him, why do thy fear to take an infant, through it is not bore [born] from thy womb now?

Of thy need at the present time, and of thy surgery which is planned in the future — yes, we see this, yes — corrective surgery shall be done of the tubular area of the same. And therefore, this sperm may be planted into the same in the future.

Yes, we see this.

We find — yes — [dirithical-type] [discoblastula?] growths of this area and blockage of the same, scar tissue of this area and blockage of the same.

Yes.

We find a cyst of the right ovary — yes, we see this. This in itself could be taken care of without surgery at the present time. We find other adjustments that the surgeon shall find.

Yes — we see that the uterus at the present time is not in the proper position for receiving the same, and therefore, [could] reject these things, the egg of the same.

Yes.

We find infection in this area; this shall be corrected with the surgery of the same. We find, therefore, that the high use of antibiotics on the [Cesarean] area [are] that of thy known antibiotic of [its] time. Therefore, we say unto thee, these things shall be granted, and the healing that thy have asked for shall be given. And therefore, we say unto thee, for thy blessings unto your Lord — and therefore, thy Lord shall kneel before thee and place into thy womb in the future a soul that thy desire.

That is all on this soul at the present time.

November 26, 1971: **Thy have many questions, ask.**

*"Yes, Aka, 'I wonder if you could give us some help as to what can be done to assist S____ H_____'s husband, B___, in his health problem?' We don't seem to be getting anywhere with it."*

As we have said before, the assistance that was needed shall be given.

As we have said before, we see thy doubt. If in the manipulations had done, been done correctly by the chiropractor, the stones of the same would have been dissolved. Yet, this has not been done. There is still hope that this could be done correctly. But the gall bladder, in itself, has become, as you would know it, to the stage of gangrene into the same. Soon, this shall have to be removed surgically.

You must understand, in the suggesting of certain doctors, we do this only that they should meet both of your financial and mental needs. We do not do this to violate your free will. But we cannot create; only our Father may do this. Therefore, we would further suggest, go to any good osteopathic doctor. Have the same to examine in the gall bladder area; you will find, therefore, infection of the same.

November 23, 1971 [in Life Readings]: **Thy have other questions, ask.**
*"Yes, Aka. [N____ D____]...she says, 'I am searching for help to find myself. Why can't I concentrate on my studies?'"*
Yes, we see thy need, and therefore, we shall go into the records of time to answer thy question.
For at the present time, as before, thy have approached womanhood, and therefore, the yearnings of the body are very strong within thyself. And we see thy need.
Yes.
And once before, in your other life, as thy would know it, thy were the sister of Hastings, or [of] that king of Curia of the same. And thy took unto thyself a lover from the Roman [guard] of the time. And because this one was not of the faith of your own, thy grew fearful that thy brother would slay of thee, and therefore, bring war unto thy time and country. And therefore, as these things did happen and war did come, destruction into thy country, thy felt that it was thine fault, and therefore, did destroy thyself.
One moment, please.
Yes, we see this need; therefore, we should say unto thee, we shall continue this reading at another time. Soul Ray grows very weak, and therefore, we shall give healing into the same.
Awaken soul Ray from his slumber.

November 26, 1971: **Thy have other questions, ask.**
*"Yes, Aka. Last week you were giving a reading on N____ D____, and she was asking for help in her studies. She said she could not concentrate on them, and you gave part of the reading that had to do with a life reading. Do you have any more on this for her tonight?"*
Yes, we see thy need. Therefore, we should say unto thee these words. Go, in the morning, upon thy awakening, and use of the meditation of the same. Open thy mind. Take from it all the worldly things. Therefore, let God flow in to thy mind. As thy should finish thy meditation, then take thy moment for prayer, asking for guidance. We shall be there. We shall assist thee.

November 26, 1971: **Thy have other questions, ask.**

*"Aka, R____ E____, who is here tonight, her home is…in Phoenix; she has had a sickness after surgery and she has a pain in her side, and she asks for assistance or affirmation regarding this."*

Yes, we see thy need. Therefore, we have before us the body, the soul, the spirit, and therefore, the immortal body of the same. Yes, we see thy need.

First, we should say unto these words, we see no sin in this one. We see thy need for love.

Yes, we see this.

You must remember, therefore, for the mind to work well, it must have a good body, therefore, and the necessary nourishment of the same should be fed into it.

First, we should say unto this one, change of thy diet.

Of thy morning meal, we would suggest the drinking of one ounce of safflower oil into the same. We would suggest, therefore, the eating of no more than three pieces of toast. Therefore, the coffee or tea may be drank. We would further suggest of the drinking of the sage tea for the morning meal.

We would suggest, therefore, for thy luncheon meal, the eating — yes, we see this — the eating of two bananas per day for the first week, the drinking of the sage tea in the same manner, taking one ounce of safflower oil in this manner. For the second week, the luncheon meal could consist still of one ounce of safflower oil and as many good, fresh vegetables of any kind as thy desire to eat, drinking still of the sage tea of the same.

Of thy evening meals — yes, we see thy need — for one meal, each of the evening meal, eating still of the fresh vegetables, adding to this diet of the seafood. None of the fried food should be eaten. For the second meal, [the] eating once a week of the liver of the beef, with still as many good vegetables. This should be done for the third meal, the eating of either the lamb, in this manner, still eating of as many fresh vegetables as the body desires. For the remainder of the week, thy may eat as thy desire. Do this [until] the second week. Of the second week, change only in this manner. Take one evening meal per week and fast in this manner.

Add to your diet a good, natural vitamin of the multiple type. Add to your diet of the vitamin C, D and E in this manner; add to thy diet of calcium — all into [the] adult dose of the same. We would further suggest the taking of the Lydia E. Pinkham in the adult dose of the same.

We would further suggest the taking of the hot olive oil packs, therefore, placing them in the evening before thy should slumber into the same area for periods of 15 minutes each time. Do not overstrain this area at the present time.

Do not take any alcoholic beverage into thy body for the present time, for at this time, it is poisoning thy body. You must realize that due to the surgery of the same your body chemicals are changing quite radically.

This is all on this soul at the present time.

November 26, 1971: **Thy have other questions, ask.**

*"Aka, B____ E_____ wants to know if her uncle, T____ G____, is all right, and if there is some way we can contact him? He has been missing for some time."*

Yes, we see thy need. We should say in this manner — in the manner in which you speak, this one, we should say unto thee, has departed. Therefore, his need upon your earth is no longer. Pray that he may see the light of our Father.

November 26, 1971: **Thy have other questions, ask.**

*"We have a request for a life and/or health reading for [6-9-70-004] from Yuma."*

Yes, we see thy need. But as our time grows short, we shall put this into another time.

November 30, 1971: *"At this time, can you give us some information concerning good insurance, health?"*

Yes, we see thy need. And the healing that is needed shall be given unto the same.

November 30, 1971: **Thy have other questions, ask.**

*"Yes, Aka. In the past few weeks, Ray's [4-3-70-001] dizziness has been getting worse. Is there anything I can do to help that?"*

Yes, we see thy need; therefore, we should say unto thee in these words. As we have said before, we may mend the damage that is done, but we cannot create. Therefore, we shall say unto thee, we shall give such healing as needed unto this one, at the present time. But remember, even though he may re-channel those proportions of the brain that is needed, if these are overtaxed in any way, the dizziness shall reoccur. This blow he received upon the head, this shall be taken care of.

November 30, 1971: *"We have a request for a health reading concerning her vision, for [11-30-71-002]; she is here with us this evening."*

Yes, we see thy need. And we should say unto thee in this way, and in this manner. That as man is born and born again, and as was said unto this one known as Jesus did say unto man, that man must know of heaven to be of the earth, and man must know of the earth to be of heaven, in your later years your eyes shall grow worse, but for this reason, so that thy soul may see. But fear not. [For] if you should give praise unto this one known as Jesus, and give praise unto God, your Father, and think of the words of Aka, that we may enter, we shall do so and give healing as needed. This must be done for three days and three nights. At the end of this period, your eyesight shall commence to heal itself, and at that time, thy shall be able to see with thy soul, thy spirit, thy immortal body, and thy physical body.

December 3, 1971 [Note: This is also in the Philosophy document]:
[**Aka is here.**

*"Does Ray stand with God?"*]
**Soul Ray stands with God.**
**Yes, we see thy need. Thy have many questions, ask.**
*"Aka, [4-6-70-003] asks for soul Andrew, if there is anything that should be done for his shoulder that he is not doing?"*
**Yes, we see thy need, and therefore, we should say unto, to thee in these words. Forgive of thy enemy, and therefore, thy Father should hear of thy prayer, and give healing into the same. For as we have said before, if thy should walk and give an offering unto thy Father, and therefore, have hatred in thy heart for thy brother, then take back thy offering, and go and forgive thy brother. But forgive thyself first, that thy brother may forgive thee also.**

**For we see thy need, soul Andrew — and as you were chosen unto the twelfth, we should say [of] these words unto thee. Come forth that we may wash of thy feet.**

December 3, 1971: **Thy have other questions, ask.**
*"Yes, Aka, [12-3-71-00]...She asks, 'What can be done to help cure my depression?'"*
**Yes, we see thy need, and therefore, we should say unto thee in these words. The mind was created by God, and therefore, created in perfection of the same. All things that are taken into the body must be as pure as the mind itself. Therefore, take nothing into the body that would cloud the mind. Take only that of the natural powers that was placed into man. For remember, your Father has forsaken you nothing. He created you "in our kind, of our image." He did hide nothing from His children; His children have hid from themselves the natural ability to use all [of] your mind, not part.**

**Develop that psychic ability that thy possess, but develop it in such a manner that you would in truth be of our kind, of our image. Use it in such a manner that it can serve mankind and God, for in serving mankind, you are serving God, and therefore, shall build the temple of God in man.**

**Your confusion is of this in itself; you are searching for a home for your soul. Therefore, as a good farmer should cultivate a field, cultivate your friends, for there are those around you who care not for you, but care only for their own selfish needs.**

December 3, 1971: **Thy have other questions, ask.**
*"Aka, [ _-__-__-___] was here last week and asked for help for her hearing, do you have any —"*
**Yes, we see thy need. And we shall give such help as is needed, for this shall come as raindrops upon the desert, a little at a time, and as your**

faith grows stronger, so shall your hearing grow stronger. We shall give thee a gift, for the sounds that thy hear now, we shall add to these, and we shall enter into the spiritual world, but we should send those [to] you that is needed to guide unto the same.

December 7, 1971: **[Aka is here.]**
[*"Good evening, Aka.*] *Where is Ray?"*
**Soul Ray stands with God.**
**We see thy need. Thy have many questions, ask.**
*"Aka, [6-8-71-010?] is ill, and his mother wants to know if there is anything that she should do specifically for him?"*
**We see thy need; therefore, healing shall be given unto the same.**

December 7, 1971: **Thy have other questions, ask.**
*"Yes, Aka. [11-26-71-003] asked recently about her uncle, [11-26-71-004], who had returned to the other life, and she wishes to know more information about him."*
**As we have said before, without the permission of the soul involved, we may not give of this information. But we should tell thee in this manner, for those who have sinned against this soul, the soul has forgiven unto the same. And as it has used its free choice to be born again upon your earth, we should say unto this one, look into your own family at the newborn, and there you shall find a newborn baby girl. And this shall be your uncle of before. For the choice, and through your prayers, have been answered unto the same.**

December 7, 1971: **Thy have other questions, ask.**
*"I have a request for a life and/or health reading for [6-9-70-005] of Yuma."*
**Yes, we see thy need, and therefore, we have before us the body, the soul, the spirit, and therefore, the immortal body of the same.**
**Yes, we see this.**
**First, we should say unto this one, go unto your physician. For we find spasms of the heart vessels of the same. This, in itself, should lead unto the disease of a [cardirary] [cardiac?] area, and therefore, could cause the respiratory system to slow down into such a manner that eventually could cause death, as thy would know it.**
**We further find — yes, we see this.**
**Yes, we find migraine headaches of the same, and therefore, this is caused from low blood pressure of the same. We further find large deposits in both lungular [lung] areas caused from the overindulgence of tobacco. We would suggest that this one that this one should use of the [saunic] baths to remove and stimulate the blood flow of the same.**
**We find damage, therefore, of the bowelular [bowel] area.**
**Yes.**

We would further suggest that a radical change of the diet, therefore, within the subject, should take place. We would suggest, first, that for the morning meal, the eating of a good, sound breakfast of the same. We would suggest for the morning meal the eating of two poached eggs, one glass of milk, and one piece of toast within the same. For the luncheon meal, one glass of milk, and as many green vegetables as you desire. For the evening meal, for one day of one week, we would suggest including as many green vegetables as is desired into the diet.

Yes.

We would suggest that no fried food be taken into this diet. Either broiled in its own juice, or baked of the same in its own juice, as much [new] beef as this subject would desire, taking away from the diet your starches. For one week, of one day, the eating of the liver of the beef. For one, the eating of — yes, we see this — of the fresh water fish should be added; of another, the sea fish of the same. We would further suggest into this diet, coffee at 10 o'clock in the morning, no more than one cup, and one cup with the evening meal. We would further suggest that the taking of one ounce of safflower oil before each meal. We would further suggest that a good supplement vitamin of the natural type be used into the same. You may add as many cooked vegetables as you desire to the evening meal, but try to substitute them with more of the green vegetables.

Yes, we see this.

We find arthritis throughout the bonial [bone] area of the body,

Yes, we see this.

You must understand that this is a virus, and should be treated as the same. Therefore, we would suggest the use of the saunic [sauna] baths be used. We would further suggest — yes, we see this is not practical, yes, we see this. Therefore, we would suggest that the drug known as [cortisone] be used. This should be used and adapt into the body itself. We would further suggest that the drinking of the sage tea be done between each meal of the same.

This is all on this subject at the present time.

December 7, 1971 [in Life Readings]: **Yes, we see this.** [6-9-70-005]

Therefore, we have before us — yes — we have before us the records of time.

Yes, we find this soul in that proportion of Atlantis of the third planet of the same.

Yes, we see this — of the island known as [Platazone]. We see this one — yes — as a printer, for as was known at that time as the Devil's mechanic, this, you must realize, is only a phrase used in their work. This was done as this one did mix the ink that was used in the printing of their newspaper at that time.

Yes, we see this.

And, as your wife was of the [woman] of the temple, and as a conflict grew between thee — and as your wife did have you brought forth, and therefore, slain for your slander against the God of One at the time; you must realize that our Father has never sanctioned the killing of another. Therefore, she bore your karma.

Therefore, we do not find this again until that proportion (cough), into that proportion — yes, we see that — of what at this time is called the British Isles, but at that time was part of your European continent. And therefore, we find you again in the same trade of the time, but in this time, you only write what is favorable for the administration of the [ten] [time?] of the same. And we find, one moment, please.

Yes, we see this.

We would suggest the balance of this reading be done at a different time. Soul Ray grows very tired. Therefore, we would suggest that you should awaken soul Ray from his slumber.

December 10, 1971: **Thy have many questions, ask.**

*"Yes, Aka. I have a note here. Can blessings please be given to the friend of [12-10-71-001]? The friend has broken his back and is in traction."*

**Yes, we see thy need; therefore, healing shall be given unto the** same.

December 10, 1971: **Thy have other questions, ask.**

*"Aka, [12-10-71-002] of...Blythe, California...he has asked, 'Will a physical problem that seems to be heredity develop in me? And have you any advice?'"*

**Yes, we see thy need. The possibility of the same could be very strong, but, in your case, it shall not happen. We shall say unto thee these words. Give that that is God, God's. Give that that is man, man's. Give that that belongs to yourself to yourself.**

December 10, 1971: **Thy have other questions, ask.**

*"Aka, [12-20-71-003], she was born...1907, in Paradise, Arizona, and she asks — 'I am searching for what I believe' — or wait, she says, just a minute. 'What is going to happen to my son-in-law and how long until it happens?' This is her question."*

**We see thy need. As we have said before, we cannot give information regarding another soul. But in your case, we shall say unto thee these words. Your son-in-law shall receive his just reward, both on earth and in heaven, and this shall come very soon, within the six-month period.**

December 10, 1971: **Thy have other questions, ask.**

*"[12-10-71-004], born...1918, in Bayview, Texas, has asked, 'Will my husband contact me, and what was accomplished by his early death?'"*

**You must realize — one moment, please, permission must be given.**

Yes, we see thy need, and therefore, we should answer in this manner. Thy husband's departure was of his own free will. But you must realize that with his early departure and the shock of the same to himself, he has had a needed time to find his own way. We should say unto thee, pray that he can see our Father's light; pray for guidance unto the same. And your husband shall make contact in your dreams of the same.

December 10, 1971: **Thy have other questions, ask.**
*"Yes, Aka, [12-10-71-005] of...Yuma, Arizona, says, 'I need to understand myself and to know why I am as I am. I am very confused. I need guidance desperately, need to realize my wants and feel confident, useful. I need to relieve my frustration. I want to know more of myself, know how I am. I want and need guidance and assurance that I am loved and needed.'"*

Yes, we see thy need. **You must remember that you never walk alone, that the spirit of God walks within thee. Soon there shall come into your life a mate of the same, and your union shall come before God. We have given unto you a task. Perform it and the reward that thy seek shall be given. In your meditation, if thy could say our name. that the door could be entered, we shall enter, and therefore, give thee guidance in thy daily life. And we should leave those with thee to guide thee and give thee counsel.**

**Remember, you are a child of our Father. You are the most important person you know. For remember, as it has been said before, the last shall be first and the first shall be last. But stand before God, and the blessings of the same shall enter and guide thee. In your meditation, think of our name, and then listen. Listen well.**

December 17, 1971: **Thy have other questions, ask.**
*"Yes, Aka. [4-3-70-002] asks, should she see — asks about a health reading. Should she see a doctor, or is she just tired?"*

**Yes, we see thy need. And we should answer in this manner. We would suggest three days of rest and meditation, and healing shall be given into the same.**

December 17, 1971: **Thy ask other questions. Ask.**
*"Aka, J____ N____ lost a considerable sum of money and she is very disturbed about it. Can you help her with where this is?"*

**Yes, we see thy need, and therefore, we should answer in this manner. The one who has taken this money now thinks of returning the same. Proportions shall be returned, but not all.**

December 17, 1971: **Thy have other questions, ask.**
*"Aka, [11-15-71-002] asked for a health reading one time and was delayed on it. She is concerned about her diet and weight problem. Can you help her at this time?"*

We have answered this question once before, but we should answer again in this manner, for it is necessary to add to. We would suggest the drinking of no alcoholic beverages. The only alcohol that should be taken in is three ounces of wine should be drinken [drunk] before each meal. At a different time if additional information is asked for, we should give a more elaborate diet of the same.

December 17, 1971: **Thy have other questions, ask.**

*"Yes, Aka. [11-26-71-003] who is here tonight asks for blessings for a friend who has been ill for a long time and was recently been injured in a car accident."*

**Yes, we see thy need, and therefore, we should answer in this manner. For healing should be given into the soul.**

**Yes, we see this.**

**And thy must realize that man cannot harm the soul, only man himself.**

# 1972 Health Readings

January 1, 1972: [Aka is here.]
*"Good evening, Aka. Where is Ray?"*
**Soul Ray stands with God.**
**Yes, that is better. Now all is in accord.**
**And we shall say again, for hark. For those who have ears to
listen, and for those who have faith, both in their selves and in God, our
Father, let them bring the bread that is needed, and the bread shall be
the body of the same. And let them pray over it, and ask for healing of
the same. And the healing shall be given, for as we have said before, we
shall furnish the wine that is needed, and we shall turn the bread into
yeast, that the healing may grow outward and inward.**

**From this day forward, your medical readings shall not be
needed, for those who come in faith shall be given the healing that is
needed.**

**And we say these words unto soul [1-1-72-001], we see thy need,
and therefore, should give healing into the same.**

**And we should say unto soul [4-6-70-003], we see thy need, and
healing shall be given into the same.**

**But we should say unto thee these words. We may only give what
is needed for those who should ask. And for those who do need shall
travel forward and come unto us that we may administer into their needs.**

**But there shall be some who should not have the faith to heal, and
to receive healing. For those, we shall continue your health readings, but
only for the specific need of the time....**

January 1, 1972: **Thy have other questions, ask. But we see this
need; one moment.**

**Yes. yes, yes, Father.**

**Yes, we see this. And we should say unto Luke, go back unto this
land of thine; go unto the one that is needed and say unto her these
words: For healing shall be given, for our Father should promise of the
same. And we should say also in these words, for there has been the entry
of the other sister, for this sister has psychic powers. We shall not allow
this entry. But remember, also, we cannot interfere with free will. If it is
the free will of the other sister to let her other sister dominate her, we
cannot stop this. We may only give the healing that is asked for. We may
only give the guidance that is asked for.**

January 1, 1972: **Thy have other questions, ask.**

*"Aka, in regards to health readings, I had a request for* [1-1-72-002] *of Globe; he was born... 1969; he's three. And he has been having problems with convulsions, coma, muscular spasms. And his home is in Kellner Canyon. His family has requested a health reading. Do you wish to speak on this at this time?"*

**We should say, we see thy need. If the help they seek is strong enough, let them come here and ask themselves. At such a time, our Lord shall decide.**

**Thy have other questions.**

*"I have no other question, other than the family had asked if they should move, and I think you mean for them to come here with their questions."*

**Yes. We see thy need. But we should say unto thee, soul Paul, we have empowered in thee to give healing of the same. This healing shall come from our Lord. But the healing would do no good unless they could believe of the same. Can you understand of which we speak?**

*"Yes, Aka."*


January 1, 1972: **Then we should say unto thee, soul Paul, fear not. There shall be many who shall venture to your door. Give your blessings freely. Some shall accept and some shall reject. For those who reject, take back your blessings and go forth to the next. But do not be fearful that they are not healed, for the Lord has given unto thee the power, as He has done unto all of these disciples. There shall be some that we shall wish that you should bring before our presence. But our presence shall be within *thee*. Lay hands upon the same, and the healing shall come.**


January 7, 1972: **[Aka is here.]**

*"[Good evening,] Aka. Where is Ray?"*

**Soul Ray stands with God.**

**Yes, that is better; now all is in accord.**

**Yes, we see thy need.**

**Thy have many questions, ask.**

*"Aka, last week I asked for information for the* [1-7-72-001] *family, who are here tonight, and they have...."*

**We see thy need. Yes, we see thy need, and we should say unto thee, you must realize — yes, we see this — the healing that is needed shall be given. But we cannot create; therefore, this one shall remain an epileptic, as thy would know of the same, for the remainder of its life. But with the product known as Dilantin this may be controlled. The other damage done to the body unto the brain of the same, the healing that is asked for shall be given.**

And we say unto these, thy parents, go unto thy home and pray unto thy Lord, thy God, unto three days, and the healing that thy ask for shall be given. But as all things must be planted before they can be harvested, thy faith unto the power of God remains within thyselves. Only if thy have the faith that our Father shall give this healing can it be given unto the same. Therefore, we say unto the parents, for as it is written before, "Honor thy father and mother," and we say unto thee, honor thy father and mother unto thyselves, and so it shall be unto this child. But first, let the father and mother honor the child, and believe into the God, our Creator, of the same.

Of the father's question, we should say unto these words. Thy have thought of other employment; this would be good. Thy have thought of moving to another land. This would not be good at the present time. Thy have planted thy seed upon the land that thy live. Harvest your own crop and let the seed grow again, and when thy harvest it again thy shall find only good fruit.

Thy have other questions, ask.

*"Thank you, Aka. 'M_____ 2' has asked for healing of an infection on her chin, and also a life reading."*

Yes, we see thy need, and therefore, the healing shall be given. The life reading shall be given at a different time.

Ask thy other questions.

*"[1-7-72-002] has asked for a health reading, Aka."*

Yes, we see thy need, but we say unto thee, thy have the faith unto thy Father, thy God. And we see thy offering, and thy offering shall be served up into our Father. And the healing that is needed shall be granted, for as the wife of John, these things thy should ask in our Father's name shall be given.

January 15, 1972: **Thy have other questions, ask.**

*"Yes, Aka. D____ S____ asks, he says, 'I am concerned about my mother's health and well- being. I request blessings and healing for my mother, [1-15-72-001]. Also I request guidance in doing my best to help her.'"*

Yes, we see thy need. And therefore, the offering thy have offered unto our Father should be given unto Him, and the healing that thy should desire should be given in the same manner as thy offering.

January 15, 1972: **Thy have other questions, ask.**

*"Yes, Aka.[1-15-72-004] of Yuma asks for healing in regards to bursitis in her right shoulder. And she also asks, 'Would a move from my present address this year benefit my husband, daughters, and my grandsons, and allow me to use God's purposes for my talents more fully?' And she asks — just a minute; this is essentially it, she asks for help in regards to bursitis in her right shoulder, and should she move this year?"*

We see thy need, and therefore, we shall say unto thee in[to] these words. For as the first shall be last and the last shall be first, thy have planted thy seed; stay there and harvest the same. Be as a mirror unto your family. Give unto what is given unto thee in the same manner, with love and understanding, and compassion of the same.

If a man should ask to borrow thy right arm, give him of your left, but do so in love and understanding. But if a man should ask for thy right arm for a selfish reason, give him not neither, but let him walk alone.

We should give of the healing thy desire. But we should ask into you in this manner; go forth and give into our Father three days of prayer. And upon the third day of the third hour of the third moment of your time, so should you receive the healing.

January 23, 1972: **And now, we should give a moment unto the healing unto soul Ray, and then awaken him from his slumber.**

January 28, 1972: *"Yes, Aka,*[1-28-72-001] *of Globe, she was born...1918, in Richmond, California.... She has asked for assistance in regards to her health. She says she is overweight, and she wonders if you can give her assistance?"*

Yes, we see thy need. You must remember, that because of thy overweight thy have a heart problem, fatty tissue passing through the coronary area. Therefore, we should give thee the healing that is necessary. But thy must have the faith.

But first, we should give unto thee, diet. And we would suggest the drinking of one glass of milk unto the morning meal, and one piece of toast; there should be no margarine or butter placed upon this.

For thy luncheon meal, one glass of milk. As many of the green vegetation as thy want thy can eat for foliage. Before the meal, one ounce of safflower oil.

Of thy evening meal, eat no fried foods. Thy should eat beef for one meal, and as many fresh vegetables as thy desire. Thy should eat of the fresh water fish of one meal, and as many green vegetables as thy would desire. Thy should eat of the salt water fish of one meal and as many green vegetables as thy should desire. Of one meal, thy should eat only of the cottage cheese and of the green vegetables of the same. Of one meal, thy should eat the beef, the liver of the beef, and cottage cheese. Of one meal each week thy can eat of what thy desire.

Before each of these meals, thy should have one ounce of safflower oil before each of these meals; thy should take a good multiple vitamin in supplement to the same.

If further assistance is needed this should be asked for, and it should be given.

Thy have other questions, ask.

January 28, 1972: *"Yes, Aka. My daughter, K____, has had a recurring health problem, Aka, and I wonder if you can help her with knowing what to do about it?"*

Yes, we see thy need. The healing that is needed shall be given. We should make one suggestion, reduce the amount of vitamin intake. In her case the vitamins are poisoning her system. We should further suggest, in her case, the taking of the Lydia E. Pinkham in adult dosage, but by reducing unto one-fourth the amount of other vitamins that she is taking at this time. Further readings on this subject shall be given as asked for.

Thy have other questions, ask.

January 28, 1972: *"[4-5-70-003] has asked for healing, Aka."*

Yes, we see thy need, and the healing thy ask for shall be given. But we should say unto thee, tilt thy head in prayer to thy Lord, and say after our words: "Lord of Isaiah, Lord of Moses, Lord of all, I ask thee, oh, Lord, unto healing into my body, my soul, my spirit, and my immortal body. Cleanse my body, my soul, of Lord; cleanse my spirit and my immortal body. I promise thee, oh, Lord, to try to walk in Thy light." In these words, the healing shall come.

February 11, 1972: **And we see [1-1-72-001's] problem. And we should say in this manner. At a different time, those that are needed shall stand by thy side. But we should stay this for now, and give healing into the body of the same. But remember, we are not great; we are but the servants and messengers of our Father. We can not create. Only our Father can do this.**

**Now is the time of the Cherub.**

**Soul Ray grows very weary. Awaken him from his slumber.**

February 18, 1972: *"Yes, Aka. [12-7-70-00?]"*

Yes, we see thy need, and we should answer in this manner. Take of the sauna baths. Go unto the chiropractic doctor that adjustments may be made in the upper neckular area. At the present time the circulatory system is blocked in this area. Be careful and do not overdo this or thy shall suffer from blood clots of the same. This should be done for one month, at least one day of each of your weeks. We would further suggest the taking of a round rubber ball of two inches in diameter, placing this in thy left hand, squeezing it very tightly. Do not put all of thy pressure or bruise thy hands. This should be done two minutes of the first day, three minutes of the second day, and therefore, working upward unto 15 minutes. This should be continued for two months, at that time. We would further suggest that the taking, once daily, of the sage tea.

A follow-up reading should be needed within a two-week period. Should the same be asked for, it shall be given.

Thy have other questions, ask.

*"Yes, Aka, there is one question on this subject that was not clear to me. You said that she should take sauna baths and chiropractic, and then you said something daily. Did you mean that she should go to the chiropractor, or take saunas daily, or did you mean that she should exercise her hand daily?"*

Her hand should be exercised daily.

*"I understand."*

Thy have other questions, ask.


February 25, 1972: *"Yes, Aka, [2-25-72-001] of...Seaside, California...has asked for help in regards to a weight problem. And she says, 'I am very unhappy with myself; please get me back to normal.' She has asked for help."*

Yes, we see thy need, and therefore, should say unto thee theses words. We have before us the body, the soul, the spirit, and the immortal body of the same. And therefore, we have the records of this one.

And we should say unto thee, we see thy need, and thy need of thy husband also.

First, we should say unto this one, enter all things with love and compassion. Beware of thy jealousies, for they come not of reality. For in reality this one loves thee very much, but is shy, and does not know how to show their feelings. Do not pity thyself, for this is not for thee. Stand firm and strong.

And of thy children's needs, see to their needs, not of their wants. Give them those things that are needed. Thy have given guidance, for it is said, "Honor thy father and mother." But this must be done as thy Father honors thee, for He did give thee free choice. Do the same with these. And as a good father and as a good mother, stand firm upon your convictions. But open your mind, your real mind, that proportion of yourselves that always has known God, that the spirits may flow unto thee freely.

Of thy weight problem, we should answer in this manner. Of thy morning meal, drink one glass of milk, eat one unsweetened grapefruit, no more and no less. Of thy luncheon meals, take of the fresh water fish; thy may eat in thy proportion of thy needs. Eat all of the green vegetables that thy desire. Drink one cup of tea, no more and no less.

For the seven evening meals — eat beef of the first meal, beef with as many fresh vegetables as thy desire. Of the second meal, eat the beef liver, again with as many fresh vegetables as thy desire. But do not eat bread with this meal. Of thy third meal, eat of the fresh water fish, with as many vegetables as thy would desire. Of the fourth meal, eat of the fish of the salt; any food that comes from the sea would be good, but again, eat only of the fresh vegetables of the same. Of thy fifth meal, thy may take any combination of those we have given. But thy seventh meal, eat anything thy desire. Before each meal drink one ounce of safflower oil.

Walk one-half mile each day; this is preferably in the morning, early morning hours. In the afternoon, preferably after thy meal, walk again one-quarter mile. If this is followed in such proportion thy shall gain physically.

Before thy morning walk, take five minutes unto meditation of the same. For thy afternoon walk, take ten minutes of meditation into the same. These together should give healing mentally and physically into the same.

Thy have other questions, ask.

February 25, 1972: *"Yes, Aka.[J__] asks, 'Do I need fear threats?'"*
Yes, we see thy need, soul [J___], and we should answer in this manner. Give of thy heart, thy soul, and thy spirit into thy Father's keeping, and thy Father shall take care of the immortal body of the same. But we should answer in this manner. Take those things that are truths, and make your judgment from the same. We would further suggest, your visits to your psychiatrist at the present time, take of this one's advice, for this is good advice. But be truthful unto this one. For if thy do not, the physician cannot heal unto the same.

Thy have other questions, ask.

March 3, 1972: *"Yes, Aka.[12-7-70-00_] has asked for a follow-up reading on the problem with the circulation in her arm."*
Yes, we see thy need, and we should answer in this manner. At the present time thy are overworking your body, and therefore, destroying the damage — you are, therefore, destroying what good has come unto the body. Do not do this. Go back and start again with the rubber ball, back unto one minute per day, graduating unto the 15-minute time, of one minute longer each day. You should continue going unto the chiropractic doctor. You should continue taking the saunic baths. This should be done at least once a week. You should continue the drinking of the sage tea. In our next reading, we should give more information upon the same if it is asked for.

Thy have other questions, ask.

March 3, 1972: *"Yes, Aka.[A___ F_____] who is here tonight.... He has a problem with his failing sight and he has asked if you can tell him what can be done about it?"*
Yes, we see thy need, and therefore, should answer in this manner. The healing that is needed shall be given, for all things shall come from our Lord. Go unto three days of prayer, both of the morning and the evening. Open your heart, your mind, that we may enter. Upon the third day of the same, your sight shall be restored into the same.

Thy have other questions, ask.

March 3, 1972: *"Yes, Aka.[S____ S____ ]"*

March 3, 1972: **One moment, please.**
**Yes. Yes, Father. Yes, Father. Yes.**
**Upon your next reading thy shall ask again.**
**Our Father says unto thee in this manner. Bow before our Lord,**
**and these things that are needed shall be given unto thee. But a life**
**reading should be requested [of] this one; there is further assistance**
**needed.**
**Thy have other questions, ask.**

March 3, 1972: *"Aka, [1-21-72-002] wants...."*
**One moment.**
**We were not speaking to S_____ before. Ask this question again.**

March 3, 1972: *"Aka, [K_____ M_____] has been having pain*
*in her stomach, and general sickness off and on for a long time, and she*
*wonders if you can assist her with what to do about it?"*
**Yes, we see thy need. Thy problem is basically one of the female**
**organs. We would suggest the taking of the Lydia E Pinkham. This thy**
**do not always do, but do this as a ritual. And then we say unto thee, take**
**of six days of prayer, the healing that is needed shall be given. And fear**
**not.**
**Yes, we see this.**
**Thy have other questions, ask.**

March 3, 1972: **But we should answer one other question, of soul**
**R_____'s trip. He should not be left unsupervised, and beware of the**
**water. Take your trip, but do not engage in what thy call as horseplay**
**with the other boys. Do not go off by thyself. For if thy fail to heed our**
**warning, thy shall leave of thy body.**

March 10, 1972: *"Yes, Aka. [J___ W_____], who is here tonight,*
*of...Miami....And she asks, 'I am in doubt as to what action to take; I want to*
*know if I should have surgery next Tuesday, as the doctor wants?'"*
**Yes, we see thy need, and therefore, have before us the body, the**
**soul, the spirit and the immortal body. Yes, we see thy need, and**
**therefore, we should say in this manner. The surgery is needed, but not in**
**the same manner as the doctors think at the present time. For these**
**things that they should find should be of a minor nature and easily be**
**corrected.**
**Thy have other questions, ask.**

March 10, 1972: *"Thank you, Aka.[C\_\_\_\_ H\_\_\_\_] is asking for [M\_\_\_\_ J\_\_]. She says, 'Ever since [M\_\_\_\_ J\_\_] has been born he has been troubled with colds.... Can you advise me on this? Also there seems to be a slight problem with his right foot, how can this be corrected?'"*

Yes, we see thy need. And of the colds, as thy would know them, the healing shall be given into the same. Of the foot, we should answer in this manner. Once each day the foot should straightened and held in this position. Hold of the upper thigh of the leg of the same. Do not force the foot, bring it gradually and slowly into a straighter position. This should be done 15 minutes of the morning and the evening. This should be continued for six months of the same.

Thy have other questions, ask.

March 10, 1972: *"Yes, Aka, [J\_\_\_ C\_\_\_\_] of...Fresno, California....And she has asked, 'I need help with my problems at home and the future health of my husband.'"*

Yes, we see thy need, and therefore, should answer in this manner. This one's diet should be greatly changed. Yes, we see the problem here of arthritis.

We would suggest the drinking of the sage tea. The pulp of the Night-blooming Cereus should be added, and if at all possible, should be taken in the fresh quantity. All calcium substances should be taken from the diet for the present time. We find also that this one is a borderline diabetic; the eating of the Jerusalem artichoke of the same should be done daily. We also find that the Vitamin D should be added in extra quantities of the same, and of the Vitamin B of the same. We also find that this subject should take the tonic known as S.S.S.

A diet should be given, that of all green substances. No meat of any kind, except that that should come from the ocean, should be eaten, of the salt water variety. No other meat should be eaten. Eat as many green vegetables as thy desire. For the present time, take out of thy diet that of the natural salt. The fish, as it comes, can be eaten. [Use of] a salt substitute or that of the salt that comes from the ocean. It would be advisable if this one could move into a much drier climate.

Of thy other problem — yes, we see this — and we should answer in this manner. Each in your own way has that of karma before thee; thy have chosen this. We may guide thee, but we cannot take that that thy have chosen from thee. Stand firm, but learn to be more giving. Learn to forgive unto others.

But we should leave thee with this message. If thy right eye offend thee, cast it aside. But, thy are thy own master upon this earth. Thy are a child of God, and therefore, are a very important soul. Do nothing into the body that would harm the body, for that would only cause thee new karmas into the same. For every action upon your earth, there must be a reaction to the same. For all things of the earth must be of heaven, and all things of heaven must be of the earth. Learn of these. Take unto thyself of the past readings. Learn of these. But remember, thy can destroy nothing; thy may only build upon what is already there.

March 17, 1972: *"Yes. Aka, [5-7-71-001] who is here tonight, has asked for a health reading."*

Yes, we see thy need, then, therefore, have before us — yes — we have the body the soul, the spirit, and therefore, the immortal body of the same.

First, we should tell unto this one that Louise is well, and she sent this one greetings.

Yes, we have before us the body, and therefore, find in the lymph glands of the same
imbalance.

Yes, we see this.

In the same manner, we find an imbalance of the pineal gland, and therefore, there are many substances, one of such is the wheat germ within itself. We find, therefore, that proportion that is secreted of the [lifelong] liquid of the same. We find, therefore, an unbalance of the system. We would suggest, first, the use of a good osteopathic doctor.

We find the diet [eaten] in its present form is a good one. But unless this is corrected, we find the forming of cancerous cells; a virus, therefore, that is secreted from the same, is now fermenting into the same, and therefore, in an incubative state.

We would also suggest that adjustments be made of the upper neckular area in that proportion of the brainstem in itself. This should be done in an upward manner, for the upper proportion, of the third [digitone] [digitonin (attached at C-3 of the digitogenin)] and of the fourth [C-4] should be moved apart. We would further suggest that medication be taken for the dilating of the blood vessels into the same.

We would further suggest that good minerals be used, a mineral compound. We would not suggest any of the calcium — a mineral with this substance left out.

One moment, please.

Yes we see this.

Therefore, we would suggest — yes — a Doctor Patterson, at the present time located in the Scottsdale area.

We would further suggest the use of the saunic baths, to increase the circulatory system.

Yes, we see an infection of the vagina. We also see — yes, in this manner — this is caused by imbalance of the bladder area. We would suggest that the drinking of at least six glasses of pure water. We would suggest the taking of the sage tea, both of the morning and evening.

Yes we find this.

We also find that this subject is a borderline diabetic; the eating of the Jerusalem artichoke would greatly help this subject in this manner.

In the presence of the doctor thy should advise him of your susceptibility to varicose veins. This should be guarded.

We see thy need and we should say unto thee in these words. If thy should take of three days of prayer, rest and meditation, the healing that thy desire shall be given.

Thy have other questions, ask.

March 17, 1972: *"Yes, Aka. [4-6-70-001] asks, 'Does Andrew [4-20-70-001] have a physical ailment which needs treatment, and should I try to help him?'"*

Yes we see thy need, and therefore, should answer in this manner. Yes, soul Andrew has several physical ailments. But at the present time it would be no benefit to yourself to try to give assistance, for this should not at the present time be accepted. At a later time, yes, but not at the present time.

We should also suggest, as we have said before, do not go at the present time into any business ventures. Stand firm on those things that thy possess. If thy do not thy shall lose them all.

But the most important of all — thy would again dream of the many houses, which are your soul. Give that to God that belongs to God. Give that to yourself that belongs to yourself. But before all other, give that to your brother that belongs to your brother. And if your brother has offended thee, go to thy brother and ask forgiveness. But before thy go to thy brother, ask forgiveness of thyself. And if thy cannot find forgiveness within thyself, then go again into meditation, and therefore, find the source of thy problem. But do not denounce others; do not find fault in others, for the problem that thy should correct lies within thy own heart.

Thy have other questions, ask.

March 17, 1972: *"Thank you, Aka. [3-17-72-001]...and she is very concerned about her feelings toward her loved ones and her instability. She has left her family, and she wonders if you can give her any assistance? She is presently living in Yuma."*

One moment, please. We do not see this. We do not find this soul.

We should suggest that thy get a proper address and a proper name of the same.

Thy have other questions, ask.

March 17, 1972 [in Philosophy]: **But before we depart we should answer a question in the mind of one. Fear not, for thy husband shall walk with thee for some time yet. But prepare for a long journey. This journey shall take you over the seas, and therefore, we ask of thee, take** with thee these readings. Let the Word, for it was first in the beginning, flow into the souls of the ocean of man.

March 17, 1972: *"Yes, Aka.* [5-7-71-001] *was given a health reading last week, and there are* two questions that she *needs clarification on. She was told to see a Dr. Patterson in Scottsdale, who is an osteopath, and she can't find a Dr. Patterson, but she found a Dr. Peterson in Scottsdale who's an osteopath. Also...."*

We see thy need, and therefore, we should answer in this manner. From your English translation, Peterson and Patterson should be one of the same.

Of thy other question, we should answer in this manner. Take that that is needed into the body. Should thy feel that the body should reject the same, do not take of this.

Thy have other questions, ask.

March 17, 1972: *"Yes, Aka. [J___ H_____ ], who is staying in the Lee Hotel in Yuma...and she has left her home and family and is very distressed. She feels that she can't go back to them because she is very hateful, and she asks for guidance."*

We see thy need, and we shall say once again, we do not see this. Get, as thy would know it, the correct address and the correct name of this soul. The information shall be given when the truth is [put] forth unto the same.

Thy have other questions, ask.

April 1, 1972: And now, we should say unto this other one who has lost his way. And we see the hurt within his family, and permission has been granted to answer of this question. For he now dwells in what thy would know as the Los Angeles area. No harm has come unto this one, but you must realize, this one in his sanest moments possessed that of free choice, and that he did use. But remember, for the next one who should achieve the Christ state may be the beggar upon the street.

Thy have other questions, ask.

April 1, 1972: *"Yes, Aka.* [4-17-71-001] *has asked for a health reading."*

Yes, we see thy need, and we should answer in this manner. Go unto three days of prayer and meditation, and the healing thy desire shall be given, for in this manner, thy should open the door that we may enter.

April 1, 1972: Ask thy other question.

*"Aka, at this time this is all of the written questions we have."*

Nay, then we should answer in this manner. For the one in need, we shall give unto thee three years of life upon this earth. And take each year as a day, and think upon it as you too were laid upon the cross. Within the third year of the third moment of this day, if you have learned, if you have shed one teardrop unto our Father, we shall extend this time. If not, you shall judge unto yourself.

April 7, 1972: **Yes, we see thy need, soul [4-6-70-003], and therefore, should answer of your question in this manner. For there is a time for laughter, there is a time for sleep, a time for work, and a time for worship. For in all things there is time, and as time should heal all wounds, push this thing from your mind and grow from it. Open your door that we may enter, and therefore, feel the warmth of our Father standing beside thee, for as we have said before, the door is open for the house you have searched for; enter, and become as one.**

**Thy have other questions, ask.**

*"Yes, Aka.[5-7-71-001's] osteopath in Tempe, [4-7-72-004], has suggested that she see [4-7-72-005] here, that he could do the same. Do you have any advice for her?"*

**Yes, we see thy need, and therefore, should answer in this manner. Of these things are good. But remember, this must be done gently, working above the area and below it, above in an upward motion, below in a downward motion. This must be done gently for an eight-week period of time.**

**From time to time, as the progress is done, we would suggest that further readings be given. The healing that thy have asked for is being given. Be patient, my daughter, for all things, with faith, shall come.**

**Thy have other questions, ask.**

April 7, 1972: *"Yes, Aka. [8-24-70-001's] right shoulder is causing continuing pain. She wonders if you can give her a health reading on this particular problem?"*

**Yes, we see thy need, and therefore, should answer in this manner. Your seasons are changing. Eat of the Night-blooming Cereus. Do so in this manner; make of this into the powdered form, placing it in a glass of milk. We would further suggest, also, the drinking of the sage tea twice per day.**

April 7, 1972: **Thy have other questions, ask.**

*"Yes, Aka, one question on powdering the Night-blooming Cereus, how should this be done?"*

**Dry it in the sun.**

April 7, 1972: *"Thank you, Aka. Aka, [4-7-72-002] who is visiting our group and who is presently ill has a very serious financial problem, and she is wondering if she should get a loan, or if you have some other suggestion as to how she can solve her problem?"*

We would suggest, at the present time, of obtaining a loan. Your other financial problems shall come to an end. But remember, we shall provide your needs, not of your wants.

Thy have other questions, ask.

*"Yes, Aka."*

One moment. Yes, we see this; yes.

We would suggest that this one check back with her physician as soon as possible. We see slight infection in the lower bowel area. The healing that is asked for shall be given.

Thy have other questions, ask.

*"Yes, Aka, you're speaking of* [4-7-72-002]*?"*

Yes.

April 7, 1972: *"Thank you. Aka,* [2-19-71-002]*, she is wondering if the spray that she was exposed to when she lived here will cause her to have a child that is other than normal?"*

Yes, we see thy need, and we should answer in this manner. Nay, these things shall not happen; thy child shall be born completely normal. We would suggest for this one the taking of a good multiple vitamin at the present time. We would further suggest — yes, we see this — this subject is anemic. We would suggest the vitamin B complex, preferably to be taken into the vein itself in the liquid form.

Yes, we see this.

Thy have other questions, ask.

April 14, 1972: **[Aka is here.]**

*"Good evening, Aka. Where is Ray?"*

Soul Ray stands with God.

Yes, that is better; now all is in accord.

And first, we should say unto thee these words. We shall give healing into this one, of soul Jan [4-6-70-003?]. But it shall come as raindrops, for we have given warnings before, and these within themselves have not been heeded. Therefore, she should need time to wander in the between land. And as she should learn, then we should call her back.

April 14, 1972: *"Yes, Aka.* [4-14-72-001] *asks, 'We are planning a move to the southeastern United States and would like your advice on this; it seems we are being directed to this move.'"*

And we should answer in this manner. This move should not be good; it should divide, and therefore, conquer all in your family. Stand together. Stand as the children of God, and the light of God shall shine upon thy footsteps and show thee the way.

Yes, we see thy other needs, and we should answer them in this manner. Thy daughter should soon marry, and therefore, bring forth a good son.

Of thy son-in-law and his vision, we should answer in this manner. There are those who should use of this work to meet their own selfish needs; do not listen to this.

Thy have other questions, ask.

April 14, 1972: *"Thank you, Aka. [4-14-72-002] says, 'I have two skin problems that no one knows how to cure. Will you help me?'"*

Yes, we see thy need. And we should answer in this manner. Go unto the chiropractic doctor. Adjustments should be made in the upper neckular area. This should bring a balance of thy body chemicals into normal. Take then of the soda, take of thy bread, take then of the white of the egg; dampen all of these with boiled milk. Apply them to the infected areas, and the healing thy ask for shall be given in the same manner. Should follow-up readings be necessary, and they are asked for, they shall be given.

April 14, 1972: **Yes, we see thy needs**, [5-7-71-001].
**Yes.**

[5-7-71-001]. **And we should answer your question in this manner. The treatment as has been given is good. We would further suggest the working in the lower spinular area to bring this into a normal completion of the same. We would further suggest the taking, as we have said before, of the sage tea twice daily.**

**Thy have other questions, ask.**

April 14, 1972: *"Yes, Aka. [4-14-72-003] asks, 'Is there a chance that [4-14-72-005] will come home, and when? He is the husband of [4-14-72-003's] sister, [4-14-72-004]. He is a prisoner of war.'"*

Yes, we see thy need. Many should think of this one as being dead, as you would know it, but at the present time he still lives. His health is not well.

And we should answer your question in this manner. Death, in itself, as you would think of it, is but passing from one room to another. There is this time — as you would call it, purgatory — this time when thy should relearn thy problems of thy earth plane, and then for passing onward, beyond this. Here we call it, a time of sleep.

**Does this answer your question?**

Yes, we see thy need. And we should give prayer unto our Father. One moment.

You must realize that neither our Father, nor His servants, as we stand, can interfere with free choice. But come back one week from now, and that the final decision shall be given unto thee. But give prayer each day unto your Father, and give meditation unto the same.

Thy have other questions, ask.

April 14, 1972: *"Thank you, Aka. [3-6-71-002] has asked for a diet. She also asks, 'Should I rent my house or plan a move in May?'"*

Yes, we see thy need, and we should answer the last first. Plan thy move, as thy would suggest it. The renting of the house would be good to supplement thy income.

Of thy health reading, we should answer in this manner. This should be done in a special meeting; there [are] information that should be for thine ears only.

Thy have other questions, ask.

April 17, 1972: **Aka is here.**
*"Good afternoon, Aka. Where is Ray?"*
**Soul Ray stands with God.**

Yes, we see thy need. And we should answer in this manner. With thy emotional problem as it is, this in itself would cause this one to be overweight.

But, you have still another physical problem. This within itself is uremia poisoning. Kidneys within themselves are not at the proper time functioning as they should. We would suggest the drinking of six full glasses of water daily. This should be done for a period of seven days. Drinking as many other liquids as thy desire, drinking before each meal, approximately of 30 minutes before each meal, that of the sage tea of the same.

For thy morning meal, take before the meal one ounce of safflower oil, one piece of toast, and one glass of milk. Do not, at any time, skip any meal. Take them properly and on time.

For thy luncheon, as many green vegetables of any variety that thy desire. Soon you will be able to buy that that is known as the cantaloupe; take of as many of these as thy desire. Use of the salt that comes from the sea, none other.

For thy evening meal, still again one ounce of safflower oil before the meal. For one meal, take that of the fish foods that comes from the sea and again of as many green vegetables as thy desire. Of another meal, take of the liver that comes from the beef with as many green vegetable as thy desire. Do not cook any of these vegetables; eat them raw, as they come in their natural form. Of thy third, eat of the fresh-water foods and again as many green vegetables as thy would desire. Of thy fourth, take of the lean of the beef with again as many green vegetables as thy desire. Of thy fifth meal, thy may eat anything thy desire. Of thy sixth, again of the fresh-water fish variety. Of thy seventh meal, again of the salt-water fish of thy variety.

Remember before all meals, taking of the safflower oil, one ounce of the same. This should be continued for a three-month period. At such time, we should give further readings.

Of that that is in thy heart, we see thy need and thy longing of the same. We shall answer your question in this manner. Give that unto your God that belongs to God. Give that unto your brother that belongs to your brother. But just as important, service thy own needs. Do not cage your emotions. And thy were not born into chastity, therefore, give that unto your body that is needed. If you do not, your family and your self shall suffer from the same. Worry not again upon this one who waits in selfish need, for we have heard thy cries in the darkness, and we shall be there and serve thy need. But give unto this one what is his, no more or no less, for him demands come in selfishness, not in grace and not before God, therefore, as the journey of his should flow unto the river, and therefore, should flow unto the pit of the same.

Thy have other questions, ask.

April 17, 1972: *"Aka,* [5-7-71-002] *is concerned regarding the mining activity up the stream from their ranch. She wonders if you have any advice as to what they should do to protect their water or themselves from contamination?"*

Yes, we see thy need. And as the time that shall come when the water shall be contaminated, protect thyself with other sources of land. But do not sell at the present time. We shall serve thee and tell thee of the correct time to sell, for as you have walked before your God, your God has walked before thee. And for those who should serve their God in serving this work, we shall take care of their needs. Have the water tested on a monthly basis from this point forward. Register these tests at the present time before witnesses of the same. Say nothing to anyone. Do not hide this, but do not take it forth unto others of the knowledge thy shall possess. When the time comes, those who should offend thee shall pay for it tenfold. Can thy understand of which we speak?

*"Yes."*

Thy have other questions, ask.

April 17, 1972: *"Yes, Aka, I have one other question. Soul Ruth is concerned about a conflict in a planned trip to Miami and also the trip to Yuma. Do you have any, can you shed any light on this for her as to what will happen or what she should do?"*

Yes, we see thy need. And as you have given honor unto your God, your God shall give honor unto you, and this honor shall be before men and women of the same. Fear not, for we walk before thee and guide thee, for thy have opened thy door that we may enter. Thy have given that unto thy Lord that is thy Lord's. Do not reject the idea of making this trip, but let them give you more than ample notice. This they have not done. And this they will do. So worry not upon it. Let us take care of this need. Can thy understand of which we speak?

"*Yes, Aka,.*" [She says].

April 21, 1972: "*Aka, last week* [4-14-72-003], *who is here tonight, asked about the husband of her sister,* [4-14-72-003[, *who is interned in the war. And you said that you would tell her this week whether or not he would come home or when or something about it? Do you have more that you can tell her tonight?* [4-14-72-005] *is his name.*"

We see thy need, and we should answer you in this manner.

This one should come home, for new strength has been built within the same.

Thy have other questions, ask.

One moment.

Yes, yes.

Upon the eight month this should happen.

April 21, 1972: **You have other questions, ask.**

"*Thank you, Aka.* [4-21-72-001] *has asked, 'Will my son,* [4-21-72-002], *go into the service after graduation from college this June?'*"

One moment.

Yes, we see this. And we should answer, nay, unto this. But fear not, for this one should make thy proud of thyself.

We would suggest unto this one that she should request a health reading into herself. Can thy understand of which we speak?

"*Yes, I will.*" [She answers.]

Thy have other questions within thy mind. Come unto soul Ray in his awakening state and we shall give unto him the knowledge to answer your questions.

Thy have other questions, ask.

"*Yes, Aka.* [4-14-72-001] *has — just a minute.* [4-14-72-001] —"

We see thy need. And we should answer your question in this manner. The healing that is needed shall be given. We would suggest at the present time the swirl baths be used to this injury. We would further suggest the use of what thy would know as the sunning lamp, starting with three- minute intervals and going forth. We would further suggest massaging at least eight times a day. This must be done very gently.

Thy ask in thy mind of this that the doctor suggests at the present time. We would suggest going unto a specialist, for what is said is not needed at the present time.

We have answered your other questions in prior readings. And we shall say unto this one once again, three days hence from this day, go unto three days of prayer and meditation. Open thy door and we shall enter.

Thy have other questions, ask.

April 21, 1972: *"Aka, [6-9-70-005] has asked for guidance."*
We see thy need and we should answer in this manner. Give unto your Lord, God, that that is His. Give unto your fellow man that that is theirs. But give unto yourself that that is yours. Give unto thyself self-respect, and those things that thy desire, of wedlock, shall come in fulfillment.
Thy have other questions, ask.

April 21, 1972: *"Yes, Aka. [4-21-72-001], and he says, 'I do not fully understand why I have undergone a recent experience.' He is asking for help in this respect."*
Thy have three experiences at the present time within thy mind, and we shall answer them one at a time. Of your first experience, this is your psychic self, that that has been buried beneath the surface, coming forth. Of your second experience, (chuckle) the ways of love and the affairs of the heart are often confusing, even to us. But be patient in this, and your patience shall be rewarded. Of your third question, that of your financial needs, give unto God what is His and He shall give unto thee what is thine.
Thy have other questions, ask.

April 28, 1972: Thy have other questions, ask.
*"Yes, Aka, [5-7-71-001] has requested a life reading."*
Yes, we see thy need. We would suggest, because of the lengthiness of this reading, that this be done at a different time.
Thy have other questions, ask — one moment please.
Yes, yes. Yes, Father.
Yes, we should say unto thee in this manner. Of the treatments unto which she has received, the later adjustment of the same has been done incorrectly. This must be done in a gradual, downward manner. The relieving of the third and fourth vertebrae would greatly relieve the pain unto the same. Unto the eighth and ninth vertebrae — yes, this should be adjusted also. This would greatly relieve the pain. But these should not be done with force; very gradually. If force is used it could cause permanent damage unto the same.
We would suggest that the use of hot olive oil packs be used nightly. This should be done into first, 5-minute intervals, increasing unto 30-minute intervals.
Yes, we see this.
As we have said before, the healing that is needed shall be given.
Of the life reading, this should be asked first, at thy next reading.

April 28, 1972: Thy have other questions, ask.

*"Yes, Aka. I have two questions that bother my mind, even though they seem perhaps trivial. One of them is, I am disturbed if I should continue to go to church because of the problems it presents, but I want to do what is right and that which will make me grow spiritually. The second thing is, I am disturbed about leaving my children so long when I go to Yuma, and I wonder if you could give me any guidance in these matters?"*

We should answer in this manner, first of thy church. You are growing spiritually in the attendance of the same. Fear not, for we shall walk before thee and prepare a way.

Of thy leaving of thy children, we would suggest that an adult be with them. Can you understand of which we speak? This shall be provided at a no material cost unto you. Fear not, for we walk before thee, soul Paul and soul Ruth, for those things that thy should need for the fulfillment of the same have already been done.

May 19, 1972: **And now, of thy question in thy mind, and that of the health of soul Ray — we warned unto thee many times of the strains that could come from mental pressures. We have prepared unto this body many times. Of thy request, this is in God's hands; give unto it prayer. If our gift unto thee has been good, then ask for the healing and it shall be given. If it has been bad unto thee, then do not ask, and it shall not be given.**

**And we shall say unto soul Luke and soul James, and soul Jude, we did not implant in this one we have called a prophet lies, nor has he spoken any unto you of his health. Look within thyself for the truth. It rests there; the knowledge has always been there.**

May 19, 1972: **Thy have other questions, ask.**
*"Yes, Aka. [C____ H___] — "*
Yes, we see thy need. And we should answer in this manner. First, the healing shall be given, if this one can believe in the same. If there is doubt in their mind we may not violate the free will. Yes, there *is* a small, non-malignant growth of the breast area. This could be extracted surgically, and should be done so if there is any doubt of the mind of this one. We would suggest the drinking of the sage tea four times daily. We would further suggest the taking of the Night-blooming Citros [Cereus], at first in quarter-by-quarter cubes, of your inches. We would further suggest the taking of the herbs known as Lydia E. Pinkham in the adult, prescribed of the same.

Of the rash of the same of the vagina area, we would suggest the changing of the washing powder of the same. But, we would say unto this one, thy have proved thy principle, now forget and forgive of the same. And forgiveness shall go before thee.

May 19, 1972: **Thy have other questions, ask.**

*"Yes, Aka.* [4-21-72-002], *the son of D____ T_____ who is here tonight, has received a draft notice."*

We see this. Yes, we see thy need, and as we have said before, there *are* medical reasons that could exempt this one from the draft, as thy know it. By asking with faith these reasons could be removed, or left. But this is of his free choice, not of yours. Let him who wishes ask. Can thy understand of which we speak?

Nay, not fully. Then we would suggest the asking of soul Ray in the awakening state.

May 19, 1972: **And thy say unto us, "How can we stand if this one should be taken, of soul Ray?" But as we promised, he shall be with thee in either form for as long as thy needs shall be.**

Soul Ray now grows weak and tired. And we shall [put] healing into his body.

Awaken soul Ray from his slumber.

June 2, 1972: **Thy have other questions, ask.**

*"Yes, Aka.* [6-2-72-001] *has been having a problem with her husband in that he hides legal papers from her and is abusing her, and she says, 'Could you advise me what to do about my property? Is it in my name only. Can he touch it? It is my living, and I would like to know.'"*

Yes, we see thy need. But first we should answer in this manner. As a man and a woman should come together in wedlock, they should share all things in truth. They should hide nothing from one another. For if love, as thy should know it, should be complete, it must be a thing of sharing, one unto the other.

Of thy legal documents, nay, thy husband cannot, as thy would say, touch this, for the laws of thy land are set up in such a manner that yours is sole and separate property.

But we should say unto this one, thy have guarded this to keep the thieves from thy door, yet, the thieves have crawled beneath the door and still taken. Open thy door in truth. Lay these things before man in truth. And in the light of God, and in the light of man, what lays in the light, a thief shall not steal. Cover it, and the thief shall steal.

June 2, 1972: **Thy have other questions, ask.**

*"Yes, Aka.* [6-2-72-002] *asks, 'I have had an ear infection for over four months, and doctors haven't been able to help me. I am very allergic to foods, drugs, and plants. Can you help me? Any pertinent information would be greatly appreciated. There are other problems that I would like help with, also.'"*

Yes, we see thy need, and we should answer in this manner. Thy body, as each body and the body chemicals should change daily, was not made to live in the climate thy are living in. Therefore, the plant life, the air thy breathe and the water thy drink, is poison unto the same. Go into the higher climate, and thy [current] problem shall take care of itself.

Of thy other problem, we shall answer in this manner. If the heart guides thee, sometimes it should tell thee lies. Let the mind guide thee. Use meditation, both morning and night. If thy should remain where thy are, go unto the [saunic] baths. Graduate these, first, at 5-minute intervals, up to 30-minute intervals.

Thy have problem in backular area, in the menstrual periods of the same. This is due to the organisms of the same not being properly used. These should be brought into adjustment by either osteopathic or chiropractic treatment. Swimming would be a good exercise for this one.

Of thy other question of thy mind, we should say in this manner. Those who would advise these sometimes would speak with false tongues. Do not let this happen. Soul Ray in his awakening state would give unto thee much guidance and advice. Come unto him. Let him speak, that we may speak through him in this manner.

June 2, 1972: **Thy have other questions, ask.**
*"Yes, Aka. I have one other question. [6-2-72-003] says, 'I would like to know if the physical problems I have been having have a physical or mental cause, and what should I do about it?'"*
First, we should say unto this one, go unto thy physician. These can be treated. Proportions, yes, are of a mental nature. Thy have tried to develop thy psychic abilities alone; this is not good. Come into group form and go unto soul Jude for direction and advice. We shall light the way before this one and prepare a haven unto you.

June 14, 1972: **Thy have many questions, ask.**
*"Yes, Aka. I have a number of questions for [9-16-71-001], that is here tonight, and I'd like to ask them one at a time.*
*Her first question is, 'Has the time come that I should change my job, and how could this be done?'"*
This in itself must come from thyself. But we should answer your question in this manner, that that thy seek stands close at hand. Take from it the things [of life] that thy need. Give into others the love that is within thyself to give, and so it shall be returned. But at the present time, should thy change thy job, thy shall find chaos and unhappiness.

Thy have received of one gift. Many shall come, but only as you stand where you are. Can you understand of which we speak?

Nay, not fully.

Then we shall answer in this manner. As your oak stands strong and tall, and forceful against the elements of the same, it gathers much moss. As a willow should bend with the elements, it also should gather much moss. But that that thy seek must come from within thyself. We have opened a door for thy studies of self-development. We have provided unto thee this prophet. Yet, as we have said before, the blind may see, and the deaf may hear, but only if they want to.

June 14, 1972: **Thy have other questions, ask.**
*"Yes, Aka, she [9-16-71-001] asks, 'Should I remain with realistic painting, or should I go into abstract action painting this month?'"*

**Thy should remain with the realistic painting. That of the abstract must belong to a different mind than your own. There are none of the spiritual world which waits to guide you in this other manner. Of the realistic painting, there are many who wait at your fingertips to guide you and give you psychic knowledge of the same.**

June 14, 1972: **Thy have other questions, ask.**
*"Yes, Aka. She [9-16-71-001] has one final question. "Could you recommend a diet for me so that I could lose weight, about 25 pounds?"'"*

**Yes, we see thy need, and we should answer, first, in this manner. Of thy thyroid, this thy should see a physician, for this must be corrected within its same.**

**Your main weight problem is that of loneliness. Therefore, we shall answer further of the diet. First, we would say, for three meals of each day, drinking of one ounce of the safflower oil before each meal.**

**Of thy breakfast, soon shall be of your melon season, eating either of one cantaloupe of the breakfast meal [or of] one glass of milk.**

**For thy luncheon, eating as many of the green vegetables as thy desire, and one glass of milk.**

**Of thy evening meal, once of one day, the green vegetables — yes, this is good — meat, that of the beef, one meal; liver, one meal; of the ocean salt-water fish, one meal; of thy fresh-water fish, one meal. These may be repeated as often of the evening meal as thy desire. One slice of bread may be eaten of each meal. Of one meal each week, thy may eat of that which thy desire, but do not overeat. Always, at all times, leave thyself a little hungry. Take unto thyself a good natural multiple vitamin twice daily. This should supplement of the other thing.**

**That thy breasts should not become, as thy would know, loose, exercises must be done. These thy already know of the same, the cupping of the breasts, first, with the left hand and then of the right, bringing forth and upward and releasing of the same. Of thy thighs, that they, as the weight should be lost, should not drop away, walking at least one-half mile, of the morning, should be done. Of that of the excess that should remain and the sagginess that might appear of the stomach area, taking of the pillow, rolling it into a tight knot, placing it upon the floor and laying upon it, rocking back and forth 30 times each day. In this manner, these muscles shall become firm and come unto thy desired measurements of the same.**

That of the sagginess of around the throat area, this can be done with massage — slowly, easily, do not bruise of this area, in an upward position. We would further suggest that for further health, seeing of a good chiropractic doctor. We find within the backular area strains because of the excess weight into the 8th and 9th vertebrae of the same. This could be easily corrected.

Of thy mental health we should answer in this manner. We have given unto thyself knowledge. We have placed before thee, work, that that should be done unto thy Lord, God. We have shown thee that that that thy desire can be given unto thee. We asked in return your love unto thy Father, and one hour's of work unto this work per day.

June 14, 1972: **Thy have one other question, ask.**
*"Aka, my daughter, [2-4-72-001], has been having a problem with her lips swelling, and she wonders what is causing it?"*
**Yes, we see this. This is because she is allergic to certain growths that has come back anew since your spraying, We should answer in this manner, the healing that is needed shall be given.**

**Remember also, thy daughter is becoming of a full blossom unto the woman form. Part of this swelling has come about during her monthly cycles. Fear them not. As we have suggested before, take of the Lydia E. Pinkham in its natural form, of the adult form, once, and as prescribed daily.**

June 14, 1972: **Now, soul Ray grows very tired. That we should not overtax his body in its present condition, we shall give healing into the same.**
**Now is the time of the Cherub.**
**Awaken soul Ray from his slumber.**

June 16, 1972: **Thy have other questions, ask.**
*"Yes, Aka, [4-21-72-001], who is here tonight, would like a health reading."*
**Yes, we see thy need, and therefore, we have before us the body, soul, and the spirit, and therefore, should say but unto thee [these] words. Thy have faith within thee, for now we shall give unto thee the healing of the body that is needed. We shall reach forward and touch unto thee. All thy must do is go unto three days of prayer. This must not be a continuous thing, but as we should touch you in your slumber tonight, let that feeling grow through thy body, and the healing thy ask for shall be given.**

June 16, 1972: **Thy have other questions, ask.**
*"Yes, Aka. [12-10-71-002's] wife, [5-19-72-001], has heard a prowler around their trailer at night when [12-10-70-002] is at work, and [12-10-71-*

002] *would like to know if there is a prowler and what he should do about it?"*

Yes, we see this. And we should answer in this manner, we would suggest that the notification of your police department. But fear not, for we go before thee to prepare a way, and therefore, no harm shall come unto thy wife or children.

June 23, 1972: **Thy have other questions, ask.**
*"Yes, Aka.* [6-23-72-001] *and* [6-23-72-002] *in Miami, Florida, both have health problems and have asked for help.* [6-23-72-002] *has a bad disk in his back, and can you give any kind of a health reading on him?"*

Yes, we see his need, and therefore, we should say in this manner, we have before us the body, the soul, the spirit, and therefore, the immortal body of the same.

We should answer in this manner. Surgery on this one should be done; the sooner, the better. The problem that lies within can only be corrected in this manner. Relief of the same can be taken within the sauna baths, but it should be only of a temporary thing. For there are pinched nerves within this area that are blocking off other areas. Therefore, only by the opening up and the removing of the same can these be extracted.

Of the other question, we also have before us, the body, the soul, and therefore, the spirit of the same. Yes, we see thy need; then we should answer in this manner. First, of thy emotional problem, thy have not found within thyself the peace of mind to live within thy own body, and therefore, seek that that is on the outside. Thy have also sought to live sometimes beyond thy means, and this, within itself, is a karmic thing. We also find within this one other difficulties. We find that the area thy now dwell in is too moist for thy health.

We also find that rheumatic problems of the same have set forth. This within itself is a virus. This could be taken from this one in this manner — first, with the use of the rays that should come from the sun. This should be done in small proportions daily and building into larger proportions. But you should also realize that these same rays can increase the aging process, if over taken. Therefore, do not overdo this.

Second, we would suggest saunic baths, first, in 5-minute intervals and building up into 30-minute intervals. This should be done. We find many problems of the back and neckular area, therefore, should be sought out by a chiropractic or osteopathic doctor and corrected of the same.

We also find within this one the problem of the varicose veins. There — this, in itself, if thy should consult with your physician, could be taken care of by medication, quite readily. Some shall have to be done by surgery.

But more important than all of these, thy should find within thyself a mental healing, a mental rest. We would suggest that thy should take a short vacation away from thy own family, and therefore, count blessings of thy family within thyself, in this manner.

Further information on this subject will be given as asked for.

June 23, 1972: **Thy have other questions, ask.**
*"Yes, Aka,[4-6-70-003] asks, 'Is my choice of a mate the right one? Do you have any advice on my livelihood? Can you tell me where the missing tools went to?'"*

We should answer, first, in this manner. Your choice of a mate, this thy shall find within thyself. As we have said before, in your choice of a mate find the peace within yourself, your own peace of mind. Do not play one against another. Of the full content of this knowledge, we would suggest that this question be asked in privacy at a different time.

Of thy tools, yes, we see this. And thy in thy own kind already know the answer to this. Therefore, it should not be necessary for us to confirm it.

**Thy have other questions, ask.**
*"Yes, Aka, she asked also about her livelihood."*

Yes, we see thy need. This, as we have said before, has been set forth and taken care of. Thy have taken the step in thy talk with soul Ray. That that was needed to be done has been done. We would suggest further talks with soul Ray on this subject.

June 23, 1972: **Yes, we see thy need, and therefore, should answer unto this one know as [6-23-72-003]. And the peace of mind thy seek should come, but give of it meditation and guidance. Take of the time now that is needed to bring thyself into one again. Consult soul Ray on this subject. These things can be given from himself.**

June 30, 1972: **We have told thee of the things to do for those would suffer from that of the spray of your own area. Yet, these things were not done in full.** [Editor's note: The U.S. Forest Service sprayed a defoliant used in Vietnam, Agent Orange, on the Pinal mountains near Globe, Arizona, about 1969-1970.]

**And now they bring before us this child.**

Yes, we see this, thy need, and we should answer in this manner, of the child, of the [6-30-72-001] child. Yes, we see this. We would suggest that only of the pure drinking water be given unto this child. We would suggest that double quantities of vitamin E be given unto the child, and more of the vitamin A into itself.

We shall say unto thee in these words, we cannot create, only our Father could do of the same, but the healing that is necessary, and that that should come from our Father shall be given. But we should also say unto thee, that that is in the heart of the mother and father, we cannot violate, only should they come in truth and ask for the same can it be given in full.

So we say unto thee, [5-7-71-002], in this manner, we shall stand by the doorway; if it is opened we shall enter, and therefore, do the things that are needed. We can do no more.

June 30, 1972: **Thy have other questions, ask.**
*"Yes, Aka. A life reading was given on [5-7-71-001]. Can anything further be given on this soul, such as earlier or later entries? Is there anything she should know concerning her health?"*
Yes, we see thy need and we should answer in this manner. For further information bring her here, that we may reach into her mind, and therefore, give that that is needed.

Of the other information she seeks, this also can be given. But let her journey forth, and therefore, serve unto the effort of giving of the same. And we shall return her effort and her glory back into her in the manner it is given.

June 30, 1972: **And we should say unto soul Ruth these words. The healing has been given and shall be given. And fear not, for those that are needed shall stand by thy side and give the guidance. But thy must also be patient and let the healing come forth. Do not overstrain or overdo or the lesions shall form in a worse way than before.**

June 30, 1972: **Yes, we see thy need, soul [6-30-72-002], and we should say unto thee these words, of what thy have seen upon this day, the infliction that man has placed upon one another, of this word, cancer. And you say unto us, "Why is there no cure?" And we shall say unto thee, there is of such, but as man was given free choice and the will to find these things for himself, at the present time, the information that is needed for this cure is being given unto those who should listen.**

And we shall say, once again, of the secret of the transplant within the same. And this should come from the sperm of man and from the creation of man — and therefore, brought forth into chemical form, and therefore, applied unto the nervous of the same — and this in itself shall make acceptance of one heart unto another.

Can thy understand if which we speak?
*"Yes."*
Nay, not fully. But your time is soon.

June 30, 1972: **Thy have other questions, ask.**
*"Yes, Aka.[5-19-72-001] says, 'My dog has been missing since the latter part of February. Could you tell me what happened to him? Was he*

*killed, stolen, or if someone took him, can you tell me who? And can we possibly get him back now?'"*

We should answer in this [way] manner. The dog within itself became lost, and therefore, wandered from thy home. The dog may be found in the Miami area, alive and well. It has been accustomed to its new masters. We would suggest that thy should leave the dog where it is at the present time, and therefore, go forth, for there is a new soul of a dog who waits to enter into thy lives, and therefore, should give of thee the protection that is needed.

But we should answer your other question that is within thy mind in this manner. As we have said before, fear not, for we shall give into thy household the protection that is needed.

But we say unto thee, guard, therefore, of that that is in thy heart, and do not be careless with the same.

June 30, 1972: **Yes, we see thy need and we should answer unto this one, in this manner. And the one we shall not speak of in name, yet they shall know that we have touched them.**

Thy have traveled far in thy mind. Thy thoughts have even come to the thought of suicide. Thy have given of thyself in love, and had it thrown unto the ground. And thy cannot understand and have become bewildered.

And we should answer unto you, as once before.

As the disciples of Jesus did see unto that that gave love and it was thrown unto the ground, and therefore, it was crucified — yet, as this one known as Jesus did say unto men, "I have come not to change the Laws or the prophecies of the same, but I have come for this time, to show you the truth of the same." And so, within the resurrection of the same, he did show man the truth.

Yet, man did even take that and misinterpret it and cast it aside. For man was given free will by our Father. And even unto His most beloved son, our Father could not interfere with that of the free will.

And thy have reached and reached again for love. But we say unto thee in these words, thy have stumbled over thy own self. Reach out your hands and we shall provide within thee the bread and wine. And we shall plant within thy mind the seed, and thy shall provide the yeast of the same.

We know that thy do not fully understand of which we are speaking. But we say unto thee, give glory unto thy God and thy God shall give glory unto thee. Put thy God first, and thy God shall put thyself first in this manner, for thy have only to walk away from thy own karma to see the truth.

Soul Ray grows very weary, and therefore, our time has grown short.

And we say unto thee, now is the time of the Cherub.

**Awaken soul Ray from his slumber.**

August 18, 1972: **Thy have many questions, ask.**
*"Yes, Aka, [6-18-72-001} is in the Gila General Hospital with a possible miscarriage, and we've been asked for help for her. Do you have any?"*
Yes, we see thy need, and we shall answer in this manner. The healing that is needed shall be given. And we answer also in this manner, for this one, give unto God that that belongs unto your God. If this is done, then God shall give unto you and show glory into the same.

August 18, 1972: **Thy have other questions, ask.**
*"Yes, Aka. [8-18-72-002] of Sabinal, Texas....He's presently in Central Heights and he is very ill with a gall bladder problem, and asks for help."*
Yes, we see thy need and we should answer in this manner. If the faith was strong, then the healing could be given, but the faith is weak, so therefore, the healers of your earth shall give unto the healing. This should be removed in a surgical manner, but the help that has been asked for shall be given in the same manner.
Thy have other questions, ask.
*"Yes, Aka — "*
One moment. Yes, yes, yes we see thy need, yes.
And we should answer, dust to dust.

August 18, 1972: **Thy have other questions, ask.**
*"Aka, [8-11-72-003], who was given a health reading on June 23, 1972, is working in an American school in Tokyo; she's a teacher... And she has asked for a health or life reading."*
This should be given at a different time.

August 26, 1972: **Thy have many questions, ask.**
*"Yes, Aka. [8-26-72-001] who is here tonight...asks for help. He says, 'Can you give a reason for the pain in my back and recommend treatment?'"*
Yes, we see thy need. And therefore, as a child, thy had what is known as spinal meningitis. This problem was brought forth unto a fall of the same. The lower backular area has decay; therefore, as we have said before, we cannot create. But into thy own mind there is knowledge.
We would suggest that of a good chiropractic or osteopathic doctor. We would further suggest that a bar be erected that thy could barely reach, using this to stretch the backular area, at first, two minutes and increasing up to ten each day. This must be done, the increasing, over a prolonged period. Do *not* overdo this.
We further find problems in the third and fourth vertebrae. This from itself, is caused from a virus. We would suggest a changing, radical

changing within your diet. Cut down on the amount of salt within the diet at the present time. Eat more of the green vegetation. We would not suggest the use of any alcoholic beverage. The spinal fluid, within the same, is at an off-balance at the present time; this must be restored.

There are many other various problems within this soul as it is at the present time. First correct these, and come back and we should answer you other questions.

We say unto thee three words, blessed are they who should wash their clothing in the blood of the Lamb, but cursed are they who should wash it and use it as wine.

August 26, 1972: **Thy have other questions, ask.**
*"Aka, [8-26-72-002] asks for a better understanding of his problems, specifically a life reading."*
Yes, we see thy need. And we should give unto thee this at a different time, for your time is not of needs of this reading. We would suggest that at your next reading this question be asked, but we also see thy need, and we should answer in this manner.

Thy have thoughts in thy mind of a mate, yet thy have prolonged these thoughts. Why should thy be so foolish? You are wasting not only your time, but that of the other. Go forward and make of the earth fruitful unto the same. And as the fruit should come forward, it shall be good fruit.

But we should say unto you in this manner, of this that thy have in mind, our Father should give blessings upon the same. Thy fear only lies within thy own mind.

August 26, 1972: **Thy have other questions, ask.**
*"Yes, Aka. [M___ DeG_____] would like to know how she can improve her sight so she can continue her work?'"*
We have seen the need, and therefore, given forth unto the healing of the same. And we shall continue to do this. Your sight shall improve, and yet again, but we should give unto thee a different sight. That is the sight of the spirit, that thy may look within thyself, that thy may plant a rose. And as the rose should grow within thy soul, so it should grow within thy body, and as all mankind should look into your eyes, they shall find the beauty of the rose, therefore, within.

And we should say unto thee, as your Lady of Guadalupe, so you shall walk in truth before man.

August 26, 1972: **Thy have other questions, ask.**
*"Aka, soul James would like to know what can be done to improve his hearing, as he is going deaf?"*
We should answer your question in this manner. Your deafness is not a physical problem, only a mental one. Your nerves, and then within

the self, is reacting in such a manner to deafen out that which thy do not wish to hear.

As once before, we came unto your home, and therefore, did bring blessings, we shall again, and therefore, restore the house divided. And as the temple shall be built from within, so it shall be built from without, and all things shall come in fulfillment. Pick up thy staff and walk again with us.

August 26, 1972: **Thy have other questions, ask.**
*"Yes, Aka. I just have one other question. Did someone go to soul Ray's house to do him harm on Friday? And could you tell us if our thoughts on this are correct?"*

(**Chuckle.**) **Yes, we see thy need, and we should answer in this manner. For one walked, therefore, to do harm, but within your own words, and within ours, none from either side shall interfere with this work. And therefore, we say unto those, let the dead bury the dead.**

September 1, 1972: **Thy have other questions, ask.**
*"Yes, Aka. I need a health reading tonight on [9-1-72-001]. This person is bothered with depression."*

**Yes, we see thy need, and we shall say into this manner. First, change thy drinking water. Your second problem is in locale of which you live. You must realize that this area has been contaminated. We should answer also in this manner. We would suggest the moving into a different location. Your depression, within itself, is caused from negative ions within your air. If this cannot be found practical, the use of oxygen as a supplement for breathing at different periods during thy day would greatly improve within this one.**

September 1, 1972: **Thy have other questions, ask.**
*"Aka, [9-1-72-002] wishes a health reading, particularly the cause and treatment for the severe pain he is experiencing."*

**Yes, we see thy need. But we do not find this soul at the location thy have given. We would suggest more specific information.**
**Thy have other questions, ask.**

September 8, 1972: **Thy have other questions, ask.**
*"Thank you, Aka. [9-1-72-002]; he has asked for a health reading, particularly because of the severe pain he has been experiencing. He wonders if you could tell him cause and possible treatment?"*

**Yes, we see thy need. One moment, please.**
(**Chuckle**), **we should say unto thee, this is a traveling soul.**
**Yes, that is — yes, now that is better.**
**Yes.**

Yes, we have before us the body, the spirit, and therefore, the soul of the same.

Yes, we find this problem, and therefore, the healing that is needed shall be given. We would suggest that this soul go unto the sauna baths. This should be done at least once daily, for a four-week period. We find this soul should go unto either a good osteopathic or chiropractic doctor, that the corrections, therefore, that could be given would greatly relieve the pain, therefore, within the same.

We see further — yes, we see this — we should answer in this manner, that the soul in question has but little faith. Therefore, we should say unto this one, thy have come unto before us to ask for healing, and we should say unto you these words. Have the faith, of a mustard seed, and it should grow and move the mountains that thy desire to be moved. Build unto our Father a temple, and the temple shall be built within thyself.

We see great emotional problems — yes — here. Upheavals within the mind; doubts within the mind; doubts of yourself and your fellow man. Do unto the things that we have suggested, and then ask for other information, and it shall be given upon your request.

September 15, 1972: **Thy have many questions, ask.**

*"Yes, Aka. [9-15-72-001], he's almost six years old — the parents ask for healing of the asthma*

*and hay fever condition, and any instructions you can give them regarding the general health of his body in the future. Also, is he being helped from the antigen injections he is receiving, and should they continue them?"*

Yes, we have before us, therefore, the body, the soul, [the] spirit, and therefore, the immortal body of the same. Yes, the injections should be continued. But the main problem of the child, within itself, is within the area that thy now dwell. Because of the pollution of the air, this, in itself, should increase and destroy the membranes within the [nasal] area, causing infection into the sinus area, And if not corrected, could cause damage unto the [lung] area. Therefore, we see thy need, and we should provide the healing that is needed.

But we should say unto thee in these words. We are not great, we cannot create; only our Father can do this. Therefore, take the precautions that are needed. Install in thy home filters of the air. These are known to you, and should not be beyond your budget. If this is done in this manner, this would greatly improve the health of the child in general.

We would further suggest, that the taking of the sage tea, twice daily. We would further suggest the using of the Night-blooming Cereus, once daily, for one week, in quarter-by-quarter of your inches, of cubes of the same. This is all on this subject at this time.

*"Thank you, Aka."*

**Should farther —**
*"Excuse me, Aka."*
**help be needed, ask, and it shall be provided.**

September 15, 1972: **Thy have other questions, ask.**
*"Yes, Aka. We have a request for a health reading for [M_____ J__*
*H_____], Yuma, Arizona....He is eleven and a half months old. And he*
*has a rash on his face, chest and arms that is not being cleared by the*
*medicine that is being used. They have seen a doctor at some time, sometime*
*ago; he said that it was infant eczema. But it has not been cleared and is*
*spreading."*

**Yes, we see thy need, and therefore, we should say first unto these words. We have before us the body, the soul, the spirit, and therefore, the immortal body of the same. One moment, please.**
**Yes.**

**We would suggest that a skin specialist be consulted. That that has been given is not correct. We would suggest in this manner, that of the glands that provide the moisture unto the body are, therefore, producing an overabundance of the salt form. Reduce from the salt intake unto the child.**

**We would further suggest — yes. One moment.**
**Yes. Yes, we see this.**

**We find a blood disorder. Therefore, we would suggest the vitamins be given unto the child, with more of the B's. We would suggest a changing of the diet in this form, that by blending, using of the raw, natural vegetables, the blending of these, it should make them easy to digest, crushing and blending. Can you understand of this?**
*"Yes."*

**This is very important, the crushing and blending of the natural vegetation. This must be given unto the child. At the present time the child is very low in a natural vegetation. We would further suggest that of the Vitamin C, that that should come from the orange juice, this should be given unto the child, more of the same. If this is not practical, then use of the lemon juice; extract this, using small quantities of honey from your local locale to sweeten the same, using good pure drinking water unto the same.**

**We would also suggest that the child should see a good skin specialist in this area. This would require — because of your lack of doctors within the area itself, we would suggest that in your land of the mythical bird of Phoenix — yes, this would be suggested; this would be good. This would not only ease the problem of the child, but the problem of the mother. You must realize that part of the rash, that the child is picking up from the mother the feelings of anxiety, and therefore, should appear upon the mother and child in the same manner. Can you understand of which we speak?**

*"Yes, Aka."*

**Thy have other questions, ask.**

*"Aka, you mentioned pure drinking water. Is the water of the Yuma area pure enough, or should this be bottled water?"*

**For this child, we would suggest the bottled water, at the present time. Your Yuma water contains too much salt.**

September 15, 1972: **You have other questions, ask.**

*"Yes, Aka. We have a problem with another child of the same family. [D___ C_____ H_____] has been having peculiar things happen. He received a bump on his head that he said happened here at my house, grandma's house. He said that someone closed and locked a door on him. [Aka chuckles] We wondered if it was imagination, or if something did happen?"*

**We should answer in this manner. Go back unto the child's first reading, and therefore, you shall find that the child's psychic abilities are sometimes more surprising to that of the adult. The child, in slumber, should experience out-of-body experiences within the same, or as you would know it, astral travel. As a child should learn to crawl and then to walk, his experiences in astral travel, sometimes he shall fall. But he shall know where he fell. It is not of his imagination, but that within reality of the same. We know thy do not fully understand of which we speak, but as we have said before, we shall prepare the ways through the children, also.**

**Thy have other questions, ask.**

*"Aka, is there any reason to worry about someone shaking his bed?"*

**Nay.**

*"He's been awakened twice."*

**Nay. His playmates, within his astral world, he can control. As we have said before, the door is open; therefore, we shall enter and give the protection that is needed, but none but the children of God shall enter unto the same. Therefore, worry not of these. We shall stop the shaking of the bed.**

September 15, 1972: **Thy have other questions, ask.**

*"Aka, I have no further questions tonight."*

**Yes, we see thy need, and therefore, we should answer in the mind of one. And we shall answer in this manner. For that that is beautiful within thy heart, let it blossom and grow forth. Fear not.**

September 22, 1972: **And we shall answer also of the one who dwells in the valley below the sea.** [Editor's note: Yuma, Arizona.]

**Yes.**

**The healing that is asked for shall be given.**

September 22, 1972: **And now, we should answer your other question in this manner. You must realize that your air is heavily polluted with the chemicals that drift from your smelters.** [Editor's note: in Globe, Arizona.]

**This, within it same, in the quantity that it is now forced into your air, is highly dangerous to your bloodstream. This, in the same, could and is causing forms of leukemia. This is also causing the pollution of your water streams once again. This will also kill off most of your plant and vegetable life if it is not soon stopped. The damage to the respiratory system is increasing.**

September 22, 1972: *"Aka, if soul [4-3-70-001] installed an air conditioning system which he has been considering and put in a chemical filter, would this help his blood problem?"*

**Yes, this would greatly help his blood problem.**

*"Thank you."*

September 22, 1972: **One moment please.**

**Yes, we see thy need, soul [9-1-72-003], and that that thy have not obtained of the Night-blooming Citros [Cereus] within the same. And we see thy effort put forth upon the same. And therefore, we should answer in a different form then.**

**Take of the mistletoe in one part, take of the hops in the second part, taking of castor oil of the third part, mixing thoroughly, making a compress, placing this upon the child's throat and lung area. Taking of the eucalyptus leaves and mixing within the same — these must be crushed into fine pulp; it is far better if they come in their green state. But do not allow the child to eat any of this. Then, over the same, making hot compresses. This should be done in morning and evening. Do you understand of which we speak?**

*"Yes, Aka."*

September 22, 1972: **And now we speak unto soul Ruth [8-10-70-001]. And we see thy needs. And as we have said before, these shall come as needed. Fear not, for we shall see unto the safety of thy family. Can you understand of which we speak?**

*"I think so."*

September 22, 1972: **Now is the time of the Cherub.**

**We should suggest this message unto soul Ray. If there is confusion or irritation on the mind, do not attempt to reach trance state. This, within itself, is what harmed you once before.**

**Now is the time of the Cherub.**

**Awaken soul Ray from his slumber.**

October 6, 1972: **You have many questions, ask.**

*"Yes, Aka. [10-20-72-002] has been bothered by something bunching up the mattress of her bed, causing her to sleepwalk.[19-71-002] has moved the bed and put up a white cross which seems to help, but would like to know the cause of the problem and if she should take any other steps?"*

Yes, we see thy need. And we should say in this manner, take that of the ankh and place it at the head of the bed, and nothing more shall happen.

October 20, 1972: **Thy have other questions, ask.**

*"Aka, [10-20-72-001], and he has a high blood pressure problem; he's asking help with that."*

Yes, we see thy need. And we should answer in this manner. Go unto your health food centers and purchase, therefore, of the compound of the low cholesterol form of the same. This knowledge is known unto those. We would further suggest the taking of the vitamin C and E in larger quantities.

We would further suggest the changing of the diet as it is within the form. We would suggest the eating of no fried foods at all. All food should either be broiled within its natural juices, or the use of the safflower of the same. Before the eating of any meal, we would suggest the taking of one ounce of safflower oil. This can be done either of the liquid or the pill form.

For the breakfast, we would suggest the eating of no more than one piece of white bread, toasted; no more than one glass of milk. We would suggest taking out of thy diet any form of tea or coffee except that of the sage tea. This should be sweetened with the natural honey of thy own region.

For thy luncheon thy may eat as many of the green vegetables as thy desire and one glass of milk.

For thy evening meal, and this should be eaten early in the evening, that thy should have at least four hours of awakening time before thy rest, we would suggest the eating of the liver of the beef and as many of the raw vegetables as thy desire. For thy dessert, we would suggest taking of good milk and bananas. This should be taken in moderate terms.

This should be eaten at least three times per week. Of thy fourth time per week, the eating of beef of thy own choosing, but no more than one-half pound of beef, again with as many raw vegetables as thy desire and no more than one potato. Thy may add unto thy diet that of the tapioca- type puddings. This may be done for two of thy days per week.

For one day of thy week, the eating of the salt-water fish, again with as many of thy raw vegetables as thy desire, and the eating of the okra in a cooked form. Again, thy can choose either of the tapioca or the banana for thy dessert.

Of thy seventh day thy should fast of the morning, eating very lightly of thy luncheon, and for thy evening meal, that of the fresh water fish of the same. Thy may eat of any other cooked of raw vegetables thy desire with this. And thy may eat of any of thy pudding or pie desserts of the natural form thy desire.

We should further suggest the use of the sauna baths, for this one is also inclined, at times, through heredity, to contact the virus known as arthritic. This would greatly help within these areas.

We would further suggest — yes, we see this — due to a fall from a chair, the eighth and the ninth vertebrae has been dislocated. We would suggest that, through the use of either an osteopathic or chiropractic doctor, these be placed back within alignment.

There are other suggestions that could be given. If they are asked for at a later time they shall be given. This is all on this soul at this time.

October 20, 1972: **Thy have other questions, ask.**
*"Yes, Aka. [11-16-70-003] has a rash under his ears that has been bothering him, and I wonder if you can tell us what we should do for it or what he should change? What would help?"*
Yes, we see thy need. And we would suggest taking of the vitamin E, adding soda unto the same and the white of an egg, making of a compound of the same, and placing, as a salve, on these areas. This should be repeated for at least two weeks. We would further suggest that more citrus be added unto the diet of the same at the present time.

October 20, 1972: **Thy have other questions, ask.**
*"Aka, [10-20-72-002], the daughter of [2-19-71-002], needs a health reading. Her address, just a minute, she's at home, Aka, which is...."*
We would suggest that more specific information be obtained. We find within this person no radical problems.
*"It's a digestive upset, Aka."*
This, within itself, is only a temporary virus, and that of a temper tantrum within the child. We find no radical changes within this child that are needed. The only suggestion that we would make is the taking away of some of the sweet, sugary forms that have been within the diet. Too many of these are not good for the growth of the child.

October 27, 1972: **Thy have many questions, ask.**
*"Yes, Aka. Could you tell me what I should do to correct the problem of severe headaches that I have occasionally?"*
Yes, we see thy need, and we should answer in this manner. Increase thy dosage of vitamin E. Do so in this manner. Add the vitamin E to the sage tea, of one capsule per cup. Increase the amount of natural honey into the same.

October 27, 1972: **Thy have other questions, ask.**

*"Thank you, Aka. [9-1-72-003] asks for a health reading for her son,
[10-27-72-001]. She says, 'We would like to know what causes the ear and
throat infections, and how to treat them or prevent them? Also, is there any
other problem we should be aware of?'"*

**Yes, we see thy need. And as we have said before, the filtering of
the air in this location, this would greatly to help improve this child's
health.**

**One moment, please. Yes, we see this. Therefore, we have before
us the body, the soul, the spirit, and the immortal body of the same.**

**We would suggest giving the child more of the vitamin E and the
vitamin B, adding to the diet more of the raw vegetable form within the
same. We would further suggest taking of the vitamin E capsule, adding
small quantities of olive oil, warming this, slightly, to body temperature,
using an eyedropper and placing three drops in each ear once a day.**

**This is all on this subject at this time.**

October 27, 1972: **Thy have other questions, ask.**

*"Thank you, Aka. [11-27-71-005], and she needs a health
reading...She has a problem of boils."*

**We would suggest a direct location be given of the soul at the
present time. We do not find this soul.**

*"At 30 Atkin Street."* [A woman says.]
**We do not find this soul.**

October 27, 1972: **Thy have other questions, ask.**

*"Yes, Aka. [6-11-71-003], and he is concerned about his health. Can
you help him?"*

**Yes, we see thy need. One moment, please.**
**Thy should ask thy question of the last soul again.**
*"Of [6-11-71-003]?"*
**Nay.**

October 27, 1972: *"Of [11-27-71-005]. She would like to know about
her problem with boils."*

**We shall answer in this manner. The soul does not reside within
the quarters thy mention; therefore, we have found the new residence of
this soul.**

**And therefore, we would suggest in this manner, that the stopping
of the use of the regular soap for cleansing that is used at the present
time; we would suggest the using of germatic soap in its place. This can
be purchased at any of your drug stores.**

**Yes, we see this. Of thy present medication, these are good. They
should be balanced with the system; in their present form they are too
strong, and therefore, causing increased nervous condition. This must be**

determined, also that the subject in mind is a highly neurotic person. We would further suggest psychiatric treatment for the same.

October 27, 1972: **You have other questions, ask.**
*"Yes, Aka...."*
Yes, we see thy need, of [6-11-71-003]. We would suggest good, natural vitamins be used, a more substantial diet within the same, stronger within the protein of the same. We would further suggest more rest at the present time for this subject.

We see a dissatisfaction within the soul itself, a searching for the spirit and immortal body, which this soul believes has not within the same, but we should answer in this manner. We have before us the body, the soul, the spirit, and the immortal body of the same. Therefore, *all* is in accord.

October 27, 1972: **Thy have other questions, ask.**
*"Yes, Aka. [2-19-71-002], her daughter, [10-20-72-002], has been having trouble with someone shaking her bed and she's been frightened by it, and she wonders if you could identify the person or the cause of this problem?"*
We are not allowed to give identification in the manner in which thy speak, but that that was a problem has been taken care of, into some form. We have suggested the use of the ankh. This, in itself, has not been done. Therefore, we would suggest the use of the Christian cross be placed at both the front and the head of the bed. The problem, in itself, shall be taken care of in this manner. That of the shaking of the bed is but a small child of the spiritual form. It shall not harm the child. It only desires love.

We shall send those who should give it love and take it unto its Father's arms.

November 24, 1972: **Thy have many questions, ask.**
*"Yes, Aka. [9-1-72-003] asks, 'Did the Night-blooming Cereus cause the attack [11-24-72-001] had today about 3:30 p.m.? If not, what, and is there anything we should give him?'"*
We should answer in this manner. As long as thy air remains polluted and as long as the wind of the same area should carry the pollution into your area, this problem can remain. At the present time, you may treat the cause, but until this problem is corrected, you cannot achieve a cure. We shall give the healing that is needed into this one. Fear not. Have faith.

November 24, 1972: **Thy have other questions, ask.**
*"Yes, Aka. I am still having a problem with very severe headaches. Is this the same thing that is causing them?"*

Yes. This problem has covered your land. Continue as we have suggested; then this problem shall turn away from thyself. *

But we shall answer yet further. Within thyself, we have placed that of soul Paul. But not as the same, for soul Paul should overcome his arrogance. This was his karma of before. He must overcome and become humble before himself. This is a fight within yourself, a turmoil of the same and of your own making. As we have said before, give that unto God that belongs to God; give that unto yourself that belongs to yourself; give that unto mankind that should belong to mankind, in this order. If this is done, then you shall make peace with yourself. For as we have said before, there is Saul, and there is Paul; they must come into one.

Cast aside that of suspicion from your nature. If there is a sword, be patient and wait. If there is grain to plant, plant that first. But do not take up the sword until the grain has been harvested.

We know that thy do not understand fully of which we speak, but the healing that is needed shall be given. But the knowledge that is needed shall be given also. For three days we shall enter into thy mind and implant new knowledge. This shall come in your awakening state and your dream state. At first, you shall feel confused and sometimes bewildered, but fear this not, for as we have said before, now the brook shall flow to the rivers, parts of all things shall flow into the ocean, and there the seed shall begin to grow. And soon it shall be ready for harvest. But do not harvest too soon, but wait until God has placed His hand upon the kernels of grain and they shall be in full blossom of the same.

*Editor's note: The U.S. Forest Service had sprayed Agent Orange on Pinal Mountain near Globe, Arizona. Those who lived in the canyons below received much water runoff and contamination and had serious health consequences.

December 15, 1972: **Thy have other questions, ask.**
*"Aka, [5-7-71-002] asks what they should be doing at this time in regard to their water situation at their ranch?"*

We have already answered this question in a prior reading. Do these things we have asked of you and your problem shall be no more.

December 22, 1972: **You have other questions, ask.**
*"Aka, [2-19-72-002]'s mother, [10-29-71-002], is in the hospital.... Do you have any advice for her health?"*

Yes, we see thy need. And we should answer in this manner. The problems within this soul, the body of the same, are many and numerous. For there is a time for birth, and a time that dust should go to dust. There is a time for waiting, and a time when the soul and the spirit and the immortal body shall join in fullness. This is not a time of sadness. We should suggest that kindness be given unto this one; that is the best medicine of all, and love and respect for that that has been given unto you.

December 29, 1972: **Thy have many questions, ask.**

*"Yes, Aka. Soul Ruth has noticed a change in her chemical balance. Is this some change you are making, or should she seek to readjust this?"*

**Nay, we should answer in this manner. The body chemicals are changing. We shall make the adjustments that are necessary for this time. At a later time you should seek out a physician, for soon your time shall come for other chemical changes. But we shall see the balance is kept within the perspective of the entry we have placed within the same.**

December 29, 1972: **Thy have other questions, ask.**

*"Aka, [2-19-71-001] is having trouble with soft corns growing between her toes. Can you tell her what she should do for this?"*

**Yes, we see thy need. And we should answer in this manner; the healing thy ask for shall be given. Go unto three days of prayer, and upon the third day, your illness shall be no more.**

# 1973 Health Readings

January 5, 1973: **You have other questions, ask.**

*"Yes, Aka. [8-24-70-001] is having trouble swallowing air, pain in her diaphragm. Can you —"*

**We see they need, and the healing that is needed shall be given. We should say unto you in this way, words. As your spray has happened, and as the deformities of the same within the land, so it did infect the animals. Your spray is gone, but the infected animals remain in your household. Remove these, and your problem shall end.**

**You have other questions, ask.**

*"Yes, Aka. I don't understand which animals you mean. Do you mean our dogs, our goats, our cats?"*

**Nay, none of these. The fowl.**

*"The parrot, Aka?"*

**Yes.**

January 5, 1973: *"Yes, Aka [from 1-21-72-002]. I don't mean to be faltering in what I am asking, but when you spoke of our parrot, he is a very dear friend of mine, and I'm willing to do what I should, but do you mean for me to kill him? What may I do with him that would not be harmful to others?"*

**We should answer your question in this manner. We have told on you and your household to take of the sage tea. Should you deny this soul that that you should take upon of yourself to cleanse of his body? Do of the same unto the parrot, and the parrot's age shall increase and health shall increase. Give unto the parrot that of the vitamin E within its food, and the problem should soon disappear, and the healing shall come in complete into your household.**

**Deny not one creature upon the earth that that our Father has given unto you.**

January 5, 1973: **And we should say unto this one known as Peter, we shall give healing into the same.**

**And we should say unto this one known as Ruth, we should give healing into the same. And we should say unto this one, of thy children's and thy family, we shall give healing. Increase thy doses of vitamin C and E into your family usage.**

**Awaken soul Ray from his slumber.**

January 5, 1973: *"Aka, [2-19-71-002] asks, 'Will a child be born of this marriage?'"*

As we have said before, we see thy karma and we shall answer in this manner. Give that unto your Lord that should belong to your Lord. Give that unto your husband that should belong unto your husband. And therefore, prepare the way for the coming of a soul into your household.

January 12, 1973: **You have many questions, ask.**

*"Yes, Aka. I have a request for a health reading from [1-12-73-001]. She says that she is having a cough which the doctors have been unable to help her with. Can you tell her what could be done for this?"*

Yes, we see they need, and we should answer your question in this manner. The pollution of your air has caused permanent damage in the bronchial area and also permanent damage into the sinus area. We would suggest that at the present time that this soul should take up residence by the ocean. That of that salt water would clear this. We should also suggest for a period of time staying away from all chemical form, such as thinners for your paint. Only rest at this period shall clear this problem up. If this is done, within a two-month period you could return back unto your homeland.

We find other physical problems within this soul. Therefore, we should say that these should be inquired about at a different time.

If it is impractical to remove yourself from this location, then filter your air into which thy should dwell. Bring forth of the salt water, that this should be added through your heating unit and mixed with your air.

February 9, 1973: *"Yes Aka. It's awfully good to have you back with us tonight. Aka, soul Ray asks for a health reading."*

We should answer in this manner. Soul Ray has gone through the ritual of asking for a health reading. But he does not want the words that we would say, said before all, so therefore, we should give a health reading into himself at a different time.

*"Thank you.. Aka, [2-09-73-001], [1-21-72-002]'s father, has asked for a health reading. He's asked for help in regards to his health."*

One moment, please.

Yes.

One moment. Yes, now we have the subject. Therefore, we have before us the body, the soul, the spirit, and the immortal body of the same. Yes, we see this.

We find, therefore, minor problems of health within this one. Most of these are brought about by over worry, and overweight. At the present time, we would suggest unto this one the use of sauna baths for the circulatory system.

Yes, yes, we see this.

We find, as you would call them, fatty growths in the backular area. We do not see, at the present time, that surgery should be needed to remove these. But from many hours spent sitting (tsk), the whole backular area needs work. We would suggest a visit to either an osteopathic doctor or a chiropractic doctor. We would further suggest — yes, we see thy need, yes — that more exercise be used. But this should be done on a gradual basis, starting with five to ten minutes per day and increasing a little more each day. If this subject should require one, we should give diet of the same at a later time.

We find the problem of varicose veins, left leg. We would not suggest the massaging of these, nor packs. We would suggest the use of banana oil before, in a poultice be made and laid to the area before his slumber. This should be continued over at least a six-week's period.

But we should answer one other question unto this one, and that, of the dragon that lays within his work area. The fear of this one is within yourself. Do not allow the fear to grow.

Strike away the fear, but do so within yourself, not into others.

But we should answer your other question in this manner. Give unto yourself that that is yours. Give unto your brother that that is his. Give unto your God that that is your God's. If these things are done in this order, your God, who has waited long, shall help you in the giving and in the protecting of both.

This is all on this subject at this time.

March 2, 1973: *"Yes, Aka. My first question, [2-4-72-001] is worried about her head. Can you give any information to ease her mind or hasten her healing?"*

We shall hasten the healing that is needed. Soul Ray should go unto this place and give healing in our Father's name, to give healing, to bring glory unto our Father, and our Father should give glory unto this person you have spoke of. And the healing shall come.

But let her listen well unto the words we should place unto his mind.

March 9, 1973: Yes, we see they need. And we shall say unto this soul who is present these words, for thy possess within thyself a secret question.

And first, we should answer in this manner. If good came from the field of good, and righteousness came from this same field, would you cast it aside, or would you bring it forth and become a better man yet still? For a marriage to blossom forth, it should take two in the making. But we should answer your question in this manner. Too many hands in the dough should spoil the batter.

March 30, 1973: You have many questions, ask.

*"Yes, Aka. I have one question about the depression. When will this come, and how long will it last?"*

**We shall tell of thee things. But first, pick up your hoe, and show us the faith.**

March 30, 1973: **You have other questions, ask.**
*"Yes, Aka. I would like to ask blessings for* [12-4-70-001] *who is in St. Joseph's hospital in Phoenix. Also,* [2-19-71-001] *has been upset and is unable to keep on her diet, and she asks help with this and with finding a suitable place to live for her mother."*
**Yes, we see thy need, and we shall provide within the same.**

March 30, 1973: **You have other questions, ask.**
*"Yes, Aka.* [3-30-73-001] *who is here tonight…Do you have anything that you can say to him on his health? Can we have blessings for him?"*
**We see thy need, and we find, therefore, the body, soul, and the spirit, and therefore, we find the immortal body of the same. And we find, therefore, within this, great confusion, because of the injury you have suffered.**

**Yes, we see this.**

**But we should answer in this manner. We shall place the wine before you. Take it up and drink it. And the yeast shall come forword, and therefore, provide the bread.**

**We should answer in this manner, your injury is but a fleeting thing. New tissue shall be provided within the damaged area.**

**But you ask of your spiritual growth and of your confusion within the same. And we say unto thee in these words. Give glory unto your Father. Give thought and meditation unto the righteous path and it shall be provided before you. Cast aside your doubts, and the needs of yourself shall come forth. But we say unto you, see to the needs of others also.**

March 30, 1973: **You have other questions, ask.**
*"Yes, Aka. Is there anything that we can do to help* [3-3-72-001] *in Gila General Hospital?"*
**We shall answer in this manner. For the passing shall come, and there shall be no pain. But give prayers unto this one that he may forgive himself. If he should do unto this, first forgiving unto others, then he should open the door once again, and within his vision of the passageway of the one known as Jesus Christ, then he shall be the messenger that should go up into our Father's kingdom.**

April 13, 1973: *"Aka, soul Ruth and soul Ray have been experiencing intense prickling. Can you give them the cause and treatment of this condition?"*

Yes, we see thy need. Of soul Ruth's problem, she has been picking up mental messages from soul Ray. The problem is within the medication taken. It would be suggested that soul Ray reduce the amount to one capsule per day.

It would also be suggested that the eating of more meat in his diet. He should eat smaller amounts, but more often. It is needed at this time of the red meat of the beef. It is also suggested that he do less strenuous exercises for a short period of time. We have seen the need here.

April 13, 1973: *"Aka, soul Ruth asks about faith, especially in relationship to working out karmas."*

We shall answer in this manner. We have told you the parable of toil. And toil shall be faith. And faith shall be love. And love shall be God. For as all things in the beginning were of God, therefore, all things were of good. Yet, as time passed, even before the first entry, some brought forth harmony that was not good.

Therefore, karma is like harmony, as though you had strung a bow, yet had a weakness within the bow and fear of shooting the bow that it might break. But if the bow is repaired, the arrow shall go straight and true and pass through all waste. But faith, without that faith the bow could not be repaired. The arrow could not be shot, and therefore, you would stand in the same place that you stood in the beginning and have climbed not to nowhere.

April 20, 1973: *"Yes, Aka. [4-20-73-001] is having a glandular imbalance and skin and back problems, and she asks for help to improve her health."*

Yes, we see thy need. And first, we should say in this manner, we have before us the body, the soul, and the spirit. But we should answer in this manner. Let this one go unto meditation and ask again, and we shall give the healing that is needed. The position of the body at this time does not permit a reading.

April 27, 1973: *"Aka, [5-7-71-001], who is here tonight, is concerned about her plans to retire, and if it's all right. She says, 'Should I plan to retire from my job this coming September?'"*

Yes, we see thy need, and we shall answer your question in this manner. Plan to do so, but also plan to fill your garden, that the mind and the body can become abundant. You have long sought out the spiritual needs of others. Now become a part of the same. Fear not that you should be [radical], or ridiculed, for your knowledge within the spiritual realm has become of great value. Sow this seed, and reap its harvest. Fear not for your health, for when you reap the harvest your health problem shall end.

May 4, 1973: *"Yes, Aka. [5-4-73-001] asks three or four questions. She asks for both health and life. She said, 'How can I best work for God and my fellow man? How can I cure the red spots on my arms, legs, and feet? And also, should my daughter sell their house in Tucson or rent it? If sell, how soon?'"*

First, we shall take the last, and we shall answer within this manner. The house should be sold. Do so immediately. A fair price shall be given for the same.

Of the healing, we shall answer in this manner. Go unto three days of meditation, and the healing shall be given. All you must do within thy mind is see that the red spots would disappear from thy body. If you shall provide the faith, we shall provide the wine and the yeast, and the healing within the body shall be complete.

Of the life reading, we would suggest this be asked at a different time.

May 4, 1973: *"Aka, [4-20-73-001] who is here tonight has asked for a health reading. She has glandular imbalance and a skin and back problem, and she has asked for recommendations to improve her health."*

Yes, we see thy need, and therefore, we have before us the body, the soul, the spirit, and the immortal body.

Yes, we see this.

We find a great imbalance within the diet of the same. First, we would suggest a diet. We should suggest that this one does not drink of the safflower oil, but this one should take of the safflower tablets, two before each meal. We would suggest that this one should eat as much of the natural green vegetation as possible. We should also suggest that this one should use — yes, we see this — a salt substitute. We would also suggest that this one eat a very minimum of sugar within the diet.

We would further suggest that this one go unto the sauna baths. This should be done in a gradual manner, no more in the beginning than five minutes at a time, increasing this up to 30 minutes in a day. We would further suggest the third and fourth vertebrae be adjusted within the backular area.

We find — yes — lacking of the vitamin E and A.

We would also suggest — yes — one moment, please.

Yes, we see this — problem in the vagina area — yes — infection. We would suggest more often washing of this area, preferably with the, not an acid-type wash, very mild wash. That that is being used is very dangerous. It is causing irritation, could cause cancerous-type growth if continued.

We would suggest increasing — yes — of the vitamin B; great lacking in this. We should add, within thy diet this should be supplemented. We would suggest eating four meals per day for a short period of time, building content. We would also suggest that this subject is a borderline diabetic; we would suggest eating of the Jerusalem artichoke. This should be done immediately, eating as much as you desire. Do not, in any way — we would also suggest that the charring of wood, preferably oak wood, charring and eating of the char itself. Do not eat a great amount of this, very small amounts.

Yes, we see this.

We should also add magnesium to the diet. We would suggest being very careful in the amount of calcium; we see an over amount of calcium in the diet at this time.

We would also suggest the rinsing the skin in a light vinegar and honey together, rinsing the skin, sponging the skin, taking away the moisture in this manner. This should be done for at least one week because of the high acid discharge that shall come from the body during this treatment.

If further information is needed, we would suggest a follow-up reading on this subject in a two-week period.

May 4, 1973: *"Thank you, Aka. Aka,* [5-4-73-002 of Tucson] *asks, 'What can I do to get rid of this fungus on my feet?'"*

We should answer in this manner. This one should take of the chaparral. This could be bought locally at your health food stores. We would also suggest that at least four capsules be dissolved in one quart of water and the feet be soaked in them. We would further suggest that the taking of baking soda, the chaparral, vitamin E, and the white of an egg, mixed together, making a poultice for the feet at night, if this is done, within one week this problem shall be no more.

We also find on this subject [a] problem that is common within your teenagers, too much sweets, causing blemishes within the complexion area. We would suggest that this same compound be used on the facial area. This should clear this up.

We would further suggest that more of the vitamin E be given unto this person. We also find an imbalance of iron. We would further suggest that more of the vitamin A and D be given, and pantothenic acid.

Yes, we see this.

May 11, 1973: *"Yes, Aka.* [5-11-73-001, of Tucson, Arizona] *who is here tonight...has asked for help in regards to his health, specifically diabetes, asthma and eye problems, and has asked for guidance in what he can do about these?"*

Yes, we see thy need, and therefore, we should answer in this manner. First, we should say unto this one, behold, for we bring healing from our Father into thy soul, thy body, and thy spirit, and therefore, the immortal body shall come whole again. We shall take from thee thy karma. But we leave in you these words, and remember them always — for what we have given, give unto others.

Therefore, we have before us the body, the soul, the spirit, and the immortal body of the same.

Yes, we find in this subject that of the dry sinus. This is caused by too dry a climate into which he dwells. It would be first suggested that this subject go into a higher altitude to dwell. The altitude and climate, both, of this land that is polluted — the air is polluted, the water is polluted of the same.

If this cannot be done financially within the family means, we would suggest, first, that sea water be brought forth and a humidifier placed within the home; second, the filtering of the air within the home. Third, we would suggest the changing of the diet — and if the diet is not changed, all that we can do will be undone.

First, the subject should have much more of green vegetation. Place before the subject of the green olives that the subject should be encouraged to eat them, [as] much as the body should demand. Second, adding to the diet that of the Jerusalem artichoke, this should be eaten whole and raw. We would suggest the eating of two to three whole of this daily for the subject.

We would further suggest, we find within the subject — yes — great deficiency in the vitamin and mineral substance of the same, of the chemicals. We would suggest much more of the vitamin E. We would suggest at least 1,000 units per day.

Yes, we see this.

We would further suggest more of the vitamin C, adult dosage. We would further suggest that meat, of the beef, be given into the subject at least three times weekly. This should be given as raw as the subject could eat it. Can you understand of which we speak?

Nay, not fully. This within itself is very important into the diet. Before each meal, the subject should be given in capsule form that of the safflower oil, one to two tablets before each meal. This should be done 30 minutes before the meal is eaten.

We would also suggest that breathing exercises be used. But this can only be done in clean air. The breathing exercises should go in this manner: first, breathing in, very, very deeply, filling the lungs [to] capacity. Do not hurt or damage the lungs. Let this subject breathe in till he feels within himself that the lungs are full, and then out, increasing this daily. We find a lack of oxygen in the blood, therefore, a lack of oxygen being fed unto the brain itself. This is not good. We would suggest within the diet the eating of more of the green vegetation. This will place within the blood system itself of the oxygen in which the body needs at this time.

We see the fear within the parents of the child's health problem. As a result from the same, this has placed fear within the child. This is not good. It would be suggested that this child should be encouraged in his health, told, quite often, of his improvement in his health. This will feed the mind the medicine that is needed, helping the mind to overcome the obstacle of the health problem.

Of the eye problem, this in itself can be corrected. We should suggest that the child be taught to meditate. If the child shall go unto three days, of 15 minutes of meditation, we shall restore the eyesight. It shall never be restored into what you would call 20-20 vision, but it shall be more than adequate to serve his lifetime.

We would further suggest that the subject be encouraged in both of the art, of the drawing of obstacles [objects?], subjects, buildings, and such. In a prior lifetime this subject was a renowned architect. His desire now is a carryover from that time. He would excel himself in this area.

Yes.

This is all on this subject at this time. Should further information be needed, it would be suggested that a follow-up reading be given on this subject in a three-week period.

May 16, 1973: *"Aka, [5-16-73-001], she's presently at home, she has asked for a health reading, specifically she has been having a problem with a bladder infection."*

Yes, we see of this, and we should answer in this manner. We have before us the body, [the] soul, the spirit, and the immortal body. First, we should say in this manner. The subject in mind is not at the location which has been given, but we have before us the knowledge needed.

First, we should answer in this manner, change of your drinking water. Your heavy chlorination is causing cancerous growths within this area.

Second, we would suggest the taking of the Jerusalem artichoke, using this in small proportions twice daily. We would further suggest the use of what you would know as the sage tea. This should be taken in, at least four times daily. We would also suggest that this be sweetened with your native honey.

We find other problems here in this subject, yes.

We find inflammation in the left lung area. We find that the overuse of tobacco in this subject, this should be cut down. We would not suggest that this subject completely stop this, because of overacting nervous system. The tobacco in small amounts would not hurt the system.

We further find in this subject — yes, yes — ulcers, lacerations, two old scar tissues in the upper tubular area, that in which is to enter the stomach itself. We find a new growth starting. We would suggest a more stable diet. But most of all, in this subject, we would suggest a vacation, rest, removing yourself from your present problems for at least a two-week time — during this time, staying into the liquid diet form.

This is all on this subject at this time. If further information should be requested, we shall answer.

May 16, 1973: *"Yes, Aka.* [5-16-73-003]*, she is 75-years old, and she has a heart condition and cataracts, and she would like help with these.* [There is a knock at the door.] *One moment, Aka.*

*"Could someone go around and bring the...oh, I see, all right.*
*"Yes, Aka."*

One moment, please. Yes, that is better.

We should answer in this manner. We have before us the body, the soul, the spirit, and the immortal body.

First, we should answer that which is most important unto this one. We see thy karma, and therefore, that the time that thy have upon this earth should be used in a manner which is most beneficial to you, we should give of this first. Thy have — yes — one moment.

Thy problem comes from before time, that of learning to forgive, mostly of yourself. Our Father sees you as you see yourself. And as you speak to Him, speak to Him as you would unto yourself. Therefore, you would forgive God, and God would forgive you.

But you have not learned to forgive yourself. This is the most important part, for you are your own judge.

In the judging of yourself, see that into which you have done. Learn from it. Blame it not upon others. But blame it not upon yourself. Take from the knowledge of it and advance onward. But do not repeat that which you have done. You think in your mind that falling down is a sin. It is not the falling down that is the sin. It is the not wanting to get back up; that in itself would be the sin. Rise above this.

Of the eye problem, the problem in itself could be taken care of with minor surgery. But for the relief of this, taking first of a castor oil pack, placing the castor oil, warm, upon a cloth, not hot, not at any temperature that should irritate the eyelids, taking also that of a raw potato of the white [stead], crushing this and placing this over the eyelids themselves, then the warm castor oil pack. This would greatly relieve this area at the present time.

Of the heart condition, we can say unto you into these words. We are not great. We cannot create; only our Father can do this. We should answer your problem by saying unto you, walk onward in this lifetime as you have. Let God see thy need and serve it.

But we should also say unto you, we do not sleep. Yet, we are not bound by your earth or your universe. We pass from door to door. Yet, when we walked upon your earth in earth form, we thought within our minds that we saw all there was. Yet the vastness we see now is beyond all vastness, for they are the many wonders of our Father.

May 16, 1973: *"Thank you, Aka.* [5-16-73-004] *and she has asked for a health reading — wants to know if cancer is recurring?"*

Yes, we see thy need; therefore, we should answer in this question — the healing that thy have asked for shall be given into thyself. Give forth faith unto thy Father. Go into three days of prayer and meditation, and that unto which you seek shall be given.

May 18, 1973: *"Yes, Aka. I would like to ask for a health reading on [12-7-70-001] tonight...She has been having abdominal trouble and also a skin problem on her arms and hands, and she is quite concerned."*

Yes, we see her need. First, we should say unto these words. We have before us the body, the soul, the spirit, and therefore, the immortal body. Yes, we see this.

First, we should say unto these words; she should go immediately unto her physician. The reaction she is receiving is that of belated reaction from the cobalt treatment. If treated it should clear up. I am sure that this matter shall be taken care of. Therefore, we should not give unto you further information. Have trust in this of her physician.

We see also that this one should go back unto the [sauna] baths, as was suggested once before. We find — yes — impurification in the circulatory system. We should also suggest that this one go unto the chiropractic doctor for adjustments of the backular area.

This is all on this subject at this time. Should further information be needed, ask.

May 18, 1973: *"Thank you, Aka. Aka, [5-18-73-001], he is here tonight, has asked for a health reading so that he can write and type better. He says, 'Can anything medically or otherwise be done to cure or improve the stiffness and awkwardness of my right arm and hand? Can Dr. Hulls help?'"*

First, we should say unto these words, yes, your doctor shall help a great deal. Second, we should answer in this manner. Take into thyself of the Night-blooming Cereus, one-inch cubes daily. Take into thyself of the sage tea, sweetening with local honey. Take unto these areas of the safflower oil, warming it and placing it on the swollen areas, doing this nightly before you go unto slumber.

May 18, 1973: *"Thank you, Aka. You said earlier of [5-16-73-001]; do you want me to say anything more on that at this time? Her name is [5-16-73-001]."*

Should this one desire a health reading, let her submit the proper information. You have other questions, ask.

May 22, 1973: *"Yes, Aka. [5-22-73-001], she is here tonight....She has asked a number of questions. She says, 'I have a throat problem, have had a throat problem for approximately a year now. I have seen a doctor and it was diagnosed as an allergy. Can you tell me please what the problem is? Is it truly an allergy? Is there any other health problem that should be brought to my attention?'"*

Yes, we see thy need, and first, we should say unto you, we have before us the body, the soul, the spirit, and therefore, the immortal body of the same.

First, we should speak of your throat problem. We find an underdevelopment of the bronchial glands. This has been caused from birth.

Second, we should speak in this manner, you live in a polluted land. Therefore, we should make the following suggestions. Take first, unto the natural honey of your area, adding one drop per teaspoon of vinegar into the honey — taking this twice daily, allowing rest afterwards, at least 30 minutes. Do not speak during this 30 minutes. But see in thy mind's eye thy throat and the problem before you. Think only of the healing of this area, the growing of the bronchial tubes, the growing of the bronchial glandular area, and third, of the increasing of the blood flow unto these areas.

We further find other difficulties within this soul.

Yes, we see this.

Because of a long period of stays in this polluted land, this has caused problems in the circulatory system, the blood flow within itself. First, we would suggest taking of the [saunic] baths. If this could be done once a week, this would greatly stimulate this in itself.

Second, we find within this one into the third, fourth and eighth vertebrae area — yes — we find that this has damaged — yes, yes — quite badly as a small child. We further find that that you would know of as a tailbone was broken at this time. Therefore, we would suggest searching out of a good chiropractic doctor. This should be done in a very gentle manner. At no time should this one force any of these. This can be done with gentle massage upward, then downward, going to the base of the spine.

We would further suggest that in the neckular area, this would help if this area could be massaged daily, going clear to the front of the forehead, slowly gracing this area in a forward position and then in an outward position, working slowly, gradually toward the back of the head. You will find an indentation at the back of your head. Work this indentation downward toward the spinial [spinal] area gently, at no time forcing any of this. Laying also, it would be preferred around the bronchial glandular area, the using of hot olive oil packs in the evening. Yes. This would help.

We also find this subject has been bothered by headaches quite frequently. After the above has been taken care of, you will no longer have the headaches.

We would also suggest the adding unto your diet first, twice daily two safflower oils before, 30 minutes before each meal — at the last, reducing this into one tablet. Yes, this would help.

We find that the taking of more of the green vegetation — it would be suggested that this subject find and locate vegetation to eat that has not been sprayed by your insecticides, only using that of the garlic spray. This would be good.

We would also suggest that an extra meal be added unto the diet. This should be of the green vegetation and sliced hard-boiled eggs.

We find also a problem within this one of varicose veins.

Yes, we see this.

We would suggest that hot olive oil packs be added to this. Now this must be done, not hot, lukewarm; it must be very carefully done. If within your mind you are not sure that you will follow these instructions exactly, do not do this. Unless it is done properly, you could cause great harm unto yourself. Warming the castor oil to where that you can put your hand into the oil — laying the cloth over the area and gradually seeping the oil into the cloth, keeping your oil warm that this can be continued. Then, after a 30-minute period, wrapping this area, not tightly, very loosely, that it may remain on overnight. You will soon find that this problem will take care of itself.

We find other small problems within this soul. We would suggest if further help is needed, she should have a follow-up health reading.

May 25, 1973: *"Aka, I have a question from[5-25-73-001].... She has an illness, and she would like information and correction for pain in the leg, tumor or any other problem. 'Any information I need to know, or to correct the situation,' she says, 'that I may be able to overcome this illness. I need to know the cause and what to do about it.'"*

We shall answer in this manner. You have a fear of medical doctors. Overcome this fear. If you do not, and seek the assistance *now*, your condition shall become worse. We are *not* creators; only our Father may create. We have placed upon your Earth doctors who are healers. If you should have the faith to go unto the medical doctor, we shall provide the healing that is necessary.

Yet, you shall say in these words, "How could this be true? How could these words be true?" And you shall deny us. Yet, we shall answer that you should know that we speak unto you the truth.

First, we should say unto you, there are many paths to our Father's house. Yet, you worry all the time of serpents at your door. Take from us the philosophy given in the first of this reading. All your storehouses shall do you little good if you are not upon the Earth to eat them, and share them.

For those who should do the work of God in truth, our Father shall provide for their needs, but not their wants. Soul Ray spoke unto you certain words, and he did place unto your body healing. This healing, at his request, was given from us also. Show us the faith you had in the beginning. Walk forth, as David did. Lay your hands upon the sore and speak unto your Father as you would speak unto yourself.

This is all at this present time on this subject.

You have a soul in the city of Phoenix, Arizona. Ask this question. *"Aka,* [5-18-73-001] —"

This is not of the soul we have spoke of; this soul is in meditation.

May 25, 1973: *"One moment, Aka.*[5-22-73-002]*, one moment.* [5-22-73-001] *says she has changed her major, as you suggested Tuesday, and has applied for nursing school. She wants to know if she will be accepted? Also, if you have any other suggestions for her, she says she is receptive."*

We see her need, and we should answer in this manner.

First, we should give the healing that is needed. This, in itself, was more important than your question. We shall take from you this virus within you, and we shall place healing into your body.

We shall take care to see your acceptance shall come. Be patient.

June 1, 1973: *"Yes, Aka.* [5-18-73-001] *has asked for a problem, a health reading or assistance concerning a lack of blood circulation in his left foot and leg. His question, he says, 'My left leg and foot at some times seem quite cold and has a very disturbing tingling sensation as if blood circulation is being impaired. During cold weather it feels uncomfortably cold. The arch is weak, almost flat. Should medical attention be sought, and can Aka offer any remedial suggestions? Thank you.'"*

Yes, we see thy need. And we should say unto thee, we have before us the body, the soul, the spirit, and the immortal body of the same.

Yes, we see this problem within the same. Medical attention should be sought immediately. Do not, at any time, treat this with either hot or cold packs. Do not take any warm baths, only lukewarm baths. Massaging this area that you shall find directly above the groin area, you will find therefore, within the same damage unto the artery. You shall further find that the rubbing of cold, skin — not very cold — skin temperature, of the castor oil above this area. We should further suggest the taking of the vitamin known as Lipo-Flavonoid. This can be bought at any of your drugstores without prescription form.

We would further suggest that this one seek out, first, of a medical doctor; that of a regular M.D. could see to the problem within itself.

But we would suggest further because of the need of adjustment unto the backular area, into the eighth vertebrae, you shall find damage there causing nerve damage into the legular [leg] area. Adjustments should be made. This in itself should greatly improve this area. But you must realize that these treatments within the same must be done over a prolonged area. You must also realize that if this is done too suddenly, the adjustment within itself, it could cause further damage. Therefore. the seeking out of an osteopathic doctor would be wise.

We further find within this subject arthritic condition, which has not at this time become a problem, yet if the use of the body-temperature castor oil upon the joint areas at this time [were to] improve this. Because of the condition, we would not suggest that any type of strong antibiotic be used onto this subject because of the chemical make-up of the body substance would react quite strongly against this.

We should further suggest that follow-up readings be given at the subject's request.

June 1, 1973: *"Yes, Aka. k, who is here tonight, says, 'I am doing a story for my newspaper on Ray Elkins and am personally interested in his work.' He has a series of questions I would like to ask. The first one, 'I have been having headaches recently. What is the cause, and is there something I can do to prevent them?'"*

Yes, we see they need. First, we have before us the body, the soul, the spirit, and therefore, the immortal body. We would say unto this one, the headaches are not of a recent thing. The headaches are from overtaxing the body, not enough rest. But we would also say that the use of vitamin E within the diet would greatly relieve this. The growth of the headache substance within itself is more from nervous exhaustion, nervous tendencies not released. Therefore, we would suggest thy should either dwell into the desert or into the mountains. Say unto the desert or unto the mountains that which is within thy heart. Release these tensions. The headaches shall go away.

June 1, 1973: *"He asks, 'Do you have any other advice about my health?'"*

Yes, we see thy need. First, we would suggest the changing of the footwear, more of the orthopedic type. Because of thy height, thy are causing a problem within the spinular area. If these shoes were made in such a manner that should throw the weight to the front of the foot more than to the heel, this should cause this person to walk in a more upright manner.

We would further suggest changing of the diet, adding to thy diet more of green substance. We would further suggest adding to, before thy meals, approximately 30 minutes before, taking of the tonic substance known as S.S.S. This can be found in any of your local drugstores. Because of a deficiency of certain minerals within the body, if this substance is found foul to thy taste, we would suggest, therefore, the taking of Lydia E. Pinkham in the capsule form, adding to this more of the vitamin B, A, and E.

Thy have had in thy mind a fear of other illnesses. We cannot see of this. Add more pleasure to your diet, and you shall find reward within the same.

June 8, 1973: *"Aka, I don't have a question on this, but* [10-29-71-002], [2-19-71-001]*'s mother...has had a hemorrhage in her eye, and she has asked for healing.*

We shall stop the pain. But we are not allowed to interfere. The choice has been made within this soul. The time is near. Give comfort and love, and understanding, even in this one who has given now out spiteful things. You must understand that the passing is that of choice. Yet, even in the passing there is lessons to be learned. But there is nothing to fear. The confusion within this one shall be but for a short time. Our Father sheds tears. Yet, even our Father can not interfere with your free choice. And we shed tear with our Father.

June 8, 1973: *"Aka,* [5-18-73-001] *who is here tonight...has asked for a follow-up on his health reading. Specifically he would like to know, 'Are the zone therapy treatments now being given to my feet of any benefit in relieving the poor circulation in the left leg and the stiffness and awkwardness in my right arm and hand? Should they be continued? Thank you.'"*

Yes, we have before us the body, the soul, the spirit, and the immortal body. Yes, but as we have said before, go unto the sauna baths. Use of these.

Thy have found within thyself an improvement within your health. You have also found an improvement in your mental condition.

We would suggest at this time the taking of more of the vitamin E, but not internally. Taking this and rubbing it into the joint areas and into the feet area. If this could be done, this would greatly improve this.

We would further suggest that take one day a week, using this one day and drink milk, one glass at each mealtime — placing forth three bananas at each mealtime, doing this three times in the day — this would give the body cleansing time. As we have also suggested, drinking the sage tea before and after each meal, continuing with the other suggestions we have placed before you — your healing shall come. Your faith is good. Your intent is good. Blessed be the name of the Lord. And we shall add one other ingredients, love of your fellow man, and the healing thy ask for shall be given with love.

June 15, 1973: *"Aka,* [6-15-73-002] *who is here tonight...has asked a number of questions. He asks, 'What is my mission in this lifetime, and what type of person was I in past lives?' Also, 'What do I do to make or improve my health condition where I have an incurable lung condition?'"*

First, we should answer unto thee the most important. Come forth from the polluted land in which you dwell. Second, we should answer in this manner. Change thy diet form. Add first of 4,000 units of vitamin E daily. Add second 1,000 units of vitamin C daily. Breathing exercises should be done four times daily — not over-laboring of the lung, but slowly breathing in, counting unto yourself, "one, two, three," breathing out in the same manner — doing this first for five-minute intervals.

Second, we would further suggest that more of the green substance be given into this one, that more of the protein and the broth of protein of the meat substance, of the beef. You must realize — you have thought within your mind that you detest this of the carnivorous-type animal of man, and we shall answer in this manner — as the sons of God did enter into the daughters of man, so the need for both, that the body should be strong. Each chemical within the body is a separate part of a whole; yet each part reacts as though it has its own mind. Yet, your mind controls all proportions of the same. The most important tonic that you can take at this time is positive thought, that of the thought that thy shall become well.

But yet, we shall give unto you a last ingredients — open the door that we may enter. Show unto us and our Father of your belief and we shall give healing, for we cannot give healing where there is no faith, for we would be violating your own body, and this we are not allowed to do.

June 15, 1973: *"Aka, [5-7-71-001] said that she would like to know if the vitamin E that she brought at Revco for her is safe for her to take?"*

We shall answer in this manner. You must first understand that this soul is highly allergic to artificial substances. We would suggest that taken of a natural form would be much better. There are many natural vitamins that could be found in capsule form. But we say unto this one, as we have said before, take of the vitamin E, but take of the herb substance which lies within this one as Lydia E. Pinkham. Your body is changing.

June 19, 1973: *"Thank you, Aka. Soul Mary is concerned about her skin breaking out, and she says, 'What should I take and clean my face with so that it will remain healthy?'"*

We should say unto you, use of the vitamin E. Place this lightly upon the skin, but first, taking that substance of the alcohol to sponge free the dirt from the skin, then placing this upon your skin early of the morning and late of the night.

June 19, 1973: *"Aka, [1-21-72-003] asks, is she right that a cause of Ray's blood disease — 'of the blood cells increasing is the absorption of undigested proteins into the blood stream because of ulcers and poor digestion?'"*

We would say, nay. We are not allowed to give the information you seek, for this should come from soul Ray. Soul Ray knows of the problem, and he knows within himself the cause. But we should answer in this manner. Should he become upset the problem increases. If you should give him medication give him tranquility.

July 20, 1973: *"Aka, [7-20-73-005] asks for healing for her father."*
We shall answer in this manner. We shall take that of the pain and give that unto the body and soul and spirit, and the immortal body, the healing that it desires unto the same. Glory be the name of the Lord.

June 22, 1973: *"Aka, [6-22-73-002], he's age 10, has asked for a health reading."*
Yes, we have before us the body, the soul, the spirit and the immortal body of the same.

We should answer in this manner. A changing of the diet — put more protein into the diet. Take away most of the sweetness of the food he should eat and that of which he should drink. Theses within themselves are poisoning his body.

Give unto this one of breakfast fruits; of eggs, that of the chicken; of good bread with small amounts of jams or jelly. Put more, place more of the milk substance, that of the dairy product into his food. Give of him pure butter, that that should come from the extraction from cow's milk.

Give of him into his luncheon meal good hot food. Place potatoes and other vegetables, placing corn.

Of the evening meals, placing that of the fish that should come from the sea of one meal in the week, placing beef, or lamb or pork into the evening meals.

If he should desire sweetness, let him eat of the honey. Give of him of the three meals per day that of the sage tea sweetened with the local honey of the same.

We would further suggest that for the welfare of his mind that tasks be assigned him that he should perform daily. This should teach his mind of discipline, which would be good for the body. Exercise, more of the same. Teach of the mind strength given in the form of assurance that he can stand as a man. Place forth those of his own age to associate with.

At the present time, there is a lack of calcium within the body, calcium and magnesium in daily quantities. We find the lack of vitamin E, A, and D. We find the lack of vitamin C and mineral substance of the same.

We find — yes — if this balance is not reached, this child should soon be that of a borderline diabetic. Take into the body substance that of the Jerusalem artichoke. Take away all candy substances. Place only within the body that of natural fruits. This would be good for the body.

We find that of a virus, of a slight virus, yes, within the body.

We would further suggest the changing of the drinking water. We would suggest the buying, not of the distilled water, but of the cleaner, bottled water.

If the following is done, you shall see a great change, both in his mental attitude and his physical health.

This is all on this subject at this time.

June 22, 1973: *"Thank you, Aka. One moment. [6-22-73-003], the subject is at home, and has asked for help regarding nerve damage 'to help improve the use of my hand.'"*

Yes, we see before us the body, the soul and the immortal body of the same; therefore, we have the body substance before us.

Yes.

And we should answer in this manner. We find arthritis within the shoulder, upper part of the body, but we also find, in the backular area, that of the neckular area.

Yes.

We would suggest the massaging of this area. We would suggest the, the attendance of either an osteopathic or chiropractic doctor. This area must be worked in such a manner that the neck should be slowly pulled upward. This must be done very gently. This will take at least two months of treatment before the nerves that are blocking this area shall be relieved and can function properly. This will also relieve the headaches that this soul has suffered.

We find other problems in the backular area. These also should be attended. We find — yes — we would suggest that that of the whirlpool baths be used of this subject. Of the location — yes, we see unto this — if this area is massaged daily, the use of warm olive oil packs upon the area at night.

We would further suggest that the taking of the cow's milk from this and replacing it with that of the goat's milk. We would suggest sweetening the goat's milk with a little honey; taking also of the sage tea twice daily. We shall assist this in this manner.

We find, because of an improper tooth extraction, pressure in the nervular area. This should be corrected.

This is all on this subject at this time. We would suggest that a follow-up reading be done after the following has been submitted to.

June 22, 1973: *"[2-19-71-001] asks if the fishhook feelings in her skin is because of vitamin deficiency or nerves, or how to treat it?"*

We shall answer in this manner. Because of the emotional condition of thy mind at this time, that brought forth by the care of thy mother, has caused a nervous disorder. Only time at this time shall cure this, but be patient, for the waiting time shall be but a little while. Release that unto which you are trying to hold, and let it pass, for the separation of the soul has already come about.

June 22, 1973: *"Yes, Aka, the son of [5-7-71-003's] niece, [6-22-73-001], is in the burn unit of Maricopa Hospitable in Phoenix with burns over 90 percent of his body. And [5-7-71-002] has asked for blessings for him and any comment you might have."*

We should answer in this manner. We may not interfere with his free choice. We shall give unto this one that unto which he desires; we shall take from him the pain. But the final choice must be unto him.

Glory be the name of the Lord.

June 29, 1973: *"Aka, [6-15-73-001] who is here tonight asks for healing, or health reading, if necessary, for the back of her neck and spine."*

Yes, we see thy need. And we should say in this manner, we should bring forth healing from our Father, God. Look upward, for the healing light has entered unto thy body and shall continue for three days and three nights. You shall hear voices, but fear them not. And so our Lord, God, commands. Glory be the name of the Lord; glory be the name of His children.

*"Thank you, Aka."*

One moment.

Yes.

It has been suggested that after the reading soul Ray administer further healing, and the healing shall be complete.

June 29, 1973: *"Yes, Aka. [6-29-73-003], and he has asked for health information — I have a note here — prayer for finger of left hand. And also, he asks specifically 'to find my directions in life and to learn if knowledge of previous lives and developed abilities can reinforce my life in terms of service and help to others.'"*

First, we should give the healing unto the hand. And so it shall be. Glory be the name of the Lord.

Soul Ray now grows tired, and it would be suggested that the balance of this question be asked at a different time.

He shall at first have problem adjusting to the presence of Ammie within himself, but as he has adjusted to all things, for now there shall be Ammie, there shall be Ray, and there shall be the spirits of Aka which dwell within him, each a separate part, yet all a whole.

July 2, 1973: *"Aka, [2-7-73-001] is here tonight. She has asked for a health reading. She has also asked, what should she be doing for God and humanity in this new age? And she is concerned about, should she take money from the co-op credit union and invest it in real estate?"*

First we should answer that of the health, and we should answer in this manner. We have before us the body, the soul, the spirit, and therefore, the immortal body of the same.

Yes, we see this.

We find within this body that of arthritis, the virus. We also find within this the virus of the same which has attacked unto the circulatory system of the same. This in itself has caused headaches, has also caused hard of hearing, eyesight problems. We would suggest that for this condition that the sauna baths be taken. The sauna baths should be taken first in five-minute intervals, no more. At no time should a strain be placed upon the heart. This must be understood. The virus of the same has attacked the heart muscles causing a weakening throughout the whole system. We further find in the backular area, of the 6th and 7th vertebrae, that of the vertebrae in itself being worn down. We would suggest that a bar, an iron bar, be erected approximately three inches out of her reach that she may reach up to and let the full weight of her body pull and separate these. We would not suggest traction of any type. This must be done lightly and not for prolonged periods. If this is overdone, more damage could be done unto the same area.

We further find within this subject that of borderline diabetic. We find that the subject within the same has treated this, but we would further suggest the taking of the Jerusalem artichoke. We would further suggest the taking of the sage tea sweetened with the local honey of thy locale.

We further find within — yes — of the left arm above the elbow, of small tubular-type growths. We find these also in the back area. These are nothing more than cysts; they are not malignant. If the sage tea is taken, first by bringing your water into a warm condition — do not boil the water — letting the tea steep to a strength that is good to thy taste buds, this then sweetened with honey would slowly dissolve these cyst-type growths. We would not suggest that over massaging these or heating them. We would suggest of the areas within the same that the taking of hot castor oil packs be used, not — only to body temperature, this must be understood. At no time should anything be placed against this body that is above body temperature. This would affect the nervous system. Only of the sauna baths, these may be used.

July 2, 1973: *"Yes, Aka, one moment.* [2-7-73-002] *that is here tonight has also asked for a health reading and advice regarding their house and future investments, also his future occupation or social involvement."*

Yes, we see thy need, and therefore, we have before us the body, the soul, the spirit, and the immortal body of the same.

Yes.

We find in this one that of the problem of the liver, in through and that of the problem of the digestive system within the same. This comes from abuse of the body in your early years. Yet, you have taken the steps to cleanse the body. This is good. We would suggest more of the vitamin E be added unto the diet, 1,000 units per day. We would further suggest that more of the vitamin C be added to thy diet, 500 units a day.

Yes.

We would further suggest that thy do not eat of any fatty substance, for within the digestive system we find there scar tissue of ulcer-type lesions.

We also find scar tissue of the left lung region. These have healed, yet they can be irritated with improper diet.

We also see that of worrying where worry is not needed. We say unto thee, there is the healing of the body, and there is the healing of the mind. Both must come together as one, for if there is no healing of the mind, then the mind can destroy all healing of the body. Therefore, for your treatment we would suggest, cast aside these things. Thy have thought of death, yet death is no more than passing from one door to another. Thy have thought that thy might be departed from those of your loved ones and that of thy wife. But yet, this should not come yet. But yet, we should say unto thee in these words, all things that have been before shall be again, that your love that was born in many lifetimes shall not part with the opening and closing of a door. For there has been nothing upon your earth that has not been of heaven, and yet, there is nothing of heaven that has not been of earth. Each within you have thought to make the other's way more gentle and easy. Yet you seek out that that you already have. When spring comes and a rose shall blossom, just because the earth should sleep in winter does not mean that it shall not blossom again in the spring. But you have brought forth a rose for the earth to look upon, and this has been a beautiful thing that all mankind has seen within you.

You say unto us, how do we know of these things? Yet we say unto you, you have spoken unto your God as you would speak unto yourself, and therefore, the records that you should keep and God should keep can be read. But we have spoken for your ears to hear. As we have said before, for we speak that the blind should see and the deaf could hear, for all things that have been buried in darkness shall be brought to light.

July 2, 1973: *"Aka,* [2-7-73-003] *has asked, 'I would like to know details concerning my present health condition.'"*

Yes, we before us the body, the soul, the spirit, and therefore, the immortal body of the same. Therefore, we should answer in this manner.

That of the heart condition, and the transplant within the same, the body has accepted. There is irritation in the tissue of the muscular area around the heart. This has come forth from too early abuse of the muscular tissue. This should not be done. We would further suggest in thy dietary, supplement these with those of both natural vitamin and mineral. Yet, we would suggest that the fatty tissues be removed from all meat substance in thy diet.

Thy have the circulatory system well in hand. Thy have done this with the power if the mind. We would further suggest — yes, we see this — we would further suggest that the taking of the larger quantities at this time, at least 1,000 units of vitamin E daily, adding normal dosage of A and D, and E.

We find, therefore, within the body of the headaches. These are brought on by the food substance thy have placed within thy body. These should come forward from that of what is known as the grout [gout]. Reoccurrences of this should come forth in thy lifetime unless thy change thy pattern of food. Stay away from rich food, spicy substances thy like so well, using smaller quantities of salt in thy diet.

We would suggest that a follow-up reading be given in this case.

July 6, 1973: *"Aka, [7-6-73-001] would like a health reading. She has a polycystic condition of her kidney and liver. Can you explain, can you suggest anything that might help her, and can you give any other information about this?"*

Yes, we see thy need. And we should say unto thee, we have before us the body, the soul, the spirit, and the immortal body of the same.

First we should say, come unto soul Ray for healing.

But second, we should say unto thee, change of thy drinking water. Drink only that of the bottled water in its purest form, for within the land you dwell, the water is polluted. That of the chemical substance which has been sprayed upon your land has now reached your Phoenix areas. There is no way, into which they are seeking now, to extract this chemical from the water. It is attacking your body in such a manner. But second we should say unto this one, take unto the sage tea, sweetening with the local honey. Take unto this one 3,000 units of vitamin E per day. Change that of your filtering system within the house. Because of the heavy air pollution this is adding to your illness.

We should also say unto this one — yes — we see this. Of all liquids thy should drink, drink only at this time of pure water. Second, drink that juice that should come of the cranberry juice. Let this flush out the system. Third, because of the heavy pollution within the circulatory system of the same, we should suggest sauna baths. But these should not be overdone. Too much heat upon this soul could destroy the chemical balance of the same. Take no more than five minutes per day of this — never any more.

Third, we find a hernia of the stomach area, a lesion within the same. The tissue, which is to hold intestines up, there is lesions there also.

We would not suggest that this soul lift anything more than ten pounds at the present time until the healing can take place.

July 6, 1973: *"Yes, Aka.* [7-6-73-003] *at the time of her request for a health reading was carrying a deceased child within her. Do you have any — can you give any assistance on this in regards to her health?"*

Yes, we see thy need. Yet, you have not given us sufficient information upon this. One moment.

We should answer in this manner. Go unto thy physician and take of his counsel; it has been good. We shall give the healing that is needed unto this one. Glory be the name of the Lord.

July 6, 1973: *"Aka,* [7-6-74-003] *has asked for assistance on his health, a health reading. He asks, 'What is the matter with me? Why do I always feel dizzy, why is my mouth always dry? Can you tell me anything about my health? Is there something wrong you can tell me how to correct it?' And he'd like to know what course his future holds."*

We shall answer in this manner. We have before us the body, the soul, and the immortal body of the same. Therefore, we see thy need.

First we should say, of your ill feeling, you must understand that within each soul is that much like the tide of your ocean. When it sweeps out it leaves upon the land many fish and other eatable things. Some of these things it lays upon the land should they be eaten should destroy you. And this within itself has been your problem. Your greatest problem has been that of an emotional one; therefore, an unhealthy mind makes for an unhealthy body. Thy have sought out and found no rest within your mind and within the people you are now with.

Yet, you say unto us, "Even if this were so, what could I do to change it?" And we should say unto you, change unto yourself. Be as a mirror that should shine out and give the love and blessings of our Father. That that you should give should be returned in kind. But if you should walk forth to offer your knowledge, your bread, your wine, your goodness, and it is rejected, then walk on. Go unto a field that should grow, and that you should grow with it. Only in this manner can your future come in completeness, that of a whole and complete thing, for you are but half a person, for you have hidden the other part. Bring it forth, let it blossom. But when you see the flowers that are placed at your feet, do not walk on them, but step over them, that others may also see the flowers. Give blessings and healing into all. And this should be the commandment of your Lord.

You have long worried within your mind, it is wrong to do of this or wrong to do of that?

And we shall say unto you unto these words. Our Lord asks but very little of His children — that they should give of one-tenth of the love the Lord gives unto His children back unto Him, and give unto your fellow man in the same manner.

July 6, 1973: *"Thank you, Aka. [7-6-73-003] has asked for a health reading regarding his liver. He'd like to know the cause of [7-6-73-003]'s liver cirrhosis and what can be done at this time to heal him, or how can he be helped?"*

We shall answer in these words. Let soul Ray go unto this one; we shall go with him, and therefore, give the healing and the knowledge that should be given unto this one at that time. Arrangements should be made that this can be done. Can you understand of which we speak?

*"Yes, Aka."*

Nay, not fully. But listen to our words again and thy shall.

July 6, 1973: *"[7-6-73-004] has asked, 'What can I do to improve my health and stamina?'"*

Yes, we see thy need. Therefore, we have before us the body, the soul, and the immortal body of the same. The spirit shall flow, and therefore, all shall come in completeness.

First, we should say unto this one, thy have business at hand; complete it. Let that of the past be the past. Bring forth unto this new time.

We should say unto thee, we have come forth to prepare a way. We have seen of your need and your desire. And therefore, we should say unto you, come forth and help us prepare the way, and we shall take these burdens from thy self and place the answers before you. But we do not barter with you, for that that which we give is given, as all things, from our Father.

We find within this one only mental anxiety.

We also find that much of the questions that thy have asked thy should come unto soul Ray for consultation. He should do unto this one that, that the two men should come together and bring healing. This, in itself, would answer the remainder of this question.

July 6, 1973: *"[7-6-73-005] has asked for a health reading. One moment...."*

One moment. The records are not within balance. Go forth and read this again.

[Editor's note: The name, which had been incorrectly read, was corrected by the person in the room who had brought the written request.]
*"[7-6-73-005] has asked a number of questions. The first one, 'I have been to the doctor's to correct my problem of weight....'"*

First, we should answer in this manner, the weight problem — once again, we have placed new knowledge within Ray's mind. That he should use it in a proper manner, it would be suggested that the use of hypnosis be used upon this one, implanting of the suggestion that her own body and mind could work in accord with this.

We also find chemical imbalance that has been of long accord. The husband in question has extracted this. This soul has not extracted this. And therefore, we should give that that is needed at this time to take forth.

Therefore, we have before us the body, the soul, the spirit, and the immortal body of the same. Healing shall be given. We would suggest that the use of hypnosis be used that this chemical can be extracted in a slow manner. If this is done too fast, it could kill of the body. We would suggest large quantities, 4,000 units of vitamin E be taken into the body daily. We would suggest, no milk at all unto this soul, magnesium be added unto this one; that of the dehydrated or de-fatted milk could be used. Before each meal, the use of safflower oil; one capsule should be taken before the breakfast meal, two capsules before the luncheon meal, and three capsules before your evening meal. More of the fish, that that should come from the sea. Once weekly beef should be eaten; this should be eaten as raw as possible. Bananas should be eaten at least three times a day, at least one banana. Take all sugar from your diet and use natural honey within the same. Sweeten, all you want, all things with this substance. You must realize that the chemical in itself has caused the body to hold large quantities of water. These are also affecting the kidney and liver area. It would be suggested that cranberry juice be used in this to extract the same. It would also be suggested that sage tea be used at least twice daily.

July 9, 1973: *"Aka, [7-9-73-001] is here this afternoon...and he has asked for a health reading, and some other questions. Firstly, he says, regarding his stomach, that he has had a digestion problem. One hour after eating he needs to lie down. He has a nervous stomach, and digestive aids do not seem to help."*

Yes, we see thy need, and we should answer in this manner. First, you must understand that thy have more than what is known as a nervous stomach. Thy have one intestine which is lapped over another, therefore, causing a blockage within the stomach area, not allowing the full usage of the digestive system within itself. Therefore, we should answer in this manner. That your digestive system should work first in completeness, this must be cleansed.

That the intestine may be straightened into its proper place we should give of you exercises. First, we would suggest that this subject lie upon the floor. Relax. As soon as the body feels complete relaxation, roll to the left side, relaxing again, doing so for five minutes. Then, roll back onto your back once again. Then, rolling to the right side, staying in this position for five minutes. After this has been done, roll back upon the back. Do not try to rise until complete tranquility has entered the body once again.

Before each meal we would suggest, 30 minutes before the eating of the meal, taking that within the substance of the milk that should come from the goat. Take this, find a cool place, and then drinking it and preparing your thoughts for your meal. Your thoughts should be in this manner, that the food should taste good; second, that you have cast from your mind your day-to-day worries and chores. If done in this manner, the stomach would soon heal itself. And in healing the stomach, so the nervous system should be healed.

At the beginning of each day, take a moment that you should tell of yourself the good things that have happen to you the day before, taking that some moment and placing the things you should do that day before you. Do not worry that you should get them all done. But do them; take one at a time and doing it thoroughly. When it has been accomplished go to the next task.

We would suggest that your family enter into this same meditation with you. Therefore, their thoughts should become tranquil along with your own. This in itself would greatly relieve your nervous tension.

We have before us the body, the soul, the spirit, and the immortal body. We read from this, and therefore, we say unto you unto these words. For the mind and body to heal together, tranquility should be the greatest medicine of all. We would also suggest that this subject eat at least four bananas a day. We would also suggest that the substance known as dolomite be used, six units per day. We would also suggest that 1,000 units of vitamin E be added unto the diet.

We would further suggest — yes — one moment — that the vitamin known as Lipo-Flavonoid
be used. We find within this subject that similar to the hardening of the arteries. We find that not enough oxygen is reaching the brain. We would suggest that as much green substance as possible could be eaten by this subject. We would further suggest that these should be eaten raw, placing nothing upon them besides a small amount of salt, none of your salad dressings at all.

We find also within the subject a recurring blindness, that of the eyes not seeing fully, a spottiness before the eyes at times. This has come, as we said before, from the lack of oxygen to the brain area.

We would further suggest, in addition to this, a good multiple vitamin be used and mineral substance. This preferably should come of the natural sources. Any of the above can be purchased at a health food store.

July 9, 1973: *"Yes, Aka. He mentions back trouble, arthritis. He says the vertebras go out and need adjusting when he exercises or lifts."*

We have seen this problem. This, in part, is of the exercise we have already suggested. We have also suggested the dolomite, that of calcium and magnesium, to add to this area. We would further suggest that a chiropractic or osteopathic doctor be consulted, that treatment upon the same, into the 8th and 9th vertebrae. This in itself would greatly relieve this area and give immediate relief unto this subject. But this subject, in the relieving of this, this should be done in a gentle manner. We would also suggest that a bar be placed in your doorway at home, if possible placing this bar two to three inches above your normal reach, letting the full weight of your body hang from this. Do not do this over a prolonged period; do this only for at least one moment, one minute in one day, no more. In the evening before you go to bed this could be done. This would help the separation of this, and therefore, the healing within the same, in this manner.

July 9, 1973: *"Yes, Aka. He mentions low blood pressure. He says he becomes dizzy if he stands up quickly after sitting for an hour or so, like in church."*

Yes, we have already answered this. That of the respiratory and the problem of the blood pressure we have answered within the same.

We also find a problem within the respiratory problem, area. This is due to the polluted air into which you dwell, into the land into which you dwell. It would be suggested that frequent visits into mountainous areas be done. If this could be done periodically, this would give the lungs a chance to bring in the extra oxygen and the cleansing of the same. We would suggest that swimming exercises be used. None of the others; it's more strenuous. This should only be done as the body, in itself, should grow in strength.

Of the circulatory problem which you have mentioned, we have already given that which was needed within the same.

July 9, 1973: *"Yes, Aka. You mentioned his visiting the mountains. When he goes to his cabin in the mountains he says he does not get enough oxygen."*

This should be supplemented in this manner, the use of a small oxygen container. But we would suggest that you should not go into the high altitude; go that into the four or five-thousand feet area only at the present time until the healing has had a chance to take effect. As the healing begins, the problem shall end, that of the same.

July 9, 1973: *"Aka, he mentions a hemorrhoid problem."*

Yes, we see this. Therefore, we would suggest the taking of the substance known as Bag Balm. This is a salve tissue which can be purchased at any veterinary supply. It is used, in common use, for that of the treatment of a cow's urine [udder]. In this case, the salve within itself should be, some placed upon the finger and inserted directly into the rectum. This should be done at least three times daily. It also should be that this area should be washed with soap and water at least three times a day before the salve is applied. We can see the busy nature of this subject, but this could be done by carrying the same with them, with a clean cloth, three clean clothes, that the same cloth should not be used to cleanse the second time. This in itself is a virus, infecting-type virus. It is very similar in course to that of cancerous growths, but it is *not* of cancerous growth; it is not a malignancy. Yet, in likeness it is much the same as could occur upon the skin. If this was done in this manner that this problem should be literally cured, it must be done promptly. Set a time and follow through these instructions in their exact form.

July 9, 1973: *"Aka, he mentions his elbows have tendonitis, or he has tennis elbow. Can you suggest what to do for these?"*
This in itself is a lacking of green substance within the body. This we have already seen. This we have already given, that which should give relief and cure the same. We would further suggest within this the using of Jerusalem artichoke, eating one a day raw. Cleanse this substance well before eating. You may also use that of the Bag Balm salve on the elbow areas.

July 10, 1973: *"Aka,* [7-10-73-001] *who is here tonight, has asked a number of questions; the first one, 'How is my arthritis and what can I do for it?'"*
First, we should say unto thee into these words. Of the arthritic condition, this in itself is not the virus type; it is caused from the nervous system. We would make this suggestion in this manner. More rest should be given unto this soul in this manner, for we have before us the body, the soul, the spirit, and the immortal body of the same. We should say, go unto the desert, and therefore, find unto this one known as the Night-blooming Cereus. Take of this in quarter-by-quarter-inch cubes, three times daily. Take unto thyself of the sage tea sweetened with local honey. Steep of this, do not boil of it. Drink of this and let it flow unto thy body, and therefore, go into the circulatory system of the same.
We further find within this body certain nerve damage. The nerve damage within itself was caused from this soul, as a child, falling from a chair, striking the back of the neck and the headular area; therefore, we find problems within the backular area of the same.
The hearing problem could be rectified. Also the improvement of the eyesight could be improved by chiropractic or osteopathic treatment of the same. This should not be done, not at one time, because of the weight of this subject. It should be done in a gentle manner, therefore, causing no pain.
We find — yes — problem of the lymph gland area. Yes.

Problem of the thyroid. Yes.

We would suggest — low sugar — yes, we see this. Therefore, we would suggest the eating of the raw Jerusalem artichoke within the same.

We find the lacking of the vitamin A. This has caused increased aging beyond years. This vitamin, within itself, should be taken at least four times daily, adding the vitamin D once daily. In this particular case, these two vitamins should be taken in separate quantities; increasing the vitamin E input, that that has been taken orally, unto 1,000 units per day. The vitamin B, therefore, for the correction of the circulatory system, this should be taken in what is known as B-plus, added quantity of vitamin B.

Yes. We see this.

We further find — yes — a problem of that similar to the hardening of the arteries in the legular and hip areas causing swelling and pain within the same, of the lower limbs. This could also could be rectified partially by osteopathic treatment of the lower spine area. We would also suggest the taking of the vitamin known as Lipo-Flavinoid with [serocone][serotone?] within the same.

Yes.

We would further suggest — yes we see this.

We would suggest the diet of this soul, that more of the green substance be placed in the diet. This would be good. We would further suggest that less calcium be placed in the diet, more of protein. We would also suggest that before the eating of each meal, 30 minutes before, the taking of one capsule of that of the safflower oil, or the drinking of one ounce in raw form.

We would further suggest — yes, we see this — correction of the footwear. This is causing problems within the backular area within the same. This should be done as soon as possible. At all times this one should use the proper footwear. If this is not done, a permanent crippling condition shall arise at a later time.

July 10, 1973: *"Yes, Aka. One moment. The operation she had last fall, 'Was it necessary? Was it good or was it harmful,' she asks."*
The operation was, in itself, was good within itself, but not totally necessary.

July 10, 1973: *"Aka, [7-10-73-002] who is here tonight asks, 'I have been working with, for eight years, somebody's leg that is very sore, and will I be able to heal it?'"*
We shall answer in this manner. First you must be able to see that which you are healing. You have caused a lessening of the pain, but not a healing of the same. Therefore, we should say unto thee, go unto the light; walk from the darkness into the light that thy may see the injury that thy are healing. Reverse the cycle of thy own body. You must take on this injury unto your own body and dissolve of the same. We would not

suggest this at the present time, for within you is not the ability or the knowledge to do of this at this time; therefore, pray of healing. This would be good.

July 10, 1973: *"Aka, he asks, 'Could you give me any help or advice to improve my neck?'"*

Yes, we see thy need. Therefore, we have before us the body, soul, the spirit, and the immortal body of the same.

Yes, we find this problem. We find a fusion of a vertebrae.

Yes.

This must be done over a prolonged period of time. It must be done with the use of magnesium in capsule form, 250 units, three times daily. We would also further suggest that thy should consult an osteopathic or chiropractic doctor that massage treatments could be given unto this area, first, that the loosening of the calcium deposit within the same.

We further find nerve damage within this area. You must realize we are not great, we cannot create that that has been destroyed. Only our Father may do this. This damage is permanent. We shall give forth unto this one the healing that is needed to take of the pain.

We find that of ulcerated condition of the stomach.

Yes.

We find — infection of the liver, inflammation within the same. We find — yes — infection of the uterine canal within the same. This could be rectified by the use of the tonic known as S.S.S. It may be purchased at any of your local drugstores. We would further suggest that the taking of 500 units of vitamin E, A, D, in normal dosage, a good multiple vitamin and mineral, preferably of a natural source — yes — more of the fresh vegetation should be eaten with as little seasoning as possible upon the same.

July 12, 1973: *"Yes, Aka. [7-12-73-006], who is here tonight, has asked, 'Should I go through with my plan for Anaheim doctor exam and therapy?'"*

Yes, we have before us the body, soul, spirit, and therefore, the immortal body of the same. We should say, this should be good in one respect. But there is other knowledge that should come forth. This subject should be asked at a different time, not in public.

July 13, 1973: *"Yes, Aka. [7-13-73-001], he's asked for, in regards to health . 'Dear Aka, please heal me, or advise how I may be helped or healed of my present mental and/or physical condition. The doctors have been unable to help or even pinpoint my problem. Please offer to those who love me and are responsible for my well-being any advice or help you can concerning decisions they may have to make about my life.'"*

Yes, we have before us the body, the soul, the spirit, and therefore, the immortal body of the same. One moment. This soul must be located.

Yes. Yes, we have this before us now.

Of the physical nature we should answer in this manner, that of a mental state, first, we should suggest that the dental work necessary be done immediately. The infection from the same is poisoning the whole body *and* the mind.

Third, we have that which would be known as brainstem damage, damage in a form that should affect complete nervous system of the same. We would suggest that saunic baths be used. This in itself can increase the circulatory system. We would further suggest that a good diet, a sound diet be used. We should add protein unto the diet. Three meals per day, this should be done; not in such a manner that thy should [gorge] thyself, but in a sensible manner. Take forth upon that of the salt water fish at least one meal per day. Take forth that of the beef, of the liver of the beef, of one meal in the week per day. Take forth that of the other parts of the beef; this should not be overcooked. Take forth that of the raw vegetation, as much as thy can consume at thy luncheon meals. Take forth that of the fruit, both of the pear, peach, of this type, adding a little milk unto the substance, sweetened with that of the honey.

We would further suggest — yes, we see this — a chiropractic treatment should be used. We find a deformity of birth in the spine within the same. We would suggest that this, that x-rays be used before treatment be given. The chiropractic or osteopathic doctor should know in detail of the injuries unto the spine.

We find that — yes — infection unto the kidney area, infection that of the liver area. We would suggest that no alcoholic beverages whatsoever enter unto this one, of no kind. We would suggest — yes — that that of the sage tea be used, sweetened with natural honey.

Yes. We find, therefore, a fracture, that which would be known as a hairline fracture, of the left side of the [labonial] [mastoid?] area. We find that this within itself has caused an imbalance. This has irritated the nervous system within the same. We would suggest that in your visit to your osteopathic doctor that the substances known as antiverts be used to stabilize the equilibrium of the same.

We would also suggest that a follow-up reading be done unto this soul at a different time, should it be asked for.

July 13, 1973: *"Yes, Aka.* [7-13-73-002] *who is here tonight...has asked for a health reading. He says, 'Peripheral stagnation and swelling of feet, lack of balance, can't stand on toes.' One moment. He says, 'The balancing of my body when standing is one of my difficulties. Then when I first start walking or exercising I am somewhat short of breath, but this leaves quite soon upon easy exercise. Also have a mucous condition of throat, and nasal system. Otherwise I am fairly well.' He asks for help in this, Aka."*

Yes, we have before us the body, the soul, the spirit, and therefore, the immortal body of the same. Yes, we see thy need, and we should answer in this manner. First, we would suggest that no salt at all be used in this one's diet, obtaining that of a salt substitute.

We further find that of a borderline diabetic. That, in itself, we would suggest the use — yes — of the Jerusalem artichoke, preferably two to three of these be eaten raw per day.

We further find — yes — that of retaining, over-retaining the water substance within the body.

Yes.

This in itself is not caused from the usual substance, that of the deterioration of the kidneys within themselves; this is coming from a heart condition, therefore, within the circulatory system within the same.

First, we should answer in this manner. This condition can only be worsened by too much exercise. Therefore, we would suggest a form of exercise less strenuous. We *would* suggest that of swimming as much per day as the body will allow. Do not overdo this, but it should be a daily exercise. This in itself would allow the pores of the body to discharge these fluids and bring that back into a normal balance.

We also find that of an inner ear infection. We would suggest that thy should go unto the eye, ear, nose specialist and therefore, unto the left ear, have this examined. This has been caused by the breaking of the eardrum at an earlier time in life, the healing over and granules of foreign substance being left within. It would be suggested that surgery be used to remove of this. At the present time, that this condition might be overcome, the use of the antivert substance within the same; we would also suggest that the stabilizing of the equilibrium could be used by the substance known as Dilantin. These subjects should be brought forth unto your doctor.

We would further suggest that 3,000 units of vitamin C be used daily for a short period of time, for at least four weeks, then going back to 1,000 units per day. Also for the four-week period, we would suggest 1,000 units of vitamin C [E?] be used in the same manner, and then at the end of four-week period going back to 500 units. We would suggest the vitamins A, D, B, C and E be used in that order. The vitamin B should be that of the thermal type, in such a manner, that that you would know that would stimulate the white corpuscle growth within the body, that that should act as an antibody to fight off and ward off the disease form.

We would also suggest — yes, we see this — we would suggest the massaging of the head area for ten minutes per day, that of the temple area, of the top of the head, throughout the whole area; this should be done.

We would also suggest for the blemishing, that of the small growths in the facial area, that the use of vitamin E be used, rubbing into these areas [through] over the skin. This would greatly help in the healing of the same.

This is all on this soul at this time. A follow-up reading can be obtained upon request.

July 13, 1973: *"Aka, [7-13-73-003], who is here tonight...has asked, 'Do you have any suggestion that could help my husband's health problems?'"*

We should answer this question in this manner. Bring forth unto thy husband, permission, and your answer shall come forth in the same manner. Thy have health problems within thy own body that should need rectifying. We shall give healing both unto your husband and unto yourself. Glory be the name of the Lord. For the Lord giveth in this manner, that your free will should not be violated.

We would suggest, since soul Ray now grows weary, that this same subject should bring forth further questioning at your next reading, in further detail.

July 17, 1973: *"Yes, Aka. (B____ G_____)...has asked for a health reading. She would like to know, 'What is wrong with my health, and is there some treatment?'"*

Yes, we see thy need. And we should answer in these words — we have before us the body, the soul, the spirit, and the immortal body of the same — yes, we should answer that first that is most in mind, of the [backular] area. We find, therefore, fusion of the same. This has come forth from surgery, calcium deposits. We also find within this area that of crimped nerves. The upper proportion, sixth - eighth vertebrae, distortion. We find disease unto the nervous system attacking of the same.

We should answer in this manner, this can be corrected. We should suggest the blood therapy: first, the taking of the sauna baths; second, in the dietary, the removal of calcium from thy diet, magnesium added to the diet within the same, 1000 units of vitamin E per day, 500 units of vitamin C per day. It would be suggested that the vitamin B-[N, in]X complex be used; this taken orally would not be sufficient. It could be in large enough dosage. It would do much better if this was injected into the vein itself, into the circulatory system.

We further find the lacking the vitamin A and B.

We would suggest that surgery be done to remove the calcium deposits and the fusion of the [bonular] area. If this is not done complete fusion shall take place.

We further find that, within this soul, kidney problem. This in itself is nothing more that the lack of exercise. We would suggest that the subject, the use of swimming exercises, that of a floatation unit be placed around the body that the legs and arms could be exercised in this form. This would stop the fusing, breaking loose the calcium deposits within the same and they could do this, naturally dissolve with into the body. This also, as the muscular areas have become no longer in use they are slowly deteriorating. This should be done daily. This in itself as a therapy would be the greatest medicine for this one.

July 17, 1973: *"She asks, 'Will I stay in Arizona or return to my place of birth?'"*

We would suggest at the present time, due to your medical condition, that you remain in a drier climate, that of the Arizonian. We would also suggest that due to a slight sinus condition the taking, therefore, of the sage tea, sweetened with local honey, would relieve of this.

July 17, 1973: *"One other question, Aka. She asks, 'Will I be crippled the rest of my life, or will I be made well? And if so, how soon?'"*

We shall answer your question in this manner. We have given unto your hands that that could heal of you. Go forth and do of these things that e have asked. And we shall place the healing within thy body that is needed. You stand before you now, two roads to follow. One, you could remain a cripple, as you would call it; yet a cripple is only in the mind. The other road you could follow should bring unto you partial, not complete, healing. This in itself is but another road to follow. And yet we say again, that that of being crippled should be only of the mind. For God has placed forth before you — for those who should lose of a hand, those who have lost their hand before you should stand beside you, and therefore, show you in a manner that you may use of one hand as two. We shall take from you the pain of the body. You must do the rest.

July 17, 1973: [Bob says]: *"One moment. [Mrs. V____ L_____] has asked for a health reading, Aka."*

[Speaking louder, Aka says]: **Yes, we should answer of your question in this manner. We have before us the body, the soul, the spirit, and therefore, the immortal body of the same.**

[She whispers]: *"What did he say?"*

We find [more] nerve damage unto the [bonial, the boney, labonia?] area, that of the mastoid, which has caused deafness unto the same. We would suggest, therefore, surgery be done unto this area, replacing that of the damaged third center in the [curricular (cochlear)] area of the ear itself. This could be done quite simply, and inexpensively.

We would further suggest, this one, because of high blood pressure, we find therefore of a low sugar count. Therefore, we would suggest, in this particular case — and this must be understood — that the taking of the sugar *from* the diet should be necessary — only small amounts, replacing it with that of the natural honey.

We would further suggest that a chiropractic doctor be sought out, or osteopathic doctor. X-rays should be taken. The numerous injuries to the backular area is too — at this time, are too many for us to discuss at the present time. But this problem could be solved quite simply with adjustments through the spinal area for this one. This would also relieve, greatly, of the pain, of the headaches this one has had. It will also increase the circulatory system in such a manner to add to this one's hearing.

We would further suggest — yes — that of the vitamin, Lipoflavonoid, be used to expand and relax the [veinliar (veinous)] system within itself.

We would further suggest that this soul — yes, we see this — that an osteo, osteopathic doctor, at the same time advice should be sought out on that of the feet. Corrective shoes could be placed upon these enabling this one much relief with this area.

July 17, 1973: *"Yes, Aka. [M_____ U_____] who is here....and she has asked if she has a heart condition? She also wants to know what is wrong with her back? Can it be cured? And can her arthritis be cured?"*

First, we should say in this manner, we have before us the body, the soul, the spirit, and therefore, the immortal body.

We find no heart problem here. We do find high count of the white blood cells causing the heart to overwork. We would suggest the seeing of your physician as soon as possible so that the proper medication, in this, could be taken.

We would suggest that the osteopathic doctor be sought out, or chiropractic doctor, that adjustments into the lower [backular] area would greatly correct that of the problem within the same.

We would further suggest unto this one that 500 units of vitamin E be taken daily, a good multiple vitamin-mineral be supplemented. But this must be understood, take that of a natural form, not of a synthetic.

We would further suggest that this one is highly allergic to the salt unto which she has taken into the body; therefore, replace the same with a salt supplement.

Yes, We also find — tumor, non-malignant tumor, left side. This is called a fatty tissue; this was caused from an early injury in life. This has caused problems of slight pain. It is not dangerous. It could be removed, either by diet or surgery, whichever this one should desire.

July 17, 1973: *"Aka, (B H) who is here tonight....has asked as number of questions. He asks — one, 'What do you think is wrong physically with me, my leg and left ear?'"*

Yes, we see of thy need. And we should answer in this manner.

We find, therefore, the damage that was done in that of an accidental [form, fall]. Therefore, we have before us the body, the soul, the spirit, and therefore, the immortal body of the same.

*"One moment, Aka. It is his right leg he has marked, and his left ear."*

Yes, we see of this. Yet, we should answer as we have answered before. We should find, therefore, from this accident thy have had, therefore, what is known as brainstem damage. We find, therefore, in this same area scar tissue of the same, and nerve damage within the same. It would not be suggested that this area be relieved with a surgery, for the nerves are damaged in such a manner that the correction of one should cause blindness of another. Therefore, it should be our suggestion first, therefore, for chiropractic treatment of the 6th, 7th, 8th vertebrae. The slow movement with chiropractic treatment of the [bonier, labonia?] area — this can be done by the shifting of the right side of the head in a very slow motional manner. If this is not done correctly, you shall find no results from the same. We would suggest in this case that as each treatment is taken that readings be following, to work within accord. Can you understand of which we speak?

*"Do you understand the message?" Bob asks the man. Then Bob says, "I understand, Aka."*

Then we should answer further in this manner. Full use of both cannot be restored — thy have already that knowledge in thy own mind — but use that thy could go on in life in such a manner to live a full and rich life.

We find other damage within thy body. We find, therefore, the subject within the same is a borderline diabetic. We would suggest the taking, therefore, in addition to the other medication at the present time, of Jerusalem artichoke in raw form.

We further find — yes, we see this — lacerations in what thy would know as the large intestine. These, of ulcerous-type lacerations, have grown scar tissue which is blocking the tract within itself. Therefore, we would suggest the use first of a mild laxative. This, of thy would know as the milk of magnesia, would do. But this should only be used when absolutely needed. It would not be wise that the subject become dependent upon the same. We would further suggest, therefore, that milder unseasoned foods be used. We do not prescribe that all seasoning be extracted from the food, but that of a rich nature. You must realize that your taste for such foods come from that of another lifetime.

We should also suggest unto you into this manner, of that of karmic nature thy have brought forth, this in itself has caused you to seek out suffering within your own body. This, you must realize, is not necessary. This should not rid yourself of the karmic. You have already done so in your own manner. It is often within a soul that a soul should over-punish themselves, or seek beyond their own means that for understanding, when in truth the understanding lays at their feet.

We find — yes, we see this.

July 17, 1973: *"Yes, Aka, he asks, 'What can I do to remedy my condition?'"*

First we should answer further upon the same question we have already answered, that osteopathic or chiropractic treatment be sought. X-rays of the area should be taken, that in truth a doctor should see that of the movement as it is done, from time to time.

*"Of the back, Aka?"*

Of the back and [up there, upper] [neckular] area of the brainstem and the bonier area. That thy have still not fully understood of which we speak, that the skull, you must understand, should contain eight parts. It has been your theory of life that the skull has hardened and, therefore, cannot be moved. This is not true, for the skull can be moved. If this was done so that the left side be shifted slightly forward and upward, then the nerves within themselves could be relieved, and relieving this situation. As we have said before, as this is done readings must, should, be taken as the adjustments are made. Can you *now* understand of which we speak?

*"Yes, Aka."*

Nay, not fully. Then we should answer in this manner. Study of this that we have given, and then thy shall fully understand.

July 17, 1973: *"He asks, 'How is my wife's (B_____'s), health'...."*

Yes, we have before us the body, the soul, the spirit, and the immortal body of the same. Therefore, we should answer in this manner. We find first infection of the vagina area. Yes.

We should answer in such a manner that she should know. That of the washing of the area should be done so with a milder medication. It would be suggested that the drinking of the sage tea, four to six times daily, sweetened with your local honey, this in itself should flush out the kidney and liver area, [add] to that into the circulatory system.

It would also be suggested that this subject should change that of the drinking water into that of a purer form. This subject is highly allergic to that that is known as your chlorine. This subject, therefore, has that of the cramping of the lower abdomen area.

Therefore we find — yes, we see this — of the [upper] left [lungular, lung, uh,] area, scar tissue of the same. This in itself is caused from that of lung damage as a young child. We would suggest it that the filtering of the home be done in such a manner that while the subject should sleep she should breathe that of pure air. This should take forth some of the pollution.

We find — yes, we see of this — we would further suggest in the backular area, the lower proportion of the same, adjustments be made. We find that of pinched nerve, which has led to discomfort, therefore, of the arms and upper neckular area unto this subject. We would suggest that further adjustment be made within the same.

Yes. We find within this subject that lacking within the mineral substance, of magnesium, the lacking of the subject of that in of calcium. We would suggest that these be taken unto 250 units, four per day.

We would further suggest in both subjects the taking unto the body substance of 500 units of vitamin E per day.

We would further suggest — yes, we see this — a lacking of the subjects. We would suggest into this subject in particular that the eating of four to six bananas per day; this could be done by supplementing within thy meal — eating more of the green vegetation, preferably very fresh — taking from thy diets less of the heavier proteins, adding to the diet before each meal, 30 minutes preferably, that of safflower oil in the form of two tablets 30 minutes before the eating of the meal. Yes, we should go back again unto the first subject, add to unto this one unto the same. Since this reading has been given on both subjects we shall combine both of their readings unto the same. Can you understand of which we speak?

*"Ruth can."*

This is good. Therefore, we should say unto thee, thy have other questions, ask.

July 17, 1973: **And we should say unto thee unto these words. Soul John, we find therefore within thy body these substances. Thy have of the measle form, which in itself has attacked the weaker parts of your body. You must remember that that that you have, but one kidney, it must do the job of two. Therefore, we should say unto thee, go unto thy *doctor*. Take of the things thy have thought of in thy mind. But at this time, antibiotic should be sought out unto the body.**

**We would further suggest unto this one that chiropractic doctor be sought out for adjustments of the lower body. The upper necklier [neck] part should not be disturbed in any manner at the present time.**

July 20, 1973: *"Yes, Aka, [7-20-73-001] has asked — he's had a massive stroke, can't swallow solid food and only some liquids, and is having trouble getting sufficient nutrition. 'What can be done to restore health and rhythm and strength and energy,' he asks?"*

**Yes, we have before us the body, the soul, the spirit, and therefore, the immortal body of the same. And therefore, we should answer in this manner. The healing that was needed was given, and yet it was cast aside. If this one should hold onto the thread of life, those instructions it was given before must be carried out to the very letter.**

Only by bypassing those damaged parts of the brain and nervous system can this one be allowed to continue to live. This can only be done by the implanting of the thought and the placing of the healing within the same.

We would suggest there is one other therapy, that the taking of hot olive oil packs be placed around the nerve and up, covering the left side of the face and headular area. This must be repeated eight times daily. This must also be done before the subject should go to sleep at night. This also should cover the left eye which also has been damaged.

There are numerous other problems within this soul, both mental and medical. We should answer in this manner. There is yet one other therapy that could be used to re-stimulate these nerves. That is placing the electrodes that you use in starting that of the heart after it has stopped in the exact same position. This in itself would excite these nerves and start them to rework.

July 20, 1973: *"Thank you, Aka.* [7-20-73-002…Tempe] *has asked for a health reading concerning 'hypoglycemia, uterus infection, eyes, sinus, ears, mouth, infections and physical problems since we moved to Arizona.'"*

Yes, we see thy need. First, we should answer into your question in this manner. We have before us the body, the soul, the spirit, and the immortal body of the same.

Our suggestion, first, is that that is needed in a higher climate and purer air. That unto which you dwell, and unto the land unto which you dwell, has become poisonous to your system. You are highly allergic to the [mineral] substance of iron that should come against your skin.

First, we should suggest the seeking out of the area within the same known as Indian Hot Springs, therefore, using of the mud baths within the same. There is within this soil that which could neutralize your body chemicals and make them less susceptible to your surrounding area.

We would further suggest that increasing of the vitamin E into 1,000 units per day, vitamin C into 500 units.

We would further suggest, one moment, please — yes — we see of thy need, the taking therefore of the honey, one teaspoon six times per day, placing that of a natural apple vinegar within the same — taking twice the amount of honey to one part of vinegar, stirring it rapidly within a small container mixing it thoroughly, adding, therefore, one-fourth of one-fourth teaspoon of plain baking soda into this substance — adding, therefore, four parts to the one part of the compound you have just mixed of that of the sage tea and drinking of the same. This in itself would help in the neutralizing of your body chemicals, and help in the overcoming of this problem within yourself.

We find, therefore — yes, we see of this — a skin problem, that of reddish blots.

Yes.

We should suggest the taking, therefore, of the white of the egg, taking that of the baked bread, mixing within the white of the egg unto the baked bread, making a [poultice] of the same and applying to these areas.

Yes.

We find, therefore — yes — we would suggest also the taking of the tonic known as S.S.S., adding to this in this manner. This tonic may be found foul to the mouth, but yet good for the body.

July 20, 1973: *"Thank you, Aka. [7-20-73-004] has asked..."*

One moment.

Yes.

Continue.

*"...for a health reading. She has had much surgery, the last for cancer. She has allergies, early glaucoma, Meniere's disease (inner ear), bad back, arthritis and circulation problems, high blood pressure, exhausted nerves. 'Is there something else that can be done besides taking so much medication,' she asks?"*

Of the medication that thy are taking at the present time, we find no fault within the same. We should answer in this manner. Should thy change of thy diet form, add more of the green vegetation to your diet. Add that of the fish that should come from the sea, three to four times per week, into thy diet. Add that unto the raw beef form, the rawer the better that this could be eaten. Add unto the diet liver at least once weekly. Add a good natural vitamin and mineral substance compound unto the same.

Seek that unto the ocean; implant thyself into the sands of the same. If this cannot be done, we would suggest the taking that of the earth, finding that similar that could be used of a bathtub, implanting a mixture of sand and water within the same, emerging [immersing] thyself except for thy face into this. If this was done for a two-week period, once per day, your problem [in] your chemicals would return their balance unto the same.

There are many healing qualities that should come from your earth that you have ignored, for the Lord, God, placed upon the earth that that should make His children grow healthy and strong.

July 20, 1973: *"Yes, Aka.[7-20-73-006] has asked — she has hypoglycemia and rheumatoid arthritis, and asks for help concerning that. One moment. She asks, 'Will the D-cell water I am using help me to get better?' And also, 'Will I be completely healed in this lifetime?'"*

Yes, we have before us the body, the soul, the spirit, and the immortal body of the same. We shall answer this question in this manner. The healing thy seek is but at thy fingertips.

First, heal of thy mind into positive thought. We should answer of the arthritic condition, first, you must realize that partially this arthritic condition is brought forth from your own nervous condition. We would suggest the taking of Lydia E. Pinkham. We should further suggest that the taking of the Night-blooming Citros [Cereus] in quarter-by-quarter cubes twice daily. We would further suggest the drinking, therefore, of the sage tea; we would further suggest the adding to this of natural honey. If this cannot be obtained, taking unto this — yes — of the sage honey or that of the mesquite honey. We would further suggest that the taking unto that of the mesquite bean, grinding this unto a fine powdery substance; taking that, therefore, that should come from your saguaro cactus, the seed of the same, grinding this into fine powder form; adding these substances into the tea, and drinking of the same.

July 20, 1973: *"Yes, Aka. She has one other question. 'I have adhesions in my shoulder joints which are very painful. Is there a simple answer to this problem?'"*
Yes, we should answer your question in this manner. Find that, as we have said before, of the mud baths. We should say, take from the clay that should come from this area, take from the sand that should come from the area and the soil that should come from the area. You shall find between Chandler and Coolidge, Arizona, there once was a small town known as Dock. There lies soil that could be added for baths that could have great healing qualities within the same. You can either take the soil from this area or from that. Both substances contain the mineral compounds that could be absorbed into the body that could give healing.

July 20, 1973: *"Thank you, Aka. [7-20-73-008...Globe] has asked for a health reading headaches, pain in the lower lumbar region from injury. She wonders, she says, 'How much longer?'"*
Yes, we see of thy need. We should answer in this manner. Come forth, therefore, unto soul Ray for healing, and this problem can readily be taken care of.

July 22, 1973: *"Aka, [D_____McC___] who is here tonight...has asked two of three questions. The first one — she has a lump in her throat. And she asks, 'Would there be other problems coming from this lump?'"*
Yes, we see thy need. We have before us the body, the soul, the spirit, and the immortal body of the same. That of the lump that thy should speak of is that of an infected glandular area. We would suggest that this area be lanced and drained. We find a small [tumulor, tubular] growth within the same; this is a fatty tissue. It is not malignant. It should be removed; it could cause further problems. We would suggest — yes, we see this — therefore, an imbalance with the body. We would suggest, therefore, that the taking of herbs, that that should come — one moment.

Yes. Take that, that that should come, therefore, of the mistletoe; therefore, that that should come of the sage — this should be sweetened lightly — yes — with honey from the area unto which thy live.

We find the cause of this. The water unto which thy are drinking has become polluted from chemical sources, that man has sprayed upon the ground. It would be our suggestion, therefore, of the taking of 1,000 units of vitamin E per day; therefore, taking unto the system 250 units of vitamin C per day; the taking into the system of the vitamins A, D should be added unto the same. We would also suggest that in thy market, as thy should buy of the green stuff unto the same, these should be thoroughly washed. But do not use the same water that thy have at hand. Take of clean water. Buy, therefore, of what thy would know of the bottled water, that in the form which should be pure.

July 22, 1973: *"Yes, Aka. She asks, 'Do you think I need to go to the hospital?'"*

We would suggest first consulting thy physician, and therefore, arrangements should be made that the growth within itself should be removed, and the glandular area should be drained. This can be — over a long period of time, if proper medication were given — could reduce this area. But the operation within itself is very slight.

July 27, 1973: *"Yes, Aka, [7-27-73-001] asks for a health reading. She had surgery this morning. She asks, 'What kind of help can you give me?' And says, 1969 and '70 she had pain in both legs; in November of 1970 she had a spinal fusion in the lower lumbar which was to relieve leg pains, but didn't help. She has had a backache since. January 1972, she had three operations for artery transplants in both legs. The morning of June 25, 1973, 'woke up with blockage in the left leg; was in the hospital for 10 days.' For the next two or three weeks, she is on blood thinning, then back in the hospital to operate on the left leg transplant again. So she's asking for help."*

Yes, we see thy need. And first, we should answer in this manner. We shall give forth the healing that is needed, that that should make of a speedy recovery.

As the patient is released from the hospital, we would suggest that castor oil packs, not hot, but of body temperature, be placed both over both leg areas, of the upper chestular part of the body, and of the shoulder areas, that which should lead from the backular upper neckular area. We would suggest that this subject should take of 2,000 units of vitamin E per day. We would suggest that this subject drink six times per day that of the sage tea sweetened with the local honey. We would suggest that the vitamin B in multiple use form be used. We would suggest the taking thereof of the subject known as Lydia E. Pinkham.

We would suggest — yes we see this. We find, therefore, of the back, lower backular area, that proportions of the body — sores of the same. We would suggest the use of sugar packs be placed over these. This in itself would greatly speed up the healing of the same. This should be done in this manner, that the sugar should be mixed with small quantities of the white of the egg, placed over the sore portions of the body, small quantities of vitamin E be added within the same.

This is all on this subject at this time.

July 27, 1973: *"Thank you, Aka. [7-20-73-006] asks for a health reading."*

Yes, we have before us the body, the soul, the spirit, and therefore, the immortal body of the same. One moment, the subject — yes, yes, that is better.

Yes, all is in accord now. Yes.

We find, therefore, pain in the lower abdomen. We find problems, therefore, of the liver and both of the kidney areas. We find, therefore — yes.

Yes — of the ovaries.

We find the swelling of the same, that — yes.

We find — yes — problems of the upper backular area. We would suggest, therefore, that these adjustments be made, by either an osteopathic or chiropractic doctor, of the upper area that surrounds the brainstem within itself. We find, therefore, [the] protruding of nerves.

Yes.

We find this should be adjusted.

Yes — of the 6th and 7th vertebrae, this should be adjusted.

Yes.

We find curvature, therefore, of the spine.

Yes.

We find — yes — slight deformity [at] birth in this area. We would suggest, therefore, that most of these problems within themselves could be corrected, either by an osteopathic or chiropractic doctor. We would suggest that x-rays be taken of this area, that the doctor may be readily advised, therefore, of the problems existing.

We find — yes — that of a rash [upon] the vaginal area, irritation in the same.

Yes.

We would suggest, therefore, that the cleansing of this be done by adding small quantities within your wash you are presently using of that of the apple vinegar within the same.

Yes.

We find a problem, therefore, within the respiratory system — nervous condition, highly irregular.

Yes.

We find, for the circulatory system, this highly irregular. These are being caused both by that of the backular area and that — yes — we find therefore, pain, upper left side of the [labonia] [mastoid?] area.

Yes.

Corrections should be made in this area also at this time. We would suggest, therefore — yes — that none of this of what you call your nerve relaxers be used. This is only increasing the problem as it is within itself. We would suggest, therefore, that after this of the osteopathic and chiropractic doctor has made the proper adjustments, you should seek out that of the assistance of soul Ray in the awakening state.

July 27, 1973: *"Thank you, Aka. [7-27-73-003] asks for a health reading. She has backaches and heaviness in her legs."*

Yes, we have before us, therefore, the body, the soul, the spirit, and therefore, the immortal body of the same.

Yes.

Therefore, we have before us the body.

Yes.

First we should, it should be understood, the lack of that of blood. The vessels [for] the main arteries are that quite similar to that you might call to the hardening of the arteries. This is causing great pain. We would suggest that of the seeking out of the Lipoflavonoid-type vitamin. We would suggest — yes — the use of body-temperature castor oil packs on the hip, upper back, and lower backular area be used.

Yes.

We would also suggest the use and the drinking, therefore, of the sage tea, therefore, sweetened with slight amounts of honey.

We find — yes — the subject in mind is that of a low blood sugar.

Yes.

We would suggest, therefore, that that of the natural honey be with the subject most of the time, that the subject shall have urges, therefore, to take of it; do so readily, it shall not harm you.

Yes.

Adjustments of the back — yes — this should be done.

We would further suggest that this subject seek out that of a clay that should come from this area, and therefore, use of baths of the same, that the lower proportion of the body might be emerged [immersed] within the same. This in itself would greatly help in that of the arthritis that is now creeping into the body. The hands also should be immersed within the same, hands and elbows. This should be done repeatedly for a three-week period. We would further suggest that small quantities, that proportions of one ounce might be taken internally, mixed with small quantities of milk, be taken daily of the same.

We would further suggest that more of the vitamin A and E [D?], and vitamin B, be taken into the body. We would further suggest the taking of at least 1,000 units of vitamin E be taken. We would further suggest — yes — that the taking of either of the S.S.S. Tonic, or that of the Lydia E. Pinkham in capsule form or liquid.

Yes.

This is all on this subject at this time.

July 27, 1973: *"Yes, Aka, could you — one brief questions about this clay. Could you tell me what it contains that makes it beneficial to peoples' health?"*

Yes, we shall answer in this manner. First, there is magnesium, that of the copper extract, that of your, both your vitamins A, B, C, that of dolomite, that — yes — your clay within itself holds that of an antibiotic, that that of yet you are to have placed a name upon. You shall find that the antibiotic can be used in many forms. You shall find that the clay within itself may be used in that of treating ulcers. You may [be] find that that of the clay may be used of that of heart condition. You will find also quantities of radioactive material within the same. These you shall think might be harmful to the body, but they are not. In that proportion that the body is lacking, it shall bring forth and excite the antibodies within the body to fight off disease within itself.

We could give you much more lengthy descriptions of the question unto which you asked. We shall say unto you unto these words. Only as suggested should this clay be used, and only within the amounts that we should give, and in the manner unto which we should give. Soul Ray in his awakening state shall know of these things and should be capable of giving to those in need that knowledge that they need at the time.

July 27, 1973: *"Thank you, Aka. Aka, [7-27-73-004] has asked for a health reading and other information. He asks, 'What is the cause and solution for the stiffness and pain in my upper back and neck?'"*

Yes, we see of this. The cause within itself was caused as a fall as a very small boy, injury to central nervous system, causing that of rheumatoid arthritis within the body. The solution should be that of the taking of the Night-blooming Citros [Cereus] in quarter-by-quarter cubes. We would further suggest the use of the same clay, and immerging of the body in the same manner. We would suggest the taking of that of vitamin E. We find that of too much at this time of the vitamin C within the body. Therefore, the use of the same should be avoided for the present time. Substitute this with orange juice in your early morning and late evening hours.

July 30, 1973: *"Aka, [7-30-73-001], who is here tonight, has asked for a life reading and also for a health reading. In regards to her health reading, Aka, she has two questions. One, 'What was the cause of the headaches in the spring of 1965? And what caused the accident I was involved in May 1966?'"*

First we should answer of the last. And the last, as thy know within thy own mind, was carelessness.

Of the headaches within themselves, you must realize that you [are] within thyself a form of epilepsy. The form within itself could readily be corrected with the use of biofeedback machinery. This within itself would relieve the hypertension within the body, also relieve that of the high blood pressure. This also could bring forth your full personality if it were used in a correct manner. At the present time, the machinery in the form and in the use that we have proposed only lies within Ray's mind. The treatment within itself could bring forth your full personality. This you yourself are in great need of.

August 3, 1973: *"Yes, Aka.* [8-3-73-001]*, who is here tonight...has asked for a health reading."*

Yes, we have before us the body, the soul, the spirit, and therefore, the immortal body of the same.

And therefore, we should answer in this manner. We find, therefore, within the body that, a rheumatoid-arthritic condition.

Yes, we see of this.

We find, therefore, within the same that of diabetic. This within itself is not of a true diabetic, for it comes from an impurity of the blood within the same. We, therefore, find within the body small tumorous growths which are non-malignant. These are located in that proportion that was the uterus area. We should suggest, within the same, increasing of vitamin E to 1,000 units, the taking of therefore of that of the Lydia E. Pinkham. We would further suggest the taking of the Night-blooming Cereus in quarter-by-quarter [inch] cubes daily. We would also suggest that since none have prepared and none have stored of the same, of your Jerusalem artichoke, that you should substitute these with that of the fruit that should come from the saguaro cactus, taking of the small seed and grinding of the same, using it for seasoning within this one's food. This at this time would take the place of the same. The eating of the fruit would help in the thyroid condition that lies within the same.

We would further suggest that should soul Ray give healing into the body, this would greatly help.

We would also suggest the taking of the clay which we have mentioned before, the adding of the vitamin E unto the substance, moistening this clay with olive oil; taking that of a warm towel, placing the moist clay in a thin layer upon the same, wrapping of the joints of these areas that are so inflicted. This would not only greatly reduce the pain and give smoothing unto the skin, but would also relieve at the present time this condition.

We find, therefore, imbalance — yes — of a glandular area, imbalance of that of the pineal gland within the same. We would suggest the use of a negative-ion machine be used while this one is in slumber at night. We would further suggest the drinking of pure, clean water, the filtering of the air unto which she breathes. We find, therefore, in a respiratory problem within the same, it might be suggested — yes — that small quantities of oxygen be fed through mask form, as the subject should respond to the same and have need of the same. We would further suggest the use of the sauna bath, but within the use of the same, if this could be done at very small intervals, no more than three minutes in the beginning, and building up into a 15-minute interval per day. This must be done with dry heat.

We shall say unto thee into these words. You have yet within your science to find the key that lies within the mind that should bring forth and stop your aging process. Within the mind lies the key to reverse the process, and therefore, taking mind and body slowly back into the youthful condition it once was.

But we should say unto thee into these words. As an old oak stands and looks upon the young, would it trade its knowledge for their youth? Thy have thy faith within God, and God has His faith within you. This within itself is the most important of all things, for the doors that shall open shall be beautiful, for roses shall be placed without thorns. [Editor's note: a rose without thorns is said to spiritually symbolize the birth or coming of the Messiah.]

August 3, 1973: *"Yes, Aka. [8-3-73-002] has asked, 'I would like a health and life reading, as my eyes are giving her a little trouble; they are dry, at night only so far, which can cause blindness. I would like very much to know how to correct this situation.'"*

Yes, we should answer in this manner. Taking, therefore, of the hot olive oil packs, placing within the same that of castor oil, mixing together, making a porous [poultice] of the same; placing over the eyes at night before slumber, this within itself shall remove the problem and remove the starting of the cataracts as they have began to form.

August 3, 1973: *"Yes, Aka. [8-3-73-004] asks for a health reading and about her future."*

Yes, we have before us, therefore, the body, the soul, the spirit, and the immortal body of the same. And the last we shall give first. Of thy internal problems within the same, these shall soon be dissolved. Time within itself is one of the greatest healers.

You ask, therefore, for your own future. This within itself shall be made by you and shall be made by you and you alone. Therefore, we should say unto you into these words. As a pool of water should flow it does not become stagnated, and therefore, the water should cleanse itself as it flows. But your stagnation, as you stand without renewal of the structure within yourself — within each soul there is free choice, that to enter or not to enter. There is free choice, that to stand as one would with their head buried within the sand, or that to walk forward into life and take of it and live of it.

We should say unto this one, and so it is written, the Lord, God, said unto these words, "OF OUR KIND, OF OUR LIKENESS, SO WE HAVE CREATED THESE AND FOUND THEM GOOD." Therefore, remember, a good father takes nothing from his child, nor hides nothing. That that you have found within yourself and thought to cast aside that was wrong could be that proportion within yourself that God, Himself, would not cast aside; then why should you?

We could speak many words. But hear the meaning of what we have given, and then we shall continue. The health reading we shall continue at your next reading.

August 3, 1973: *"[8-3-73-003] asks for a health reading to find relief from pain in her teeth for which dentists have been unable to help."*

Yes, we see thy need. First, we should answer, we have before us the body, the soul, the spirit, and therefore, the immortal body.

We shall answer in this manner. They have been contaminated with lead. Thy have lead poisoning. This within itself has settled within the jawbone area. We shall suggest that the problem lies not within the bone of the jaw as much so as treatment through the blood. Therefore, we would suggest, first, seeking out that of a good blood specialist. There are several known drugs that this could be treated by. We would not suggest the use of cortisone within this; this would only irritate and add to the problem as it stands. We would suggest the use of that proportion injected into the jawbone area of penicillin. This must be done in small quantities. If this could be injected into the basic root center in eight places in the lower jawbone area, this problem could be removed.

If this is not found feasible, then we would suggest the taking of that thy would know as Vaseline, taking that of the vitamin E, mixing to one teaspoon of Vaseline 10,000 units of vitamin E, mixing it together, taking thy own finger and swabbing the gum area on both upper and lower proportions; drinking, therefore, of the sage tea sweetened with local honey and the drinkings of as much of the cranberry juice as the body will abstain [sustain].

August 17, 1973: *"Yes, Aka. [7-27-73-005] asks for a health reading. He says he has pain in his right leg and trouble with his eyes which have made him bedridden."*

Yes, we see thy need, and we should answer of your question in this manner.

First, we should say in this manner, of the lack of oxygen we see unto the brain. Therefore, we say unto thee, we have before us the body, the soul, the spirit and the immortal body. Yes, we see of this. That within the same has caused — yes — damage unto the [labonier?] area, to the brain stem area — yes — causing much of what you would know as palsy. This, in itself, if not checked, stopped, shall continue and go forth. Therefore, we should answer in this manner. Venture forth into that which you would call this land, here. Come forth unto soul Ray and let him give unto thee of the healing that is needed.

We find damage unto the lower spinal area — yes — damage unto the liver area, improper circulation within the same. First, we should suggest that of 2,000 units of vitamin E per day be given unto this subject daily, vitamin A and D, that of the pantothenic acid should be taken, vitamin B — yes. We would suggest unto the diet more of the vegetation in its rawest form, well cleaned. We would further suggest that of the new compound that soul Ray has brought forth be used, that unto which he has created in the warm form. This should be applied, from the brainstem area to the lower proportions of the tail bone area, and done so at least once daily. We would further suggest that the eating of as many of the green olives as thy could desire to eat, purchasing large quantities, and when thy would want to snack, eat of these. Do the same with that of the banana and the milk. But for each glass of milk thy should drink, eating three bananas.

Thy have in thy mind, "Of how long a period this should take to bring about the healing?" This should largely be to the person, as the soul, as we have said before, has free choice. They can ignore our suggestions, and therefore, there shall be no healing, but the disease shall go on and increase. If the suggestions are taken, then immediate results shall be shown.

August 17, 1973: *"Thank you, Aka. Aka,* [8-3-73-004]*, and she asks for a health reading."*

Yes, we find of this, and therefore, one moment — yes, that is better — therefore, we have before us the body, the soul, the spirit, and the immortal body of the same. Therefore, we find, therefore, within this soul — yes.

First, we should mention of a problem of the vagina area. Yes.

We find small cyst-type growths upon the ovary — yes — of the right ovary. Of this within itself medication could be sought to dissolve of this.

We find, therefore, within the soul — yes — of the 4th and 5th vertebrae, separation of the same, causing lower backular pains. Yes.

Of this we would suggest the use of either osteopathic or chiropractic treatment.

We find within this soul very poor balance of vitamin and mineral substance, imbalance within the same. First, we would suggest, therefore, the taking of the Lydia E. Pinkham. Second, we would suggest, therefore — yes — of a good natural vitamin-mineral compound be taken. Extra vitamin E should be added unto this.

Yes.

We would further suggest unto this one that that of the extreme nerve condition which this one has suffered has been partially up to her own emotions, her own frame of mind. Part of this is due to the worry of an overweight condition. This in itself should not be as such. If thy should eat first before meals, 30 minutes before meals, taking that of the safflower oil, adding beef at least once meal per each week, adding the fish that should come of the sea of one meal of each week, adding that of liver of the beef once each week. It would also be suggested that that eating of the lamb should be done once each week. Eating more of the raw vegetables; this should be done with adding small quantities of salt, placing no, none of your — one moment, we must find this word — yes, yes — your dressing — yes — unto this. Drinking one glass of milk for breakfast and one piece of brown toast. For the luncheon meals, adding that of cottage cheese, fruits, and vegetables, with no other substances.

Yes, we find within this one that of a sinus condition, and therefore, we should answer in this manner. We would suggest the taking, therefore, of the sage tea, sweetening with the local honey if possible. Do not boil this, steep it. We would further suggest the taking of plain water, adding salt, that that should be extracted from the ocean, four tablespoons to each quart of water, bringing this to a boil, placing a towel over the head in such a manner to make that of what you would call a vaporizer, using this once daily to cleanse out this area.

August 17, 1973: *"Yes, Aka,* [8-17-73-001] *asks for a health reading. He says, 'I have not been able to,' one moment. 'I have not been able, to the arthritic condition affecting the joints of my body, by physical means.' I don't get the sentence."*

We can answer the question, and therefore, we should answer in this manner. We have before us the body, the soul, and the spirit of the same. First, we must advise this one that most of thy arthritic condition is caused, that from nervous imbalance. Second, we should say that you have of two forms of arthritis, one of which is a virus, and therefore, must be treated as the same. We would suggest that of coming unto soul Ray, taking, therefore, of the formula unto which he has brought forth, and placing compounds or portions [potions] over these areas. We would further suggest that, that taking of the Night-blooming Cereus in quarter-by-quarter [inch] cubes. As this plant — yes, we see this.

Therefore, we would suggest, one moment — we would suggest that the taking of the Jerusalem artichoke. We would suggest that when the crops are harvested that they should be dried and made into powder form and stored, that this may be used for medicinal purposes. At the present time, should thy take of the fruit of the saguaro cactus, eating of the same, these shall be tasty; therefore, eat all thy want.

At the present time, we shall place new thought and new formula that this problem of your searching of the cactus [Night-blooming Cereus] may come to an end. We have new thoughts we shall put forth into soul Ray's mind.

August 17, 1973: *"Thank you, Aka. [8-17-73-002], he asks for a health reading, advice for a doctor or a remedy for his back. He asks advice to grow spiritually, and he asks about past lives."*

First we should answer, that of your past lives should be brought up at a different time.

That that you may grow spiritually, we have placed the wine before you, that this may be done.

We have said unto thee, those of the group, to place at least three of your readings, the spiritual philosophy that we have given forth, in your newsletter once monthly.

We have placed the wine and the bread. We have also furnished the yeast. Thy have come to our door. We shall give unto thee that unto which thy mind shall digest at a given time.

Of thy health, we shall answer in this manner, for soul Ray now begins to grow weary, and our time has grown short. Bring forth these questions at your next reading.

And now we say unto thee these words. Those who are members of the Board of Trustees, come forth one unto another. We have said unto that unto which we wish be done unto those of your bylaws. When we said unto thee, written material, this included that of the same. For a soul to grow it cannot be placed in a cage, that souls who are bound together in a common cause they must be able to walk as one. We have said before, we shall allow nothing from either side to interfere with this work. What the Lord has giveth, the Lord may taketh away. Call your Board of Trustees together that all may be in accord. We have told you before that where harmony cannot prevail we cannot reside.

August 24, 1973: *"Thank you, Aka. [8-24-73-002] asks for a health reading. She asks what might be done to dissolve the blood clot in her one good eye so that she might see enough to get around? Also she seeks relief from the pain she has had since her stroke this spring, and whatever help is possible."*

Yes, we have before us the body, the soul, and the spirit, and therefore, the immortal body of the same. And we shall answer in this manner. We shall take from this one the pain. We shall give unto this one a sight of seeing. But we say unto you, there are many doors, and our Father has many mansions. Blessed be the name of the Lord.

August 24, 1973: *"Aka, [8-24-73-002] asks for a health reading. He states, since his head injury at age 24, he has had vision trouble, suffering dizziness, nausea and ringing in his ears, and has been told he has Meniere's disease in his right ear and perhaps a tumor. He asks for help, and asks if he will get worse as the years go by, and if so, should he have surgery?"*

First we should answer in this manner, we have before us the body, the soul, the immortal body, the spirit of the same.

Yes, we see this.

First we should answer of the ringing of the ears. This is a disease called Meniere's, or inner ear infection. It is caused, therefore, from brainstem damage, partially. It is also caused, therefore, from a hardening of the arteries, the main arteries that should feed of the brain and the inner ear within itself. We would suggest, therefore, first, a drug known as Ardelin be taken; this could be taken in 10 grams. We would suggest, therefore, that the vitamin substance known as Lipoflavonoid be used in this condition, therefore, to soften these blood vessels that have become hard, and therefore, make them more pliable.

Yes, we find, therefore — yes, we see this.

We find, therefore, of a blood condition.

Yes.

We find an infection in the lung area. We find, therefore, the blood within itself trying to coagulate within the system, and therefore, producing more red corpuscles to offset this condition of the lungs. We would suggest the taking of 2,000 units of vitamin E per day. We would suggest that the subject, the use of negative ion machine be used whilst in slumber. We would suggest — yes — that a filtering system be placed within the home, therefore, that the subject in mind could breathe clean air. We would also suggest that the changing of the drinking water in a more purified form. If the following recommendations are followed through, the subject should not grow worst, but begin to heal.

August 24, 1973: *"Yes, Aka, he had one other question concerning a problem with hemorrhoids and bleeding and asked if there was anything other than surgery that be done for this?"*

Yes, we would suggest taking of vitamin E and vitamin A, mixing together with the vitamin D, taking that of the white of the egg, mixing it into a slight compound, adding there of the safflower oil. If this placed unto the rectum area this should heal the wounds within the same and cause a shrinking of the same.

For those who have similar conditions, we would not suggest the use of this; this is for this one subject only. Because of his body chemical substance, it has been suggested in this manner.

August 24, 1973: *"[8-24-73-004] asks for a health and life reading. She says her health is poor, liver and kidney trouble, rheumatoid arthritis, colon trouble, and so forth. 'For my gout I am taking Benemid daily and vitamins and minerals. And help would be greatly appreciated.'"*

We should answer in this manner unto this subject. Come, therefore, unto soul Ray for healing. We shall place the knowledge, therefore, within the mind that this problem can be taken care of.

August 24, 1973: *"Aka, [8-24-73-005] asks for a health reading."*

Yes, we have before us the body, the soul, the spirit, and the immortal body of the same.

Yes.

One moment, this subject must be located.

Yes, therefore, we have the subject in mind. First we should answer in these words. We find within the subject matter what is known as that of Valley Fever. This could only be treated in this manner — with rest, clean air, vitamin E in 1,000-unit per day, vitamin A, [B], the taking, therefore, of that compound known as chaparral, taking each unit six times per day.

We find, therefore, within this subject — yes — that of a problem within the heart within the fourth valve, a deteriorating of the same. It would be our suggestion that the subject should seek out the help of a physician. If the heart can be slowed down and the body to function off of less oxygen and blood substance, the healing of both could happen quite easily. This could be done with what is known as a bio-feedback machine and the teaching substance within the same. At the present time, your doctors do not have the knowledge to put this into practical use. Therefore, we would suggest meditation in that form that you should lie in a very comfortable position, placing within yourself and in your mind that of God. If you should contact soul Ray, a meditation tape could be supplied that would greatly help this in the same and help you in the learning of the same.

Yes, we find — yes — within the kidney-liver area small cysts-type growths forming upon the liver itself. At the present time these could be removed surgically, or could be dissolved [with] that of the psychic.

Yes.

We find that this subject should seek out unto chiropractic or osteopathic doctor. The upper portion backular area is greatly in need of treatment of the same, 8th, 9th vertebrae. If this condition continues you shall find permanent disability within the same.

Should this subject require follow-up reading after the following suggestions have been taken, we would be glad to give unto the same.

August 24, 1973: *"Thank you, Aka. [8-24-73-006] asks for a health reading. He says, 'I have had an infection in the cavity above the upper palate of my mouth for as long as I can remember, and I have not been able to find a cure. What is the cause, and how can it be cured? Is there any relation between the infection and the tightness I feel in my chest at times? Also, what does the future hold in regards to my vocation?'"*

We shall answer unto this one into this manner. First, we should say unto thee, we have before us the body, the soul, and the spirit, immortal body of the same. One moment, we must locate this subject.

Yes. Yes, now we have the subject.

Therefore, we would answer in this manner.

Yes.

Of the infection within itself, we would suggest that the seeking out of a doctor that this substance be removed, and therefore, allowing new tissue to grow back within it same.

Of the other questions, we would suggest that you should ask at a different time, for now soul Ray grows weary.

And we should say to thee in these words. Now is the time of the Cherub. And the Fifth Angel walks upon your earth. Beware. New eruptions shall arise, close within your land this time.

August 31, 1973: *"Aka, [8-31-73-001] asks for healing. He has a small upside-down, pear-shaped obstruction that looks like a second stomach in his esophagus, which is located above the regular stomach and has a very small opening in the bottom, causing him great difficulty in swallowing food. Sometimes, he says, it is so bad he is unable to get water or liquids down for two or three days. He also asks for a health reading."*

First, we should answer in this manner. The healing that is given shall be given in this manner; surgery must be performed upon this soul, corrective surgery. The surgery within itself is not as serious as the subject should think. Therefore, seek out that that is at your hand, and use it in the same manner, and the healing thy should ask for shall be given.

August 31, 1973: *"Thank you, Aka. [8-31-73-002] asks for healing. She has a sinus problem and sometimes difficulty with her breathing. She has requested a health reading, 'if you are able to do this.'"*

Yes, we have before us the body, the soul, and the spirit of the same, and therefore, the immortal body. Yes, we see thy need. One moment.

Yes.

We should answer in this manner. First, we should suggest the taking of 2,000 units of vitamin E per day. Second, we should suggest the taking of the sea water, and therefore, bringing it to a boil, placing a damp towel over the head, that thy may breathe of the vapor that has come from the sea water. This should help in the healing of the same.

We find, therefore, within the same this that is called [of] varicose veins — yes — of the thighs, [an aspirate] area of the same, yes. We would suggest that use of the warm mud that has been perfected within the same, applied to these areas. This would help in the stimulating of the vessels and the drying and pulling forth of that of the blood substance of the same.

We find in the 3rd and 4th vertebrae area, therefore, damage within the same. We would suggest, therefore, the chiropractic or osteopathic treatment be sought, that this could be rectified quite simply.

Yes, we find that of a scalp problem — yes —that of an itching and flaking substance of the same. We would suggest, therefore, that the taking of the white of the egg, that substance known as baking soda, mixing together within the same. Add that of your liquid form, that which would come, which you would call of beer unto the same, adding, therefore, unto the same small quantities of olive oil, working this into the scalp area, leaving for 30 minutes, and then washing this substance from the scalp; this would greatly relieve this area.

Of the healing thy have asked for, this shall be given in the manner into which the instructions we have given you are followed.

August 31, 1973: *"Aka, [7-2-73-002] asked, 'Do you find evidence of cancer in my prostate? Can you see a clearing of my present blockage, and if so, how soon? Do I need a special course of treatment which has been proposed on the theory that I do have a degenerative condition?'"*

First, we should suggest in this manner, thy do have a degenerative condition within the same. But we would suggest, therefore, rather than prolonged treatment, surgery, that this could simply be rectified. We would suggest the drinking, therefore, of large quantities of cranberry juice, and therefore, of that known as the sage tea, sweetened with honey, as much as thy body shall allow. This in itself shall clear the blockage.

That of the prostate and the problem within the same is not of cancerous nature. It is not malignant within the same, but left over a prolonged period, it soon could become that. Therefore, we would suggest that this should be — that the tissue, therefore, that has grown into place should be removed by surgery.

August 31, 1973: *"Yes, Aka, [8-31-73-003] has had a problem in her right arm and hand. She says needle tests show she does not have complete use of her nerves in the arm. Doctors say she possibly had polio, but she had immunizations. She has had to give up working as a beauty operator. What is wrong, and can anything be done to correct it?"*

Yes, we see this, and we should answer in this manner. First, we have before us the body, the soul, the spirit, and the immortal body of the same. We find, therefore — yes — in that proportion known as the brainstem area damage within the same. We would suggest, therefore, that through chiropractic treatment this condition could be rectified.

We further find — yes.

We would suggest, bring this soul forth unto soul Ray, and therefore, let him project healing into the area of the same.

August 31, 1973: *"[2-4-72-001] who is her tonight...asks for a health reading on her left arm. Is it healing as it's supposed to be? Is there anything she can do to help it? She also asks, did she damage her elbow as well, and what can be done to help it?"*

First, we should answer in this manner. We have before us the body, the soul, the spirit, and the immortal body of the same. Therefore, we should answer in this manner. Come forth unto soul Ray that healing may be given unto this area, that the damage done, as we have said before, is a v-type break which lingered downward into the joint within the same. This has caused an irritation of the ligament within the arm. It would be suggested that she come forth unto soul Ray that healing should be administered. We would further suggest that that of the warm clay be used on the area. This should be done according to soul Ray's instructions. We would further suggest that for the present time this arm not be over exercised that healing can be given and that the healing should not be destroyed that *is* given. Can you understand of which we speak?

*"Yes."* [She answers.]

August 31, 1973: *"Yes, Aka. She has another question. She asks, when the goat kicked her did it do damage to her head or right ear?"*

No, we do not find of this. We find bruises, yes, but no permanent damage within the same. We should place the healing within the body, and therefore, the healing shall commence.

August 31, 1973: *"Aka, [8-31-73-004], he's in the need of a health reading."*

We should answer in this manner, give more specific information; our time is limited.

September 7, 1973: **You have questions, ask.**
*"Yes, Aka. Can you make any suggestion for [5-7-71-002]'s tooth infection? She is allergic to antibiotics."*

We have seen of this need, and we shall have given healing unto the same. That was, shall be no more.

September 7, 1973: **You have other questions, ask.**
*"Thank you, Aka. [8-17-73-002] asks for a health reading; he asks for your advice of a doctor or a remedy for his back."*
**We shall say unto these words; we have before us the body, the soul, the spirit, and the immortal body of the same.**

**Of the problem of the backular area — yes, we see of this. We would suggest thy seek out a good osteopathic or chiropractic doctor; there are many. This could be remedied.**

**We would also suggest that the taking of this one, because of an infection within the liver-kidney area, all alcoholic beverages at this time. We would further suggest the seeking out within your own religion counseling that should come of a spiritual nature. Within this you shall find that that you seek, should seek.**

September 7, 1973: **You have other questions, ask.**
*"Yes, Aka. I have a request for a health reading for [8-24-73-006]. He says, he was told to have a continuation of this reading regarding his chest. He has a problem in his chest with — one moment, just a moment here — tightness in his chest that he feels at times. And also, he wonders, what does the future hold in regards to his vocation?"*
**We should answer in this manner; we find within this soul the body, the soul, spirit, and the immortal body of the same. We find, therefore, a hiatic [hiatus] hernia within the same of the chest area. It is not a serious problem. We would suggest, take from the diet that of the rich foods. Take from the diet that of the cheese forms within the same. Take, therefore, before each meal that of the safflower oil, taking into the body 1,000 units of vitamin E per day, with normal dosage of both mineral and vitamins supplement within the body.**

September 7, 1973: **You have other questions, ask.**
*"Yes, I have a request for a health reading for [9-7-73-001]...asks for a health reading, reasons for pain across shoulder blades and back. She says she has heaviness in the chest, anxiety feelings, fear and so forth, and tremendous spasms throughout the body, head to toes."*
**We do not see of this.**

September 7, 1973: **You have other questions, ask.**
*"[9-7-73-002] asks, 'What should I do for my skin problem?' She also had asked the question, 'Should I take the job offered two days ago or not?'"*
**(Chuckle.)That decision has already been answered for you.**
**Of the skin problem, we should answer in this manner. Seek out consultation from soul Ray. A solution shall be found within the same.**

September 7, 1973: **Thy have other questions, ask.**

*"Yes, Aka. [9-7-73-003] asks for health and life readings. She has had a viral infection from flu three years ago which is localized in the semicircular canals and vasculatory system of her right inner ear causing inflammation. For a year she has suffered a strange buoyancy, a floating sensation at the slightest movement. She also is a borderline diabetic, and takes weekly antigen shots for allergy to trees, grass and so forth, which showed up three years ago. Please tell her what to do for this dizziness, she asks."*

Yes, we have before us the body, the soul, the spirit, and the immortal body of the same.

First we should say unto this one, thy have developed what is known as Meniere's, or that of an infection to the inner ear. This in itself can be treated by the use of the drug known as Antivert.

Yes.

We would further suggest that the use of warm castor oil be used to cleanse the ear. This should be left in for short periods of time and then the use of that which you would call of the peroxide be used to wash out the ear within itself.

The backular area is greatly in need of adjustment. This would partially correct this problem. We would suggest the seeking of a good osteopathic doctor; that of frontal lobal area, that unto which, therefore, within first and second vertebrae, if adjustments could be made within this area the problem within itself would slowly reside [subside].

September 7, 1973: **You have other questions, ask.**

*"Yes, Aka. I have a series of questions for [9-7-73-004]...and asks for a health reading, about her daily life, and future. She says, 'I would like a general health reading,' including, is she on the right dosage of hormones? She is also interested in knowing what to do to improve her eyesight."*

Yes, we have before us the body, the soul, and therefore, the spiritual body within the same. Yes. We see of this.

We would suggest the use of Lydia E. Pinkham to bring forth a balance of the hormones. We would suggest the use of hot — warm olive oil packs be placed over the eyes; first, of the olive oil, second, of the castor oil. Do not put the castor oil in the eyes themselves, only on the outer lid within the same. This would greatly improve that unto which you ask.

We say unto you unto these words. Now is the time of the Cherub.

Soul Ray now grows weary. That we may not overtax the body, awaken soul Ray from his slumber.

September 15, 1973: **You have questions, ask.**

*"Yes, Aka. I have a health reading request for a 34-month-old boy,* [8-37-73-004]. *His parents ask how to treat or eliminate hyper kinesis?"*

Yes, we see thy need, and therefore, we have before us the body, soul, spirit, and therefore, the immortal body of the same.

The treatment within itself, and the diagnosis within itself, is not the same. We find small non-malignant growths in the lower [lombera] [mastoid?] area, which has, therefore, placed pressure which has caused the problem within the inner ear. Therefore, should this be removed with minor surgery, the problem within itself would readily disappear. This could be determined quite simply with the use of what you call of your x-ray.

September 15, 1973: **You have other questions, ask.**

*"Thank you, Aka.* [9-7-73-004], *has asked, 'I have had a stapedectomy on my left ear which has been very successful. Would one on my right ear be advisable and successful, especially with the fenestration and plastic surgery that was performed in that ear approximately 23 years ago?'"*

We have before us the body, the soul, the spirit, and therefore, the immortal body of the same. Your present problem is not of that that you had before. The problem is that which you would call the hardening of the arteries. The suggestion would be, therefore, with medication. This could be done with either the use of nitrogen in small quantities or with the drug known as Ardelin, 20 milligrams per day once — twice daily, given orally. We would also suggest the use of a vitamin known as Lipoflavonoid, This should be taken in such a manner — yes, we see this — that the subject in mind could also use this as a vitamin supplement, therefore, taking six capsules per day.

We further see the problem — yes — problem of the left ovary — yes — pressure against the same. We would suggest therefore, come, therefore, unto soul Ray, that healing could be given unto this area.

We further find in the liver area a degeneration of the same. We would suggest the use of vitamin E in quantities of 1,000 units per day. We would suggest the use of vitamin B, preferably — yes — preferably this could be done by injection into the bloodstream. If this is not found practical, use that unto what you would call your vitamin B-Plus supplement in such a manner that you would take three times the normal dosage, or six of these per day. This should only be done for a 30-day period, no more. Then go back to a normal dosage.

We find, therefore, within this subject — yes — we see this (sigh), that of the overactive thyroid, that of which would be known as a borderline diabetic. Neither of these are serious. The eating of the Jerusalem artichoke, the taking, therefore, of the substance known as Lydia E. Pinkham would stabilize these areas within the same.

We find that of a cosmetic problem. We would suggest, therefore, that you should seek out that of the clay of soul Ray. This could be used to rectify the condition.

We find, therefore, the problem of slight overweight, therefore, pressure against the heart area. We would suggest that before the eating of any meal the taking of two capsules, units, of safflower oil — yes. This should be done at least 30 minutes before the eating of your meals. We would suggest that your breakfast consist of no more than one glass of milk and one piece of rye toast, that your luncheon meals consist of no more than one glass of milk and as many of the green vegetation as you should desire. You shall find that the breaking out, the reddish spots upon the body are caused from the lack of green vegetation. We would further suggest — yes — the taking of the vitamin A and D in normal quantities.

This is all on this subject at this time.

September 15, 1973: **You have other questions, ask.**
*"Yes, Aka. [9-15-73-001] asks for a health reading and about his job. He says x-rays show three degenerated discs in his back, and he needs to know what to do to strengthen them or bring them back to normal. He's concerned about his eyes. And he says his arms are getting too short to read by."*
Yes, we have before us the body, the soul, the spirit, and therefore, the immortal body of the same.

We would suggest, therefore, chiropractic help be sought, that that of the third and fourth vertebrae, therefore, should be adjusted, that that of the brainstem from that of the scalp or skull unit which should come into eight parts should therefore be shifted, therefore, to relieve pressure upon nerves of the same.

We find, therefore, that this soul has a great problem with the dentures of the same within the teeth. If this problem, if this soul could seek out a good oral surgeon and the gum disease within the same could be rectified, this would cure the problem of the eyesight, with the proper adjustments of the head and neckular area within the same. We would suggest that at the present time the use of vitamin E be used, rubbed in all along the gumular area. These should be massaged for at least two minutes per day. This would greatly help to alleviate this area within the same. [Editor's note: the tape that was available ran out at this point, so the rest was not checked.]

We, therefore, also see of his other questions, and we shall answer in this manner, that these too should be sought out in private consultation unto soul Ray, for they are of a personal nature too delicate to discuss in public.

September 28, 1973: **You have many questions, ask.**

*"Yes, Aka. I have a request for a health reading for [9-7-73-001]. She asks for a health reading on pains across her shoulder blades and the back. She says she has heaviness in her chest, anxiety feelings, fears and so forth, and tremendous spasms throughout her body, head to toes."*

Yes, we see thy need, and therefore, we have before us the body, the soul, the spirit, and the immortal body of the same.

Yes, we see this.

First, you should understand these words. You are going through that period of the change of life. You have the need of estrogen within the body. We would suggest that the taking of the Lydia E. Pinkham be used for the same. There are other herbs within this that should calm your nerves.

Second, we would suggest the taking of 1,000 units of vitamin E per day.

Yes, we see this.

We find, therefore, of a disease that has been since childhood. (Sigh.)This is a disease of the blood vessels within themselves, a deterioration of the same. It would be wise at this point to seek out, therefore, a surgeon, that transplants may be applied into the same.

Yes, we see this.

We would also suggest, because of the financial condition — yes — come forth, therefore, unto soul Ray that healing may be given unto thee.

This is all on this subject at this time.

September 28, 1973: **Thy have other questions, ask.**

*"[9-28-73-001] asks for a health reading, and asks, 'What should I do about my acne condition? Are there any treatments I should take?'"*

We have before us the body, the soul, and the immortal body of the same. Therefore, we should answer in these words.

Bring forth first unto more purified water unto the system, taking, therefore, into the system of 1,000 units of vitamin E per day. Of the acne condition within itself, come forth unto soul Ray, therefore, taking of the mud substance of the same, applying unto the proportions of the body that are infected in the same manner.

Yes, we see this.

We would suggest the use of calcium and magnesium that the leg spasms might be relieved. We would suggest the going forth unto a chiropractic doctor that this problem could be ratified [rectified]. You will find between the 7th and 8th vertebrae a problem within the same, therefore, nerves extracting, and contracting. This problem can be easily ratified.

We find further problems within the backular area, of the upper neckular [prebonial] area, therefore, within the brainstem area, pressure caused — yes — from that which you would call of a car accident. We would suggest that adjustments be made in this area at this time.

If other suggestions are needed, a follow-up reading would be suggested.

September 28, 1973: **You have other questions, ask.**

*"Yes, Aka, [9-28-73-002] has asked for a health reading. She says she has a buzzing sound in her head, not from high blood pressure. A naturopathic doctor found she had low iron and said she was tense and tightens up around her shoulder. Also she feels neglected by her sisters and brother and her neighbors."*

Yes, we have before us the body, the soul, the spirit, and the immortal body.

First, of the buzzing sensation within the head, first you must understand that you have that which is known as hypoglycemia. It would be suggested that you should seek out that of a regular medical doctor, that that substances of Ardelin [Arliden] be used to expand the blood vessels, the smaller blood vessels, that more blood could enter unto the inner ear in the same proportion. The problem within itself does cause, or called, Meniere's — it is quite common and can be treated. We would suggest for that of the vitamin substance known as Lipoflavonoid be used that the blood vessels within themselves may be made more pliable, and therefore, more servitude [serviceable]. We would further suggest the use of saunic baths be used in this case. We would suggest avoiding all loud noises. You will find that once this is corrected, the medical problem within the same, you will find a greater harmony within yourself, and therefore, a greater harmony within your family.

October 12, 1973: **Thy have many questions, ask.**

*"Yes, Aka. Regarding a health reading for [8-31-73-004]. He had a health reading on his hyperkinesis recently in which you said growths were the cause. And they state that the doctor's x-rays failed to show any growths. His father... says, 'How do we go about finding them and treating them?' He also has a rash on his legs."*

We shall say unto thee unto these words. With the proper use of the biofeedback, this growth could be reduced. Or it could be removed with surgery. Bring this child unto soul Ray, that he should administer healing into the same.

If that of the lower [limbordier] [limbic?] area was x-rayed, from front to rear, from the pituitary to the pineal glands, therefore, beneath the same you should find, therefore, of the growth. The growth in itself is nonmalignant. Yet, it should give, and therefore, react upon the nervous system of the same, for therefore, giving improper balance of the signals therefore sent from the mind to the brainstem, and therefore, throughout the body. That is all on that subject.

October 12, 1973: **You have other questions, ask.**

*"Yes, Aka, I have a request for a health reading for* [10-12-73-001].
*She says that she has pain in her feet which the doctors think is caused by
diabetes. She feels they will have to be removed. She also has difficulty with
her arteries. She asks for help with her feet, diabetes, arteries, including the
big artery that goes to her heart. Any suggestions of vitamins or food to her
would also be appreciated."*

Yes, we see thy need, and therefore, we have before us the body,
soul, the spirit and the immortal body of the same. One moment.

Yes.

Now we have the body before us. We would suggest the taking of
2,000 units of vitamin E per day; the taking, therefore, of the substance
known as Lydia E. Pinkham in that of capsule form 30 minutes before
eating; taking, therefore, in capsule form of the safflower oil, two tablets
30 minutes before eating, three times daily. We would suggest the use of
the Jerusalem artichoke be used, eaten raw; add, therefore, unto the
green olives, as many as you should desire of the same.

We would further suggest the use of the clay form unto which we
have mentioned before. This should be applied to the both, of the lower
limbs, feet area, and up unto the upper thigh.

We would further suggest that the taking of the sage tea and that
of the hops be mixed together in equal proportions, therefore, making of
tea form. This should not be boiled, but seeped, sweetened slightly with
natural honey, but very slightly.

We would further suggest taking of the substance known as
dolomite. Six capsule units should be taken per day — two three times a
day, one in the morning, one at the evening — two in the morning, two at
the evening meal, and two before bedtime of the same. We would not
suggest the amputation of these limbs or surgery of any kind on this
subject at the present time. This should only have cause for further
infection.

We find, therefore, into the urinary tract, of the vagina, a
problem of infection of the same. We would suggest, therefore, the use,
first, of nothing more than vinegar and clear water be used as a cleaning
substance.

We would further suggest on this subject that that of the 6th and
7th vertebrae be worked on or adjusted, therefore, by either an
osteopathic or chiropractic doctor; that of the upper brainstem area,
therefore, be moved in a upward position, deviating, therefore, the
structure of the spinal column to go in that proportion that is needed,
therefore, in an upward position. Therefore, we would further suggest
that the spleen within itself be opened, and allowing the spine, therefore,
to go back into its proper place. This would greatly alleviate the problem

of the nervous system within itself, and therefore, allow better flow of blood into this area.

October 12, 1973: **You have other questions, ask.**
*"Thank you, Aka. [10-12-73-002], this must be Phoenix; I don't see the city — one moment — asks for a health reading. Do you see this person, Aka?"*
**We do not see of this. You have other questions, ask.**

October 12, 1973: **You have other questions, ask.**
*"Yes, Aka, [10-12-73-003] asks for a health reading. She has headaches affecting the back of her head and neck, bridge of nose, and back of eyes, constant aching throughout limbs, arms and legs, lower abdominal stress."*
**Yes, we have before us, therefore, the body, the soul, the spirit, and therefore, the immortal body of the same. One moment.**
**Yes, yes.**
**Therefore, we should answer in this manner. We find, therefore, that of rheumatoid arthritis. We find, therefore, within the heart area, that which would be known unto the third valve of the same, malfunction.**
**Yes.**
**We would suggest, therefore, one moment — yes, we see this now — that of the sauna type baths be used.**
**We would further suggest that this subject should seek out, therefore, of a good oral surgeon. Therefore, we find this subject with that that is known as lead poisoning. This was brought about in early childhood. The substance of the same, the poisoning, has settled, therefore, into the gumular area. If this problem was removed, this subject would respond immediately. This is caused by what is known as a low form of constant infection feeding into the body form. We would suggest that the taking of 2,000 units of vitamin E per day. We would suggest the taking of 1,000 units of vitamin C per day. We would suggest the taking of A and D in normal adult dosage, no more. We would further suggest — yes, yes — taking, therefore, of the ginger leaf, taking, therefore, of the mistletoe leaf, taking, therefore, of the sage leaf, taking, therefore, of the hops. These should be placed together in equal proportions and tea brewed from the same, not boiled, but seeped, sweetening, therefore, with the natural honey. This in itself should cleanse the circulatory system within the same, and therefore, bring forth a cleansing, therefore, in the blood within the same. We would further suggest the taking, therefore, of the safflower oil in capsule form three, three times daily, 30 minutes before each meal, therefore, removing that of the cholesterol of the bloodstream. We would suggest taking, therefore, of the Jerusalem artichoke be placed in raw form daily.**

We would further suggest — yes — yes, we would suggest that a visit to either a good osteopathic or chiropractic doctor, that the whole backular area should be adjusted, therefore, within the same. This will have to be done not once, but repeated times because of permanent damage into the vertebras and a softening of the same. These adjustments should be done at least once a month.

October 19, 1973: **You have many questions, ask.**
*"Aka, I have a request for a health reading for* [10-19-73-001]. *She has a problem particularly on her lower spine."*
Yes, we have before us the body, the soul, the spirit and the immortal body of the same.
Yes, we see thy need.
But we should answer first in this manner, the fall, the problem in itself has originated, a fall that was taken from a bicycle as a small child. That in [the] proportion known as the tailbone has been broken. The sciatic nerve, therefore, within the same, we find damage into the same. We further find into the third, fourth [to] sixth vertebrae separation of the same. We would suggest, therefore, that this soul go unto that of either an osteopathic or chiropractic doctor, that adjustments should be made.
We would further suggest that a good bone specialist therefore be sought out, and the first problem, therefore, should be corrected with surgery within the same, removal of the same, therefore allowing the spine to protrude downward into its normal position.

October 19, 1973: **You have other questions, ask.**
*"Yes, Aka. I have a request for a health reading for* [9-7-73-004]. *She says she is following your advice. She has noticed a burning sensation the last two or three days in her upper urinary tract, she thinks, and wonders what is causing it? She asks if the combination of vitamins added to her usual Merdex synthetic vitamin and mineral complex which she has taken for years might be the cause?"*
Nay. We have before us, therefore, the body, the soul, the spirit and therefore, the immortal body of the same. The problem, therefore, lies [in] nothing more than a staph infection within the same. We would suggest taking, therefore, first of the sage tea. This should not be boiled; it should be seeped within the same, sweetened with local honey. We would further suggest that in the washing of the area, the use of apple vinegar be added into the normal washing proportion of the same. This should readily take care of this problem.

October 19, 1973: **You have other questions, ask.**

*"Yes, Aka, you mentioned some time back that you might recommend a substitute for Night-blooming Cereus. Do you have something to recommend at this time?"*

**We have placed this in soul Ray's mind. This compound shall soon be brought forward.**

October 19, 1973: **You have other questions, ask.**

*"Yes, Aka. I have a request for a health reading for [10-12-73-002]. She says, 'What is the cause of me having a low-grade fever of 99 to 100 degrees every day, and what is causing pain in the urinary bladder area? Can it be cured?'"*

**Yes, we have before us, therefore, the body, the soul, spirit, and therefore, the immortal body of the same. We should answer first of the first question. This is caused by what you would know as the — known as Valley Fever. We would suggest that rest, the taking of 2,000 units of vitamin E per day, a good natural vitamin-mineral supplement be added into the same.**

**We would further suggest, therefore, of the bladder infection of the same — first we should answer in this manner, for more care should be used in that that is placed within the same, more cleansing. Second we would suggest that she should go unto her local physician, therefore, that antibiotic could be prescribed. This would simply cleanse this area. We would further suggest the drinking of as much of the substance known as cranberry juice as possible. We would further suggest — yes, we see this — that the subject in mind, we find, therefore, into the ovary, left ovary, a small cyst, secretion of the same, which is causing the problem, therefore, into the same. This in itself should either be removed, psychically or surgery [surgically]. If further information is needed on this subject, we would suggest that she should bring this question forth at another time.**

October 19, 1973: **You have other questions, ask.**

*"Yes, Aka. [10-12-73-004] has asked regarding health reading. He says, 'I have tinnitis, nerve damage, osteosclerosis [arteriosclerosis? otosclerosis?] in both ears, arthritis, especially in my hands, and lower back trouble, and pain in my left foot. How can I regain my health?'"*

**Yes, we have before us the body, the soul, and immortal body of the same. We would suggest that in the above-mentioned areas cold packs be placed unto the same; after the cold packs have been placed into these positions, that that of a hot olive-oil pack be used. This should be repeated twice daily. We would further suggest the use of the mud substance that lies within soul Ray's mind.**

October 19, 1973: **You have other questions, ask.**

*"Thank you, Aka. I have a request for a health reading for* [10-19-73-002]. *She says, 'My main health questions pertain to general state of my health in regards to recent diagnosis of cysts in the bladder. What should have been the correct diagnosis given before coming to Arizona, also,' she says, 'the swelling in my legs that I am currently experiencing?'"*

Yes, we have before us, therefore, the body, the soul, the spirit, and therefore, the immortal body of the same.

Yes.

We would suggest that the subject seek out that of the assistance of her physician. One moment.

Yes, we see this.

The subject in question has that known as uremic poisoning, and therefore, should be treated in an according manner. If this is not corrected it could cause death.


October 23, 1973: **You have other questions, ask.**

*"Aka, she asks, 'I would like to know if I will have good health for the remainder of my life?'"*

We find within this soul a health problem. At the present time we should say unto her, come unto soul Ray for consultation.


October 27, 1973: **You have other questions, ask.**

*"Yes, Aka. [8-27-73-001] asks, 'Aka, I have made available the remedies and cures you have suggested in various readings. How do I get the people who need these things notified that they are available?'"*

First, we should answer in this manner. Those things we have brought forth unto you, patent of the same.

Second, therefore, as we have said before, a new form shall be laid before you, for new advertisement fields shall be reached. We have laid these and the knowledge within the same within that of soul Ray's mind. Now is the time that he shall show you a way to harvest your crop.

Fear not, for the sign within the heavens unto which we showed you was reward for your faith, yet further reward is yet in the making. Continue with the faith, and that of the harvest shall be plentiful, yet the seeds shall not runneth out.

You have other questions, ask.

*"I have no other questions, Aka."*

Yes, we see thy need, and then we shall answer in the mind of one. For that that thy have prayed upon, we looked upon you and gave healing unto the child. We have looked, therefore, upon the mother and gave healing. We shall also give healing unto that of the grandfather.

But for those who should ask in our Father's name upon this night, healing shall be given unto all.

Hallowed be Thy name. Hallowed be Thy name of the Lord, our Father, God, unto all worlds.

Now is the time of the Cherub.

Soul Ray now grows very weary. Awaken soul Ray from his slumber.

October 30, 1973: **Thy have many questions, ask.**

*"Yes, Aka, I have a request for a health reading for* [10-30-73-001]. *He is here tonight, and he asks what is causing his dizziness, headaches, and what can be done about it?"*

Yes, we see thy need, and therefore, we have before us the body, soul, spirit, and therefore, the immortal body of the same. We find therefore in the seventh and eighth vertebrae, therefore, protrusion of the same, damage. We would suggest that either by osteopathic or chiropractic treatment these first be placed back in their proper proportion.

Yes.

We find that which is known unto thee as sinus, or the sinus glandular. We find also within this one that which is known as Valley Fever. We would suggest, therefore, that 3,000 units of vitamin E be taken unto this unit, unto itself, daily. We would also suggest, an irritation due to the dryness is causing, therefore, inflammation within the same. We would suggest that sea water be brought forth, that it be brought unto a slow boil, and that of cloth be placed above and over the head allowing the subject to breathe in this substance. If this is impractical, we would suggest the taking, therefore, and adding to water that known as the Aloe Vera Juice or plant of the same, taking, therefore, of the dehydrated salt that has come from the sea, placing 10 teaspoons full of Aloe Vera to one quart of water and 10 teaspoons of salt into one quart of water. In this manner that which is known as a vaporizer could cleanse this area and cause healing into the same.

Yes.

We further find that which you would call as an inner ear infection of the left ear.

Yes.

We would suggest that the body in itself has become immune to the antibiotic into which it has taken unto itself. Therefore, we would suggest the use of the *Aloe vera* in liquid form, six tablespoons per day.

We further find within this subject — yes — that of hypoglycemia. The subject has that known as low blood sugar. We would suggest, therefore, that the use of orange juice be given in 8-ounce quantities three times daily unto the subject.

We would further suggest — yes — that more rest for this subject.

If the following that has been given is followed in its precise manner, the problems that have been set forth shall soon leave.

We would further suggest that a correction be made in the corrective vision lens that the subject now uses. This would greatly help. We find — yes — that of light vision problem in the retina of the eye. It would be suggested, therefore, that a slight tinting be placed in these lenses within the same.

Yes.

We find, therefore, unto the thyroid of the same an imbalance. We would suggest, therefore, the use of that known as your safflower oil with the B6 be used in capsule form 30 minutes before eating, six capsules in total in daily use of the same.

We would further suggest — yes — the taking, therefore, of the sage tea that cleansing of the circulatory system could come about. This should be done by steeping the tea, not boiling it, sweetening, therefore, with local honey of the same.

We would further suggest that the subject eat less of sugar, but be allowed to eat in proportions of honey as needed into the body.

Yes — this is all on this subject at this time.

October 30, 1973: **You have other questions, ask.**

*"Thank you, Aka.* [10-30-73-002]*, who is here tonight, asks for a health reading regarding neck and shoulder tension problem, and he would like to know what is causing it and what can be done for it?"*

Yes, we have before us the body, the soul, the spirit, and therefore, the immortal body of the same. First, we should mention unto this subject that the tension and neck problem within the same is due from exactly that which is mentioned, over tension, that of too much, causing fatigue. We would suggest that the subject take, therefore, periodic periods of rest form. This should be done in the exercising form of that known as swimming. This would relieve and allow the spine within itself to go back within its proper proportions.

We find, therefore, a slight problem of that known as rheumatoid arthritis. We would suggest, therefore, that the mud substance that soul Ray has brought forth be used. We would suggest therefore that the white substance that Ray has brought forth be used, this white substance which should be massaged into the neckular area, and lower shoulder, lower back section or proportions of the spine. We find, therefore, that the subject, due to this slight deformity, therefore, of the left leg is shorter than the right. This could be corrected with orthopedic shoes quite simply, but before this is done we would suggest that the subject go unto either osteopathic or chiropractic doctor for correction of the lower back and spine and pelvic area unto the same.

We further find — yes, yes — scar tissue, slight damage, both lungs. We would suggest the taking of 2,000 units of vitamin E per day. We would further suggest — yes — the taking of a good natural vitamin-mineral substance be added unto the diet. We would further suggest that this subject eat three, at least three, meals per day. They should not be heavy meals, and if the desire is for more, then eat more often, but this should be done skipping no meals.

The subject in mind, we find, therefore, in the large tubular area of the stomach in the stomach lining therefore within the same what is known as a nervous stomach, slight lesions or ulcer form starting within the same. Unless the tension is brought down, unless that which is kept within is allowed to come out — more relaxation.

This is all on this subject at this time.

October 30, 1973: **You have other questions, ask.**
*"Thank you, Aka. [10-30-73-003] asks for a health reading. She asks, 'What is causing my digestive disturbances, and what can I do for it?'"*

Yes, we have before us the body, the soul, the spirit and the immortal body of the same.

Yes.

We find therefore within this subject — yes — of that of lesion attachment unto the intestines. We find that of nervous stress in greater quantities. We find, therefore, within the same stress brought forth from not placing ideals into practice, great frustration from the same, lack of communication.

Yes.

We find, therefore, an upper hydroaic [hiatal?] lesion unto the diaphragm of the same. At the present time this is quite small and would not take surgery if properly cared for. We would suggest the taking of that substance known as Lydia E. Pinkham, three capsules per day, 30 minutes before eating — one capsule unit taken 30 minutes before eating, three in the course of one day. We would also suggest the taking, therefore, of the Safflower Oil with the B6. This should be taken two, 30 minutes before eating — six capsule units per day.

We would also suggest that a cleansing of the circulatory system be done by the use and taking of the sag tea unto the same.

Yes.

We would further suggest that this subject within itself is that of a borderline diabetic. We would suggest the use of the substance known as Jerusalem artichoke, eaten in its raw form. If the substance cannot be obtained at the present time, take that of the Aloe Vera in four teaspoons per day, one 30 minutes before eating each meal, one before bedtime. We would further suggest the taking, therefore, of that substance known as Dolomite, combination compound of calcium and magnesium. We would suggest that these be taken in one compound, therefore, taking three capsules of the morning, and three before bedtime. If nervous tension should build, you may increase this to nine capsule units per day, but no more.

Yes.

November 2, 1973: **Thy have many, questions, ask.**

*"Yes, Aka.*[10-19-73-003] *asks for a health reading and about his future. He asks, 'How should I prepare for my own particular circumstances?'"*

Yes, we have before us the body, the soul, the spirit, and therefore, the immortal body of the same. We [shall] therefore, see the karma within the same. And we should give of thee the last first in this manner, that thy future should be marked by many wayward lanes, yet for every door you should not enter, there shall be a door beside it that you should enter. Therefore, use that unto which the Lord has given of thee, that of free choice, and the goals thy should desire shall come forth. And a way shall be provided.

We should place before thee the bread and the wine. Bring forth, therefore, the yeast unto the same, and feed the multitudes.

Of thy physical problem, we find, therefore, of minor substance, and therefore, we should say unto thee, give glory unto thy Lord, and healing shall come unto the body of the same.

November 2, 1973: **Thy have other questions, ask.**

*"Thank you, Aka.* [11-2-73-001] *asks for a health reading...."*

Yes, we have before us the body, the soul, the spirit, and therefore, the immortal body of the same. We therefore see within the same that of rheuma — yes — a [rubella] rheumatoid arthritis. This has caused a dizziness and a thickening of the bone structure of the skull within the same; pressure, therefore, into the brainular areas; a restricting of the blood flow unto the brain as such. We would suggest, therefore, that the use — yes — taking of the substance known as S.S.S. This within itself is a tonic of herbs. We would further suggest the use of the substance known as Lydia E. Pinkham, three capsules per day. We would further suggest the taking of that, substances known as calcium and magnesium; it would be far better using this in the forms known as dolomite. We would also suggest the taking of six teaspoons of aloe vera juice per day.

We further find within this subject that of a poisoning of the liver form — yes — a problem, therefore — yes — within the kidneys of the same and bladder causing this subject, therefore, to have what is known as false urination, pressure, yet the dispensing not of the urine. We would further suggest, therefore, that the taking of the safflower oil in three capsules per day, adding within these capsules, therefore, of the B6 substance. We would further suggest the takings of 900 units of vitamin E per day.

Yes.

We find within this subject, therefore, the problem of the vision. This could readily be corrected with the replacing of the lens within the spectacle form of the same.

We further find within the subject, into the 10th and 11th vertebrae — yes — this within itself should be corrected by either osteopathic or chiropractic treatment.

We would suggest that the subject, therefore, bring forth into the home that of filtering clean air. It would also be suggested that the subject use that in slumber of the negative-ion machine.

November 2, 1973: **You have other questions, ask.**

*"Yes, Aka.[ 11-2-73-002] asks for a health reading and for spiritual guidance. She wants more spiritual improvement.."*

Yes, we see thy need, and first we should answer in this manner. Of the spiritual development within the same, come there forth and seek from within the group thy belong those who dwell near thee. This would greatly help in your development. We have provided the philosophy, yet there are many others.

We do not say unto thee, leave of thy churches. We do not say of thee, cast aside thy faith — only that thy should come in preparation, as we have come, for we have come for but one purpose, that in itself is the preparation for the coming of the Messiah. Bring forth this as intended, and thy cup should runneth over, for God dwells within all mankind. All thy must do is open the door that we may enter.

Yes, we see, therefore, of the health problem within the same. And we should answer in this manner. We have before us the body, the soul, the spirit, and therefore, the immortal body of the same. We find, therefore, within the same that of rheumatoid arthritis. We find, therefore, within the same that of a borderline diabetic. We find, therefore, within the same — yes — of an acne skin problem.

We would suggest therefore the taking of the substance known as aloe vera juice, taking, therefore, of the substance known as Lydia E. Pinkham, taking both, one teaspoon to one capsule, 30 minutes before eating.

We would suggest the filtering of thy air. This is causing within the same a bronchial condition. We would suggest, therefore, the changing of the drinking water, bringing, therefore, into a purer form.

*"Yes, Aka, [11-9-73-002], and she asks, 'Could you please give healing and cure for my father of multiple sclerosis? In the name of our Lord, Jesus, I pray.'"*

We shall answer you in this manner. We are not allowed to interfere with the free choice of another soul. For is it not written, "Ask and thy shall receive?" And for he who should ask in his own words, that that he should ask for shall be given.

November 9, 1973: **You have other questions, ask.**

*"I have a request for a health reading from [11-9-73-003]. She asks for a reading to try to find why her back pains constantly between thoracic vertebrae four and five."*

**Yes, we have before us the body, the soul, the spirit, and therefore, the immortal body of the same. One moment.**

**Yes, now, yes — now we find this soul, and therefore, we have the body before us.**

**First we should answer your question in this manner. This comes from a virus, arthritic condition. This type of arthritis eats away at the bone tissue in itself, allowing the chemical balance to deteriorate. We would suggest that this soul come forth unto soul Ray that help might be given unto the same.**

**We would suggest that as soon as possible that soul Ray obtain that of the negative ion to be used in such cases as these.**

November 9, 1973: **You have other questions, ask.**

*"Aka, she asks for help regarding her sinus condition which has been worse since moving to Fayetteville, North Carolina. She says, 'Can you tell me whether the move to a drier climate would be helpful? Is there any medication I can use?'"*

**Yes, we have before us the body, the soul, the spirit, and therefore, the immortal body of the same. One moment.**

**Yes, yes. Yes.**

**The soul has been located.**

**First, we should answer in this manner, yes, the moving into a drier climate would be very helpful, but that of pollution, into a polluted land, should not improve the situation. Therefore, we should say unto you unto these words. Obtain, therefore, for the present time that of the negative-ion machine. Obtain, therefore, that of filtering of your air. Obtain, therefore, that of clean, pure drinking water. Taking therefore of the sage leaf, preparing a tea from the same by seeping this; sweeten lightly with natural honey. Taking therefore of salt that has been dehydrated from the ocean, placing 10 teaspoons to one quart of water, therefore creating a vaporizer by bringing this water to a boil and placing a towel above thy head, doing this three times daily, that these area shall not only be drained, but healing shall come from the salt of the same.**

November 9, 1973: **You have other questions, ask.**

*"Yes, she asks, 'Why do I not have the necessary will power to lose my excess weight?'"*

**That comes from the same question you asked in the beginning, the lack of faith within yourself, and therefore, you should question the**

faith of another. Learn, therefore, to respect yourself in the body that God has given you, for remember, the body is the temple of God. Pollute it not.

November 9, 1973: **You have other questions, ask.**
*"Aka, she asks for health information on her 18-year-old son, [11-9-73-005].She is concerned, among other things — one moment, here. She says, 'He has always been and still is when at home a bed wetter. What, if anything, can be done to correct this?'"*
First, we should answer this question in this manner. As we have said before, we cannot violate this one's free will. If he himself should desire an answer, let him ask, and he shall receive the same.

November 9, 1973: **You have other questions, ask.**
*"Yes, Aka. I have a request for a health reading from [11-9-73-006]. She says, 'Please help me find a way to improve use of my hands, arms, walk better and talk better.'"*
Yes, we see thy need, and therefore — one moment.
Yes.
Yes, we see we have overtaxed soul Ray's body, and therefore, this question should be brought forth in your next reading form.
We should say unto thee unto these words. God loveth His children in many ways. For He should leadeth His children, if they should listen, each down their own separate paths.
Now is not the time for separate paths. Come unto *one* in your food storage. Be as one. Pool your knowledge. Pool your resources. Bring them together. Do unto these things and we shall see of thy needs.
Each of you have seen that unto which God has allowed within us to do. Each of you we have given healing. Each of you we have given life and purpose. Bring these together, for in truth be as brother and sister. Give knowledge unto one another.
We have placed into your keeping this one we call a prophet, who prefers to be called an instrument. We have placed knowledge for your use. Open your eyes and your ears. Your separate paths will only bring you chaos. Bring this house into one house, not divided in any way, and the blessings of God shall not be denied.
Each of you have duties to perform. Allow us to perform our duty, our function.
We can force you to do nothing. We can only ask. Study our words well. You shall find we have come not for our needs, but for yours.
Awaken soul Ray from his slumber.

November 16, 1973: **You have other questions, ask.**
*"Thank you, Aka. I have a request for a health reading, Aka, for [11-16-73-001]. She asks, she says she is worried about her 65-percent hearing*

*loss, since her husband has not worked for more than one and one-half years and probably will not again; her hearing loss is becoming a real problem. She also has arthritis in both feet and ankles which is very painful. She also asks about her husband."*

First, we should answer first unto these questions — in this manner. We may only give information unto those who should ask, for they are the ones who should receive.

For the arthritic condition, first we should answer in this manner. Take, therefore, of the white and black clay forms that soul Ray has brought forth, applying them in the prescribed manner. Take, therefore, of the Aloe Vera Juice, taking therefore eight tablespoons per day. Take therefore of the Night-blooming Cereus. This can be preserved in this form by taking that of hydraulic pressed juice forms and dejuicing the substance of the same, and cold packing as prescribed before, then therefore of taking three tablespoons of the juice form per day. We would also suggest the taking therefore of the calcium-magnesium in the form, therefore, of Dolomite. We would further suggest the taking, therefore, of the chaparral in the form of eight tablets per day.

Yes.

We would further suggest the taking, therefore, of the Lipoflavonoid vitamin substance. We suggest this because of hardening of the arteries leading therefore from the heart into the brainal area. We would further suggest that the use of the drug known as Ardelin [Arliden] and Antivert be used. This must be acquired from that of a physician.

Yes, we see this.

This should be used therefore — yes — of the Ardelin [Arliden] 10-milligram units per day, of the Antivert, units in one 10-milligram unit per day, of the Ardelin [Arliden], twice daily.

Yes, we see this.

We further find — yes — in the pituitary gland imbalance. Yes — you must realize that through this gland you have that that should secrete into the pineal gland, therefore, which should regulate the chemical form or forms of the body, causing cell growth or delayed growth, or growth therefore out of proportion, and affecting each cell as a separate and total individual substance of the same.

We would suggest, therefore, the seeking out, if possible, of that of either bio-feedback therapy or that of hypnotic therapy to be used upon this subject in above prescribed manner — that the subject in manner be regressed therefore back into such an age as before that that she has had, the present condition. In this manner, the body and the antibodies therefore to attack unto the virus of the rheumatoid substance would come about much quicker, and recovery of the same.

Yes, we see this.

We find therefore infection, therefore, of the liver area, and kidney, bladder, and therefore, secretion from that of the vagina of the self and the uterus. We would suggest therefore unto this subject the using, first, of the large quantities of that of the cranberry juice, drinking as often as thy can; the drinking therefore of clean drinking water; placing in the diet that of 2,000 units of vitamin E per day.

Yes.

We would further suggest the cleansing of thy air form within thy home. This would greatly help into this area. We would further suggest that you use that in vagina area for the cleaning of the same, using proportions of one quart of your measure to one pint of your measure of vinegar, apple vinegar, into that of the same, adding therefore 10 tablespoons of *Aloe Vera* into the same. This should be used as a washing form regularly.

November 16, 1973: **You have other questions, ask.**

*"Yes, Aka, [7-6-73-002] asks for a health reading....And she asks, 'Will I have children, if so how many? Will I graduate from school into my chosen profession this year?' She has not been specific on her request for a health reading."*

Yes, we have before us, therefore, the body, the soul, the spirit, and therefore, the immortal body of the same. You asked, will you go unto your chosen profession, and we shall answer into this manner. You will receive that of the doctrine [doctorate] necessary to enter the profession, yet marriage shall interfere in this manner. You shall have three children, two of which shall be girls and one of which shall be a boy.

November 16, 1973: **You have other questions, ask.**

*"Yes, Aka, she had asked also for anything in regards to her past lives."*

We would suggest that this question be brought forth at a different time.

*"I have a request for a health reading for [11-16-72-03-002]. He asks, 'What do you recommend for my heart condition, and what do you recommend for phlebitis and poor circulation?'"*

Yes, we have before us the body, the soul, the spirit, and therefore, the immortal body of the same. One moment, please.

Yes, we see this. Yes.

Of the heart condition, first we should answer into this manner. Of the [severe (sinus, sinistra, semilunar?)] valve, we find blockage within the same. This is caused from long overweight. This has caused of the building up of fatty tissue, therefore malfunction of the valve within the same.

Of the circulatory system and improvement of the same, we would suggest in this manner — first, of the taking that of the safflower oil in four capsule units before eating, 30 minutes before eating; this should be added with the B6 compound which should lie in the capsule unit within the same. We would suggest the taking of 2,000 units of vitamin E, added therefore with 1,000 units of vitamin C. We would further suggest the taking, therefore, within the same of mineral oil, the drinking of one ounce per day before eating.

We would further suggest that that of the sauna baths be sought out and used, first in a graduating manner, no more than five minutes a day in the beginning, and building up into a 30- minute unit. This within itself would answer all three of the questions within the same.

November 16, 1973: **Thy have other questions, ask.**
*"Yes, Aka. [11-16-73-003] asks for a health reading, specifically, can anything be done for her spinal condition?"*

Yes, we have before us the body, the soul, the spirit and the immortal body of the same.

Yes, we see thy need — one moment.

Yes.

Therefore, we have before us the body.

Yes, we see of this.

We would suggest, therefore, that either the seeking out of an osteopathic or chiropractic doctor, that if adjustments of, in an upward proportion of the eighth and ninth vertebrae are made, in the correct manner, the opening therefore of the pelvic area, allowing therefore the spine therefore room to go back in its proper proportion, this would greatly relieve the curvature of the spine.

There is permanent damage there unto the nerve center, that into known as brainstem area. This within itself will cause problems and difficulties at different periods of this one's life span. Corrective surgery could be done. If — yes, we see this — if the surgery was done in the above subscribed manner, and that is what is called the searing of the [ceverian] [cervical?] nerve, if this was done in the lower proportion of the left leg area of the spinal unit, this would [alleviate] this problem. But you must realize that as this is done, your warning signals unto this proportion of the body shall no longer be fed back into the brain, and damage could be done to you in other manners. We would suggest, therefore, that you might venture forth for therefore unto soul Ray and let him give forth healing unto the same.

November 18, 1973: **You have other questions, ask.**
*"Yes, Aka. [11-18-73-001] who is here tonight has asked a number of questions. He has asked firstly for a health reading regarding a cure for allergies, specifically sinus. Also he has a perceptive block in his mental coordination, and he would like to know how to regain and continue to grow, or what can he do to clarify his thought perception?"*

Yes, we see thy need, and first we should answer that of a physical nature.

First, we should answer in this manner. Of the allergies within the same, at first as they should attack unto the human body, they are nothing more that irritations into the membranes. But soon the body consumes into the bloodstream, and this becomes unto the same a virus. Your mankind, as it is today, has not sought forth this knowledge. We would suggest that the use of the negative ion be used, the negative ion machine, using that, therefore, within the same of a filtering system placed before it.

We would suggest, therefore, that thy should go unto this one known as T_____ O___, for there are many types of these within the same. We have placed the knowledge therefore, that [that] in the machinery that is needed could be built, and so it is being done. The wrong type of negative-ion machine would emit deadly ozones. These would kill germs, but would also destroy cells within the human body.

If this is used in a proper manner during your slumbering hours, it would allow the pollution of the positive ion which has entered the body, and therefore, formed a virus or mutate, to reverse itself. This within itself would take a matter of time. It will not come about immediately, but very slowly. Day to day, you shall notice changes within yourself.

You will also notice a great change in that of the mind. The destroyed matter within the mind will become whole again, and the problem that you now have before you shall slowly disintegrate.

We know that the answer we have given you is a simple answer.

We would further suggest that this subject take, therefore, of the sage tea, Do not boil this, but bring it forth — yes — bring this forth by steeping the same, sweetening this with natural honey, honey that is brought forth from your own locale.

We would further suggest, for immediate relief, taking that of the sea, or that salt that has been brought from the sea, placing it into water, and therefore, bringing the same to a slight simmer, placing a towel over the head and breathing of this. This should be done in one-sixth part — one- sixteenth part of salt to one quart of water. This should give the subject immediate results; it should relieve the pressure unto the brainular area, relieving, therefore, and allowing the salt substance to dry out the sinus cavities and cause healing into the same.

November 18, 1973: **You have other questions, ask.**

*"I have one final question. He asks, 'How can* [11-18-73-002] *help her allergies?'"*

We usually will not give out information upon another soul, but since the concern is real, we would suggest that the prescription in the prescribed manner that we have given forth be given unto the one you have spoken about.

And now we should say and go farther, should thy need of consultation, come forth unto soul Ray. Bring forth that that is needed, and it shall be provided for in a like manner.

November 18, 1973: [p or m?] Now is the time of the Cherub. The Dragon rests but a short period of time. We say unto you, the children of the Dragon are the children of God also, but they are a greedy lot. Beware.

Awaken soul Ray from his slumber.

December 7, 1973: **Thy have other questions, ask.**

*"Yes, Aka. I have a request for a health reading for* [12-7-73-001]. *He asks, 'My health problem is suspected heart trouble and severe chronic sinus condition. In the evening and morning I get a hoarse throat . No doctor so far has given me any relief. I don't know if anything can be done, but I hope so. I also suffer from hypertension around people and while driving. I had to give up driving in heavy traffic. I am being treated by Dr. Holmes of Maricopa County Health Clinic. My extreme nervous tension started when I had my first heart attack December 10, 1971.'"*

Yes, we have before us the body, the soul, and therefore, the immortal body of the same.

First we should answer in this manner. Permanent damage has been done unto the brain from the lack of oxygen being fed unto the brain over a prolonged period. Damage, therefore, has affected many cells within the same. We would suggest that that of the biofeedback therapy be used and that of the negative ion therapy be used in accordance with the same. But this must be voluntarily done on the part of the subject. Therefore, without this, there can be no cure. Both the irregularity of the heart and the damage within the same could be corrected under these conditions, and of the mental condition of the same.

The movement of the closeness of the moon, affecting, therefore, the fluid substance that the brain lies in, at night, would cause unto such a person great difficulties and stress within the same. Only in these manners, as we have suggested, could this be treated.

We will also suggest unto this one that if the above therapy treatment is not taken, it would be suggested that this one voluntarily commit himself into an institution, for at his present rate, he shall soon harm, bring harm, physical harm, unto the ones he loves the most. And therefore, that that thy would know of for the use of controlled voltage to the mind could reverse some parts of the pattern therein.

That is all on this subject.

December 7, 1973: **You have other questions, ask.**

*"Thank you, Aka. [12-7-73-002] asks for a health reading...She asks if there is anything she can do to help arrest rheumatoid arthritis which will not bother the diverticulosis she has."*

Yes, we see thy need. And first, we would suggest the taking into the body substance — yes — one moment. Yes — we have before us the body, the soul, the spirit, and the immortal body. One moment.

Yes.

Correction must be made here. At the present time we have — yes, yes — one moment, a decision must be made.

Yes — yes, we find this.

Yes, now we have before us the body, the soul, the spirit, and therefore, the immortal body of the same. Now we have the correct subject in matter form.

We would suggest, therefore, that this subject take into the body substance 2,000 units of vitamin E per day. We would suggest the taking, therefore, within the body substances of 1,000 units of vitamin C per day, the taking in of the vitamin substance of A and D in 2,500-unit per day. We would further suggest the taking and the use of both the white and the black clay forms, unto which has been presented unto soul Ray's mind, be used into the infected areas. The vitamin E should attack that that is flowing into the bloodstream and attack the virus into the same. The mud substance should increase and therefore the circulatory flow of the same, and therefore, attack unto the superficial and into the bone marrow-type of flow of this type of the same.

You have both types of arthritis — one that attacks the bone marrow and travels through the same; the other attacks and flows within the bloodstream of the same — both, commonly close, but yet apart. They both are a virus.

If the above subject could be placed, therefore, in direct line of a cosmic generator, or therefore, within the same of a magnetic field, north and south, this could cause an arresting of the case, and therefore, a reversing of the cycle of the same. We have given this information in prior reading form.

We would suggest, therefore, of the biofeedback be used with hypnotic therapy in regression [for] the brain cells within the same. This could be done.

Your magnetic form and field could be done by the placing of negative ion machine — two, one to the north of the patient, one to the south of the patient. This could be done in such a manner that the positive ion within the body substance which has caused the virus could be reversed.

By placing the mind form into a younger state during treatment — this must be carefully recorded by use of oscilloscope and data transcript, graphic, and be checked, the progress be checked, in a daily manner — this would reverse the cycle, but not over-reverse the cycle, only bringing it into its normal state.

All factors of the body and mind and cell change could be brought into its normal form.

December 7, 1973: **You have other questions, ask.**
*"Yes, Aka. She asks,' Last September, 1972, she had a simple mastectomy. Are there signs of problems with cancer in the future?'"*
**Other than superficial, or you would call them, skin cancer, at the present time, we find none. If the process that we have described above could be used, this could eliminate such reoccurrences of the same.**

December 7, 1973: **You have other questions, ask.**
*"She has one other question. She asks, 'Do you see other health problems to deal with?'"*
**There shall be other health problems, but if the above that we have suggested is done, this should, these should not come forth.**

December 7, 1973: **You have other questions, ask.**
*"Yes, Aka. [12-7-73-003] asks for healing for her son, [12-7-73-004]. She states as follows, Aka, 'At age seven M___ was in an auto accident and lay in a coma for six months. After patterning.....'"*
**We see of thy need, and our Father weeps.**

**We would suggest that the help needed for the child, take, therefore, of the information that we have given in the before reading, the reading we have given on the subject's prior to this one.**

**We shall give unto thee and unto thy family that that is needed.**

**We also see that this soul has sought for deliverance. Yet, as our Father weeps, we weep. But we may not interfere with this soul's progress. And therefore, we are not allowed to give that that thy ask in full, only in part. Yet, our Lord, God, sees thy needs and shall deliver into thy hands the healing that is needed.**

**Within the forest there are many trees. And yet, not one bird may fall from the tree without our Father's permission. Yet, in the nature of all things, some birds must fall to create a balance within the bird itself. Yet the beauty of the song the bird has sung never dies, for once you have heard with your ears its beautiful tones, memory shall remain forever in your heart. And so it is with some children. The beauty of his song shall never be forgotten, that he shall know where he has been, and therefore, he shall know where he is going.**

**Glory be the name of the Lord.**

**For from the heavens thy shall find within your Book is written that the stars shall fall from the heavens, and the earth shall be cleansed and a new Messiah shall be born upon your earth.** [See *The Revelation*, chapter 12.]

Soon you shall celebrate the birth of the one known as Jesus Christ.

He said unto those who would listen, "Look unto the heavens, and ye shall know that I shall return upon the earth. Therefore, be good shepherds unto your flocks and tend my fields." [See *Acts* 1:6-11 and *John* 21:15-17.]

We are here but for one purpose, that is the preparation for the coming of the Messiah.

The Fifth Angel walks upon your earth. None further need walk.

Now is the time of the Cherub.

Awaken soul Ray from his slumber.

December 28, 1973: **You have many questions, ask.**

*"Yes, Aka. I have a request for a health reading from [7-17-73-005]....She says that she has very severe pain at the base of her skull, numbness on her left side. One doctor thought she has symptoms of M.S. What does she have, and what can be done to help her?"*

Yes, we have before us the body, the soul, the spirit, and the immortal body of the same. Yes — one moment. Yes, this is better. Now all is in accord.

First we should explain in this manner. This person is highly susceptible to your pesticides and defoliant that have been used upon the ground and in the air. Therefore, nerve damage has been done.

We also find that of a — yes — of a minor stroke, or that of a blood clot of the same. The clot in itself is slowly deteriorating.

You must realize that from these toxants damage has been done, not only into the pancreas, but into the spleen itself, therefore, affecting the bone marrow.

We would suggest that the taking of 3,000 units of vitamin E per day. We would further suggest that the use of negative ion machine be used, that the patient be placed on a north-south axis, placing an ion, negative ion unit, at the head and foot at a precise north-south axis. We would further suggest that biofeedback therapy be used, but not in its present form. We would further suggest the taking — yes — of all forms of vitamin substance at the present time in large quantities; that of the C, 1,000 units per day; that of the A and D, these two should be taken together, we would suggest 48,000 units per day; the taking therefore of the pantothenic acid form be used.

There is another form of treating the subject, and this is with a blood transfer of total substance of like kind.

We would further suggest the use of both calcium and magnesium taken in equal parts.

Yes.

You have that which is known as shock therapy. If this were used upon this subject, this would help to correct electrical imbalance of the body.

All of these are all of the same of alternatives of the same, all causing the same effect.

We would further suggest the drinking of pure drinking water. This is a must. The water thy now drink is polluted with chemical imbalance of the same.

We would further suggest the cleansing of the air unto which thy breathe.

We would suggest that this subject drink at least one gallon of water each day. This may be done in different forms: preferably of just water, second of the sage tea sweetened slightly with honey, third in the form of fruit juices of the same.

This should be continued and a follow-up reading be given at a later date on this subject.

December 28, 1973: **You have other questions, ask.**
*"Yes, Aka. I have one other question on this person. You said biofeedback, but of the present form. Do you have any comment as to what would be the correct form?"*

In soul Ray's mind lies the secret of the precise form that should be used. And until such a time as his studies are complete it would be unwise for others to attempt the same.

December 28, 1973: **You have other questions, ask.**
*"Thank you ,Aka. I have a request for a health reading for* [10-12-73-003]. *She says she has headaches affecting the back of her head and neck, bridge of her nose and eyes, constant aching throughout limbs, arms and legs, and lower abdominal distress."*

Yes, we have before us the body, the soul, the spirit, and the immortal body of the same.

Yes.

We find before us here that of a malfunction of the heart, the lack of circulation within the same. First, we would suggest the taking of the Safflower Oil with B6. Second, we would suggest the sauna baths be sought out, these to be started at 15 minutes and growing gradually up to one hour, but this must be graduated slowly. This in itself would stimulate the circulatory system, cleansing that of the same. We would suggest the taking of 950 units of vitamin E per day, the taking of 1,000 units of vitamin C to day, the taking that of the Lipoflavonoid vitamin substance, six per day.

We would also suggest a radical change in the diet form in the above-stated manner, that for breakfast, one glass of milk and one piece of toast, no more; for luncheon, all the green substance the subject should care to eat and that of small quantities of cottage cheese. If hunger should impair, you may eat one banana, no more. For the supper meals we would suggest in this manner, the eating twice weekly of fish substance, three times weekly of beef substance eaten as rawly as you may eat it. Small quantities of potatoes and other vegetation may be taken into the body along with this. We would suggest the eating of the liver form once weekly. Of the last day thy may eat anything thy wish in the supper form, one meal, only.

December 28, 1973: **You have other questions, ask.**

*"Thank you, Aka. I have a request for a health reading on [12-28-73-001]. He asks for a health reading or a healing for his eyes. His doctors say he has a blood clot on one eye, and that his eyes hemorrhage, and that it's a matter of time before he loses his sight."*

Yes, we have before us the body, the soul the spirit, and the immortal body of the same. One moment.

Yes.

Now all is in accord.

The hemorrhage is caused from clogging of the blood vessels leading from the inner ear, therefore, unto the eye socket, or back of the eye socket, within the same, this allowing clotting to take place. We would suggest the taking, first, of warm castor oil packs be placed on the eyes three times daily; at night, when the subject sleeps, castor oil packs be placed on each eye, placing in the eye once daily one drop into each eye of that of the aloe vera and the castor oil mixed together in equal parts.

We further suggest the seeking out of a physician, that the drug known as Ardelin be taken to open up other smaller and dilating other smaller blood vessels and allowing more blood to flow into the same. We would further suggest the taking of that of the Lipoflavonoid vitamin substance in six capsules per daily. This must be done that the blood vessels should become more pliable. If the above is used, the problem should cease.

Soul Ray now grows weary, and our time has grown short.

We shall leave with this message. Your new Messiah now dwells upon your earth in child form. He shall be protected. Glory be the name of the Lord.

Awaken soul Ray from his slumber.

# 1974 Health Readings

January 18, 1974: **You have other questions, ask.**
*"Yes, Aka, thank you.* [11-9-73-006] *asks for a health reading,
Aka....She says, 'Please help me find a way to improve the use of my hands,
arms, walk better and talk better.'"*

**We shall answer unto these words. Come forth unto soul Ray for
therapy, and that that is needed shall be given.**

January 18, 1974: **You have other questions, ask.**
*"Yes, Aka.* [7-12-73-006] *asks for a life and health reading.
Specifically she says, 'I feel at a crossroads, both health-wise and life-wise,
and am seeking to readjust, to go forward, not back. What causes my extreme
fatigue?' There are other questions."*

**We shall not give the life reading requested at this time. It should
be asked at different time. But we should say unto her, the answer lays,
lies in the beginning of this reading. The fatigue has come from within
herself. For that into which she has seen, she has not seen, for that which
she has heard, she has not heard. For the problem itself is not a physical
problem, but a mental problem.**

January 18, 1974: **You have other questions, ask.**
*"Yes, Aka. There are a couple other questions regarding her. She
says, 'What can I do to correct clumping of red blood cells, and is there merit
in chelation therapy or chemical endarterectomy as received in Anaheim,
California?' And then she asks, 'What is the best method for me to develop
spiritually?'"*

**First, we should answer that other question thy have asked first.
And we should answer in this manner, we see not of a control of the
disease thy possess. We would suggest, therefore, the taking of 3,000 units
of vitamin E per day. We would suggest, therefore, the taking — yes. One
moment.**

**Yes.**

**The transfer of blood — taking that of three pints of blood from
the body and replacing it with good blood. This should be done over a
period of time. The transfer should be made once monthly for six months.
If this were done, the problem itself would end.**

January 18, 1974: **You have other questions, ask.**

*"Yes, Aka. She said, on July 12, 1973, when she asked if she should go through with her plan for Anaheim doctor exam and therapy, you told her it would be good in one respect, but other knowledge should come forth at a different time, not in public, and she would like to know what you meant."*

**We should say unto thee unto this manner, come forth unto soul Ray for consultation.**

January 18, 1974: **You have other questions, ask.**

*"Thank you, Aka. I have a health reading request for* [1-18-73-001]. *She asks, 'What way am I to fulfill myself by serving others, and is there a specific man involved?' Apparently this is not a health readings request; excuse me, Aka."*

**We see not of this.**

January 25, 1974: *"Thank you. Aka, [1-25-74-001] asks, his parents ask, 'What is the cause of [1-25-74-001]'s recurrent illness? Is there any cure?'"*

**Yes, we see thy need, and we should answer in this manner. We have before use the body, the soul, and therefore, the spirit and the immortal body. One moment.**

**First, we should answer in this manner. The child in itself suffers from hypoglycemia, or that of low blood sugar. Over a prolonged period, damage has been done to the brain area, a lack of blood or oxygen flow unto the brain. This in itself has brought forth a form of epilepsy in the same.**

**We would suggest that biofeedback therapy be used in accordance, therefore, with hypnotic therapy. We would suggest the taking of 2,000 units of vitamin E per day. We would suggest the taking — yes, we see this — taking, therefore, of the Jerusalem artichoke, grinding it finely that it might be easilier [more easily] eaten. More green vegetation be brought into the food substance. No sweets except that of honey in pure form. We would further suggest that the use of oxygen, developed forth into the system in mechanical means; the drinking of more of that of pure drinking water.**

**We find also, therefore, that of a sinus condition. We would further suggest the use of a negative-ion unit, with filtering system in accordance, be used while the child sleeps.**

**This is all on this subject.**

January 25, 1974: **You have other questions, ask.**

*"Yes, Aka. [1-25-74-002] asks for a health reading...She asks, 'What is the cause and cure of chronic depression?'"*

**Yes, we have before us the body, the soul, the spirit, and the immortal body of the same.**

First, we would say, environment has a great deal to do with the problem set forth. The use of negative ions while in slumber would take away that of the depression periods, allowing more and more of new body and new tissue to form into the brain substance of the same. It would be further suggested, the taking of 1,000 units of vitamin E, 2,000 units of vitamin C. A good multiple vitamin substance should be added into this. We would further suggest the greatest improvement in all would be a change of atmosphere, or that of moving from your present location.

January 25, 1974: **You have other questions, ask.**
*"Yes, Aka, she also asks what can be done about a recurrent rash on the hands, and also what is the cause and cure of recurrent severe headaches?"*
**We have just answered these questions.**
*"Thank you, Aka."*

February 8, 1974: **You have questions, ask.**
*"Yes, Aka. I have a request for a health reading for* [2-8-74-001]. *They ask, 'What is the cause of* [2-8-74-001]*'s allergy? What is the cure? Is this something that will reoccur each time that we move to another area? And is there an area we can live where this problem would not occur?"*
**We say unto thee unto these words, we have before us the body, the spirit, soul, and the immortal body of the same. Go forth, therefore, and obtain that of the negative-ion machine. Use this in slumber, and therefore, you may live in any location without fear, for the healing shall come from within in this manner.**

February 8, 1974: **You have other questions, ask.**
*"Aka, they ask if he has other physical or mental problems that they need to help him with?"*
**Yes, we see thy need. We find hypertension, but this is normal. We find no other defects within the body substance of the same.**

February 8, 1974: **Thy have other questions, ask.**
*"Thank you, Aka. I have a request for a health reading from* [2-8-74-002]. *"*
**Yes, we have before us the body, the soul, the spirit, and therefore, the immortal body of the same.**
**We find within this soul substance that of hypoglycemia. We would suggest that a high protein diet be used. We would further suggest the use of orange juice in the morning, one cup — that this subject matter should carry with him in their possession that of the natural honey from the location unto which thy dwell; at periodic times taking one tablespoon of the honey, but by not eating any other of the sweet substance. Replace**

the sweet substance with protein dietary matter. This should readily improve and cure this problem within the same.

We find, therefore, in this subject that of the prostrate, or prostate gland, inflammation of the same.

Yes.

We would suggest, therefore, the taking of the sage tea, seeping of the same, sweetening slightly with the natural honey substance. We would further suggest the taking, therefore, of 2,000 units of vitamin E per day, 1,500 units of vitamin C per day, a good multiple vitamin and mineral substance unto your natural daily diet.

We find, therefore, infection of the bladder and liver areas. We would suggest that, as prescribed, medication be used, these problems should soon disappear.

February 8, 1974: **Thy have other questions, ask.**

*"Thank you, Aka. I have a request for a health reading for* [7-27-73-005].*"*

Yes, we have before us the body, the soul, the spirit, and therefore, the immortal body of the same.

Yes.

We find, therefore, that of an arthritic condition, or of the rheumatoid arthritis type. This is attacking the central nervous system, causing, therefore, the sciatic nerve to protrude outward; further causing, with large amounts of calcium into the brainstem area, causing problems into the vision.

We would say unto this one, therefore, come unto soul Ray for consultation. If this is not to be done, then seek out that of a physician.

Thy have in thy mind that of the use of acupuncture. Do *not* do this. Permanent damage could be done.

February 8, 1974: **You have other questions, ask.**

*"Yes, Aka. I have a request for a health reading for* [2-8-74-003]. *He asks, 'What should be done to correct the problem with my knees?'"*

Yes, we have before us the body, the soul, the spirit, and the immortal body of the same. We find, therefore, that of fluid substance of the knee joints of the same. We would suggest taking that of the Aloe Vera E Earth, placing this over the damaged area three times daily, taking, therefore, of the [cream] substance of the same and applying to the same areas. We would further suggest that the use of sauna baths be used, first in short intervals. We would further suggest the taking, therefore, of 12 of the dolomite substance of the same per day, taking therefore, into the body substance 4,000 units of vitamin C a day, taking, therefore, into the body substance of 5,000 units of vitamin E per day. This should be continued for three months.

We would further suggest — yes — that the drinking, therefore, of the sage tea substance be used. We find, therefore, in this subject that of a sinus condition. It would be suggested, therefore, that the use of the negative-ion unit be used unto this person, that the body substance rebuild itself in a natural manner.

February 8, 1974: **You have other questions, ask.**
*"Yes, Aka, this person asks one other question, 'Are there other physical, emotional, mental, or spiritual disorders? She....'"*
**We have just answered that question.**

February 8, 1974: *"Thank you. Aka, [2-8-74-004] asks, 'Please, I'd like a general health reading. In particular I'd like to know if I could take a birth control pill to reduce bad pain until the digestive system is well. If so, for how long can I take the pill?' She's taking Lydia Pinkham, Safflower Capsules with B-6, Gesti-enzyme digestive enzymes, and occasionally Donatol and Camalox with a limited diet."*
Yes, we have before us, therefore, the body, the soul, the spirit, and the immortal body of the same.

First, we should answer into this manner. We find into this subject of an upper hiatic hernia of the same. This should either be closed with surgery or brought forth into psychic surgery.

We find, therefore, that of an ulcer, or of ulcer lesions, into the large intestine. We find three of such lesions and a fourth in a perforated form.

We find, therefore, into the left ovary the cyst substance of the same.

We find in the vagina area — yes — cyst substance of the same, or that of ovarian-type growths. This could be done, corrected, in two manners, either that of the psychic surgery or the surgery of taking forth one part of the intestine and alleviating this proportion and making a new opening into the stomach tissue of the same. The second proportion would be that which you would know as a hysterectomy of the same, and this would be of a total hysterectomy. Or, you may bring yourself forth and come, therefore, unto soul Ray, that he may use that of the psychic surgery unto the body substance in performing these tasks, and leaving, therefore, the female organs intact.

This is all on this subject at this time.

February 8, 1974: **Thy have many questions, ask.**
*"Yes, Aka. I have a request for a health reading for [2-16-74-001]. She asks, 'One, should I try to undergo surgery for three hammertoes on my right foot?'"*
Yes, we see thy need. Yes, the arthritic condition throughout the body at this point should take that of surgical implication. We should say

unto thee, thy think thy are allergic unto the vitamin substances which thy are not. Prepare thy body in such a manner that strength should come within, that the mind should think clearly, and the answers shall come forth one by one. We find that the healing thy have asked for shall come, but only as thy should earn it.

February 8, 1974: **Thy have other questions, ask.**

*"Yes, Aka. Perhaps you've already covered this, but let me ask what she asks. She says, throughout life she has had periods of extreme fatigue and illness. Nervous tension the last six years has caused intestinal pain and bleeding. She has been put on a strict, low-residue, no vitamin-pill diet with relaxants, relieving pain, but leaving her dull and exhausted. The doctor gives her B-12 injections, and she is wondering if...."*

Yes, we see of thy need and we should answer further in this manner.

Take, therefore, 10,000 units of vitamin E per day into thy system for 30 days. Take, therefore, that that is known as the dolomite into thy system in consistency of 12 tablets per day. Take, therefore, into the body substance and the use of both the Aloe Vera E Cream and the Aloe Vera E Earth. Use of these in the prescribed manner. Take, therefore, a general vitamin substance that should contain both of the mineral and vitamins. Take, therefore, of the A and D vitamins.

If the subject should build of tissue of the same, eating, therefore, of the liver of that of the beef three times daily — correction, three times weekly; eating of the fish that should come from the sea once weekly; eating, therefore, of the fish substance that should come from the fresh water once weekly. Take, therefore, of the Jerusalem artichoke, adding unto thy diet, eating of it in raw substance.

Yes.

We would further suggest the taking, therefore, of the substance known as the Lydia E. Pinkham; this should be started in a daily substance of one tablet form three times per day. At the same time thy should take unto thy diet of the Safflower Oil with B-6, one three times daily. This should be done for one month, then increasing unto two, and then unto the third month unto three of these two substances. At the end of this period thy body and mind should come as one, and healing should come forth.

February 8, 1974: **Thy have other questions, ask.**

*"One other question, Aka. She says that her greatest longing is to learn to serve and love God with all her heart. Will it be possible for her to have strength and alertness to meditate and to serve God through helping others?"*

We should say unto thee, there are many ways to serve unto the Lord, God. The body is the temple that God has provided for you to live in, and therefore, the temple of God. Destroy this with neglect, and the soul should have no house to live within, nor should the spirit. But by the building of this temple, you are serving God. And therefore, we say unto you, we place before you the bread and the wine. Provide the yeast. Take forth the philosophy we have given. Taste of it. Take, therefore, the proportions that should feed thy needs, and thy should know of the meaning we have placed within the same.

February 8, 1974: **Thy have other questions, ask.**

*"Yes, Aka. I have a question from* [2-16-74-002]. *She asks, 'My husband,* [7-13-73-001], *suffered neurological damage December, 1972, which doctors said would be permanent, but* [7-13-73-001] *has already recovered past the point doctors predicted.' She says that, 'Money, school, and parents dictate that we now be separated with* [7-13-73-001], *living on a farm in Virginia. I'll be able to see him only every few months for several years until I finish school, which I must do now to be able to support us. What can I do for* [7-13-73-001] *now?'"*

We should answer in this manner. Soon we shall bring forth the funds necessary for the bio-lab unto which is within soul Ray's mind. At this time, bring forth this subject, and the help that is needed shall be given for the repair of the nervous system of the same.

We would suggest, at this time, that the taking of 2,000 units of vitamin E per day, the taking, therefore, unto the system of 500 units of vitamin C per day. We would further suggest that the taking of a good natural substance, vitamin substance, such as that as the one known as Lipoflavonoids, six tablets per day, taking, therefore, unto the system. At the present time, this would greatly help the body to improve itself.

We find other factors here unto which we are not allowed to answer without permission from the subject matter. Therefore, this is all on this subject at this time.

February 8, 1974: *"Thank you, Aka. Aka,* [10-12-73-001], *who had a health reading October 12, 1973, asks, 'What will dissolve the plaque in my arteries?' Also she wishes to have help with her pain, please."*

Yes, we see of thy need, and we should answer in this manner. That of the vitamin E should dissolve the plaque within the system of the same. But this should be done in a proper manner, the taking of 5,000 units per day. We would suggest, therefore, that the taking — yes.

Yes, we see this.

One moment.

Yes.

The use, therefore, of a negative ion machine would, therefore, help greatly in this.

March 1, 1974: **You have other questions, ask.**

*"Yes, Aka. I have a request from* [3-1-74-001]. *She asks for a life and health reading, the health pertaining to lower back, menstruation problems and headache."*

Yes, we see of thy need. Yes, we have before us, therefore, the body, the soul, the spirit and the immortal body of the same.

First, you must realize the subject matter is suffering from that of hypertension, that of an imbalance in her own day-to-day life. But therefore, within the vagina area of the same we find that of — yes — nonmalignant growth of the same, that that would be more known as cysts upon the ovary. We find other cyst form within the uterus itself.

Yes.

We also find that of an infection of the bladder area and kidneys. We would suggest — yes — that the subject in mind should consult a physician of surgery, or therefore, come forth, unto healing of the same.

We would suggest the taking, therefore, within the body substance of that of the sage tea sweetened slightly with honey. We would take, therefore, within the body substance of the same 3,000 units of vitamin E per day. We would take, therefore, within the body substance — yes — of 1,500 units of vitamin C per day. We would take, therefore, of a good natural vitamin and mineral supplement into the body. Taking, therefore, that of the cranberry juice and drinking in large quantities each day.

Yes, we see this.

We find problems, therefore, within the circulatory system of the same, that of a fatty tissue substance. We would suggest the use of that of the lecithin or safflower oil with B6.

Yes, we see this.

We would also suggest that the subject take not of any fatty tissue into the body substance. Eat none of the fried foods.

We would further suggest that the use of dolomite be used in that of nine capsule units per day.

We find — yes — the source of the problem of the circulatory system, also a lack of oxygen, damage, therefore, into the lungular area. We would suggest that the subject should find that of a higher, dryer climate.

Yes, we see this.

We find the subject matter suffering from allergies of the same. Therefore, we would suggest the use of the negative-ion machine unto this subject.

This is all on this subject at this time. One moment. If the above were used, surgery would not be necessary.

April 10, 1974: **Thy have many questions, ask.**

*"Yes, Aka.* [4-10-74-001] *asks to know, 'Will our finances be increased by a better paying job for me, or will C___ be physically able to return to work soon?'"*

Yes, we see thy need, and we shall answer in this manner.

You have brought this soul unto soul Ray for healing, that of the surgery and the knowledge we have placed within his mind and through his hands. And therefore, we have brought forth and answered your prayer that he should live.

Therefore, we should bring forth your second prayer. Your financial condition shall improve, but it should come as raindrops. But soul C___ should not return to work for the present time. This shall come at a later date.

Blessed be the name of the Lord. Blessed be the gift, and blessed be those who should ask for the gift in our Father's name.

April 10, 1974: **Thy have other questions, ask.**

*"Yes, Aka.* [4-10-74-005] *says, 'My system is very run down, and there is hardly a time when I feel real well. What's causing the problem, and what can be done about it?'"*

Yes, we see thy need, and we should say unto thee unto these words. Come forth unto soul Ray for consultation, and the necessary information that is needed shall be placed before him to make the necessary repairs in thy system. We say unto you, come forth after thy ovulation period.

April 10, 1974: **Thy have other questions, ask.**

*"Yes, Aka.* [10-19-73-002], *'Where can I get a job where I can make a living? What is the problem in my left ear?'"*

Yes, we see thy need and we should answer in this manner. The problem of the left ear comes from brainstem damage of the same, the lack also of blood circulation into the inner ear proportion of the same. We find, therefore, this of a ringing sensation. We would suggest, therefore, that of the Lipoflavonoid be used, of six capsule substances per day. This would greatly help to alleviate this problem. Take therefore — yes — of the dark clay substance, this which soul Ray brings forth of the Aloe Vera E Earth, applying to the back and frontal side of the ear, and to the forehead. Do this over the entire area. We would also suggest that you come unto soul Ray for consultation and ask of the new shampoo formula which is in his mind which should help to increase the circulation in the hair follicles of the same.

You asked of a job and we should answer in this manner. There are many opportunities where thy stand at this time. Look around you and take advantage of them. But look upon it in this manner, that the toil, place love within it and love shall be returned, and the toil shall no longer be toil, but should be happiness and faith.

April 10, 1974: **Thy have other questions, ask.**

*"Yes, Aka.* [10-19-73-002], *'Where can I get a job where I can make a living? What is the problem in my left ear?'"*

Yes, we see thy need and we should answer in this manner. The problem of the left ear comes from brainstem damage of the same, the lack also of blood circulation into the inner ear proportion of the same. We find, therefore, this of a ringing sensation. We would suggest, therefore, that of the Lipoflavonoid be used, of six capsule substances per day. This would greatly help to alleviate this problem. Take therefore — yes — of the dark clay substance, this which soul Ray brings forth of the Aloe Vera E Earth, applying to the back and frontal side of the ear, and to the forehead. Do this over the entire area. We would also suggest that you come unto soul Ray for consultation and ask of the new shampoo formula which is in his mind which should help to increase the circulation in the hair follicles of the same.

You asked of a job and we should answer in this manner. There are many opportunities where thy stand at this time. Look around you and take advantage of them. But look upon it in this manner, that the toil, place love within it and love shall be returned, and the toil shall no longer be toil, but should be happiness and faith.

April 18, 1974: **You have many questions, ask.**

*"Yes, Aka, we have* [4-18-74-001]. *She would like a general health reading, especially controlling weight gain."*

Yes, we see of thy need. We should answer in this manner. Take therefore of thy, from thy diet, of that of the salt. Use in its place either that of a salt substitute or that of the salt that should be hydrated [dehydrated] **from the sea. Take therefore into thy system that of the safflower oil and that of the B6 compound unto one capsule, taking six per day of the same. Taking into thy diet form, of the morning meal, one glass of milk and one piece of toast. For thy luncheon, eat as much of the green foliage as thy desire and one glass of milk. Take therefore unto thy evening meals, therefore, of the green foliage and that of bananas for one meal per week. Take that of the green foliage and that of the fish that should come of the sea of one meal. Take that of one meal the fish that should come of the land water and the green foliage. Take therefore of one meal that of the liver form that should come of the beef and green foliage. Take therefore of thy other meals, eat them as thy would wish, only do so in smaller quantities.**

We should also suggest thy should come therefore unto soul Ray that thy metabolism should be raised and adjustments made unto the same.

April 18, 1974: **Thy have other questions, ask.**

*"Yes, Aka, we have [4-18-74-002]; 'What's my next step after I get well?'"*

We shall say unto these words. There are flowers that lay beneath thy feet. Look upon them; do not destroy them, and they shall lead thee into the land of happiness. Go not backward but forward. Know where thy have been, and thy shall know where thy are going, for the past is the present, and the present is the most probable path into the future. Therefore, the dividing line shall lay before thee. If thy stop to see the flowers, thy shall take the right path. If thy do not stop to see the flowers and give blessings unto yourself and mankind and your God, then you shall take the wrong path, and your past shall be your future.

April 18, 1974: **Thy have other questions, ask.**

*"Yes, Aka. [4-18-74-005]; 'I am experiencing a great deal of confusion affecting both my health and my work. Can you help me to perceive my present situation more clearly?'"*

Yes, we see of thy need. And we should answer in this manner. The Lord, God, has placed into thy hands a gift, yet thy have not used it in fullness. Thy have sought out artificial means to stimulate thy mind. We shall tell thee that the time shall come forth of the machines that should take of the mind the light and sound, and therefore, to repair the body, the soul and the mind within itself. Yet these are only, have only started.

Therefore, we say unto you, take the gift that God has given you. Lay aside thy other things. The problems of thy body are not that of reality. They are manufactured from thy mind because you are afraid to pursue the gift that God has laid before you.

Each, in their own way, was given a gift, some to write, some to paint. Yet, much as an animal, you look unto other pastures and think they are greener than your own. Develop the gift that God has laid before you, and you shall develop the inter self.

May 10, 1974: **We see thy grief of this one, and the sorrow of the parting. Yet we should say unto you unto this manner. We shall allow you to look to the other side. In three days you shall have full knowledge of which we speak.**

**Can you understand of which we speak?**

*"No Aka, I do not understand."* [A man answers.]

It is not meant unto you, only one [note: (5-10-74-001)]. **And this one shall know. The veil shall be lifted that your mother shall be seen unto you, that you should know that [all] love is there, both love and forgiveness.**

May 10, 1974: **You have other questions, ask.**

*"Yes, Aka, I have a request for a follow-up health reading on [2-16-74-001]. She says that the medicine makes her mouth sore and makes her constipated, and so she has cut back on the medicine to some extent, and she wonders what she should do?"*

We should only answer in this manner. Come, therefore, forth before soul Ray, that healing may be administered of the same. This is all on this subject at this time.

June 1, 1974: **Thy have other questions, ask.**
*"Yes, Aka. [11-9-73-006] asks for a health reading. She says, 'Please help me find a better way to improve use of my hands, arms, walk better, and talk better.'"*

Yes, we see of thy need. And we shall answer in this manner. That you should understand fully the meaning of our words, we shall place, therefore, your needs in soul Ray's mind. Come forth, and he shall administer to the healing of the body, the mind, the soul, and the spirit.

We have given forth much healing unto your people. That this one should know the full meaning and the full love of our God, we give, therefore, the healing she asks for.

Glory be the name of the Lord.

June 1, 1974: **Thy have other questions, ask.**
*"Yes, Aka.[11-18-73-001] asks how he should apply for disability and what disability to apply under?"*

First, we should answer in this manner. Of the question of disability, at the present time the disability should come under the factor of a mental problem of the same. He should, therefore, seek the counsel of psychiatry. The rest should come in a natural form.

But we say unto thee, soon the bio-therapy that is needed to make the corrections of thy mental process shall be laid before you. Come forth, therefore, and receive of the same.

You must realize that permanent damage has been done in the cerebella region of the brain. Only by overlap of nervous systems and the main nerves into the same can these corrections be made into the brainstem.

Of the nervous system which should go from the pineal to the pituitary glandular system of the same, damage and hemorrhage has taken place in this area, causing a malfunction within the same. This can be corrected with bio-therapy.

Do not grow impatient, for the healing thy have asked for we have given in a reading. Yet they grow [grew] despaired. Thy would not continue with the therapy that we suggested; thy cast it aside.

A disability is not the answer to your needs. New growth and health should be your answer. But since within your mind you should seek this, then follow the path we have given, and the disability thy ask for shall be given.

We say unto you, each should have free choice. It was our Father's will in the beginning. It was man's will that he should [choose] death and life again, therefore, that he should become of our likeness, of our kind.

But if a farmer should plant his crop, and go out the next day and see the sun is shining and the crop has not grown into maturity in one day, should he walk away from it? These things you have done; therefore, these things you must correct.

June 1, 1974: **You shall have other questions. You have some in your mind now, but our time should grow short.**

**For we should answer into the mind of one. Cast from thyself thy imagination, the destructive part of thy imagination. There are weeds that grow in the garden and there are flowers that grow in the garden. We should place before thee, in our own way, flowers. If you choose to eat the weeds, you shall only renew the karma.**

June 26, 1974: **Thy have other questions, ask.**
*"Yes, Aka. [10-19-73-002]: 'What is the problem with my gums? Also, how can I heal my gums?'"*
**We shall say unto you unto these questions into this manner. As has been stated before the reading, no medical questions would be asked. We shall answer in this manner. We have placed a healer among you. Come forth unto this one, and he shall administer unto the same.**

June 26, 1974: **Thy have other questions, ask.**
*"Yes, Aka. [3-1-74-001] says, 'I want to thank you for my health reading. In my reading you said I am suffering from hypertension, that of an imbalance in my day to day life. Could you please explain the cause and how I can correct this? Thank you.'"*
**First, we should answer in this manner. As we have stated before we are not here tonight to provide that of the health reading. We shall answer your question in this manner. Soon, the necessary equipment shall be made available for bio-therapy. We should say unto you, come forth, therefore, unto soul Ray, that implant, brain implant, may be done, and the overlay of nerve center into the same.**

July 7, 1974: **You have many questions, ask.**
*"Thank you, Aka. [7-7-74-001] asks, 'Will I live to raise my children?'"*

Yes, we say unto thee unto these words — for we have before us the body, the soul, the spirit and the immortal body — the healing thy ask for shall be given. Glory be the name of the Lord.

July 7, 1974: **Thy have other questions, ask.**
*"Thank you. [7-7-74-002] asks, 'Will H___'s health improve?'"*
**We have not of this, for we have not of permission of the same to answer this question.**
*"Thank you."*

July 8, 1974: **Thy have other questions, ask.**
*"Thank you, Aka. [7-8-74-004] asks, 'Will I ever get back down to my normal weight, and when or how?'"*
**Yes, we see thy need. There are certain glandular problems within the same. We would suggest that thy should go unto soul Ray for consultation and healing of the same. We would suggest that thy should write unto soul Ray, that he may answer in letter form and give, therefore, unto you a dietary substance that would help in this manner.**
**But we say unto you, all these things may be done. Yet without faith or hope — the Lord, God, placed in your hands free will. Some parts you must do yourself. We may give you the yeast, the bread, and the wine. We cannot drink it for you nor eat it for you.**

July 8, 1974: **You have other questions, ask.**
*"Thank you, Aka. [7-8-74-005] asks, 'What can you tell me about my father, whom my mother left when I was a baby?'"*
**We may only answer in this manner. We are not allowed to violate the free choice of another. One moment, permission must be given.** [Editor's note: a 15-second pause.]
**Yes, now we may answer the question in this manner. Soon there shall be born into thy family that of a girl child. It shall be of the same.**

July 8, 1974: **Thy have other questions, ask.**
*"Thank you, Aka. That's all that we have written."*
**Then we should answer in this manner. There is that among you who has come for healing. We see thy need.**
**Glory be the name of the Lord. Ask in thy Father's name and thy shall receive.**
**Now is the time of the Cherub.**

July 22, 1974: **Thy have other questions, ask.**
*"Yes, Aka. [7-22-74-001] of New York city, who is here tonight, asks, 'What have I not been able to do — why have I not been able to make my living through my psychic abilities? Or would you suggest another way to support myself?'"*

Yes, we see thy need. And we should answer thy question in this manner, in this way. Through a funnel of light thy came forth upon the earth. There have been times that thy have been jealous of thy own gift, yet times thy would rid thyself of it.

We say unto you, the land unto which you dwell is a land despoiled by man, a land corrupted by man. It is a Babylon that shall fall beneath the sea. It is part of that that shall be cut away. We say unto you, take of thy talents, of thy gift, and take it elsewhere.

You asked of other employment, and we should say unto you, it would be good to seek of this.

But we say unto you, soul Ray has worked upon the body and administered unto the healing, yet it is not complete yet, for it should come forth into the third day. Yet your mind can destroy all that we or he can do if you allow it to do so.

We say unto you, you have traveled into a different land and different people, yet they are all of God's children. You have brought forth part of those people with you that you have left behind. If you should seek other employment for your own health's sake, come, therefore, into a warmer, drier climate, that thy may flourish once again into womanhood. Care not, therefore, what others have done.

We shall place that into soul Ray's mind, that in the morn that he shall give into thee consultation. If thy should take of our advice and his, then your problem should cease, and be no more.

But we say unto you — as he sees, so do we. When you speak unto him he should show you courtesy and not say, "You are not telling me the whole truth." But we see in thyself. When thy speak, speak of the whole truth, not a half a truth, and that that thy ask for shall be given.

We say unto you, take, therefore, of thy life that God has given and thy shall be as a murderer, for thy would destroy the temple of God, thy body. You must judge unto thyself, and thy sleep would be long and painful, for thy would live again and again until thy truly saw the truth within thyself. We have opened a doorway that thy should see it now. We have answered your questions.

Glory be the name of the Lord.

But we say unto you, the Eagle flies *now*. We are here but for one purpose, that purpose is the coming of the Messiah.

July 22, 1974: **But we say unto you, who have traveled so far for healing and should wish a child, and conceivement of the same [7-22-74-003 and 7-22-74-004] — that we shall give. Continue with the treatment of the same, and the child shall be given forth from the Lord, God.**

**Can you understand of which we speak?**

**Then we say unto thee, you shall.**

July 27, 1974: **You have other questions, ask.**

*"Yes, Aka. [7-27-74-003] asks, "I would like to ask, if it is for me to know, whether or not I should bear another child in my lifetime, whether or not the motivation within me to bear again is self-orientated or is it truly what should be? Thank you."'*

We should say unto you at this time, there are certain adjustments and healing that soul Ray should administer into the body. But for the present time it would not be suggested that you should bear another child until healing should come in complete. There are other problems, that, both of your monetary value and that of your relationship, that should come into full blossom with your mate. Another child at this time would not be suggested.

July 27, 1974: **You have other questions, ask.**
*"Aka, [7-27-74-004] asks, 'What is my exact time of birth?'"*
Yes, we have before us the records. We have before us the body, the soul, the spirit, and the immortal body of the same.
Yes.
We find the time as 2:31 a.m.

July 27, 1974: **And now we should answer the question that should lie in the mind of one who has been treated by soul Ray. Continue, therefore, unto the treatment form of the same, and full enlightenment, both spiritual and physical, shall unfold. You have felt but a small proportion of the gift within.**
And yet all say unto themselves, "This is meant for me."
And we say, for the last person he treated upon this day, [7-27-74-005], this information is given.

July 27, 1974: **Yet, we say unto the others in the same manner, in the same way. For as healing has been asked for, so it shall be given. Glory be the name of the Lord, our God.**

September 2, 1974: **We should say unto this one, of soul Ruth [8-10-70-002-2], in this manner. We see of thy need, and that that is needed for the healing shall be sent forth. Only if the one in need [9-2-74-001] may accept our gift in the name of God can it come in fulfillment. Within soul Ray's mind is that that is needed for total healing and longevity given back unto the soul. We say unto you, do that unto which thy can to provide that they make a journey unto this land, that he may tender to their needs.**

September 12, 1974: **You have other questions, ask.**
*"[9-12-74-004] asks, 'Many doctors have made many diagnoses of my son's condition. What is your diagnosis and am I following the right course?'"*

Yes, we see of thy needs. First, we should answer in this manner. We may not answer questions about another soul without the soul's direct permission.

But we shall answer in this manner. Thy have asked for healing, and healing shall be given.

September 12, 1974[in Philosophy]: **You have other questions, ask.**

*"Aka, [9-12-74-007 — 'In your opinion, how important is a vegetarian diet to us and how strictly do you think we should adhere to non-animal byproducts?'"*

**We shall answer your questions in this manner. You have both the vegetarian and carnivorous animal within the man. If the genes and the ancestry that should make up of your mother, your father, your grandfather, your great grandfather, and so forth, should be of a vegetarian type, then that in itself, your body genes, that that you were born into and the...shall be of the same.**

**But we say unto you, far memory in its awakening should help change those genes. If your mind should cast back into another lifetime that you were vegetarian, then your body substance should change and body chemical, biochemical make-up, should change that the vegetarian diet could be sustained. Yet again, if the genes and the far memory is that of a carnivorous type, then the vegetarian diet, strict vegetarian diet, could kill of this one.**

**That that you place in your stomach should not make you closer to God. That that you place in your mind comes out of your mouth and is given unto another; that should place you closer to God.**

**But we say unto you, the mind is much like the stomach. Place in it only what thy can digest at one time, and in this manner good growth should come forth from both.**

September 25, 1974: **You have other questions, ask.**

*"Yes, Aka, [6-26-74-002] says, "Thank you, Aka. Do you have a message concerning my health?'"*

**Thy have come forth for healing. And the Lord, God, has heard thy prayer and healing shall be given. Glory be the name of the Lord.**

October 5, 1974: **Thy have other questions, ask.**

*"Yes, Aka. [10-5-74-004], and she asks, 'What year and month will our first child be born?'"*

**We say unto you, your child shall be conceived in the month of November of this year. And blessed be the children who should be born under the sign of the ankh, for they shall be those who should know of the Messiah first. Many new entries and many new places of entry are being**

prepared across thy earth. That that thy have asked for shall come in a bountiful manner.

October 26, 1974: **You have other questions, ask.**
*"Do you wish me to give another request for a life reading, or shall I go to shorter questions, Aka?"*
**We should say unto thee, because of soul Ray's health, we would suggest the shorter questions at this time.**
*"This one comes from [8-24-73-003]. On August 24, '73, you answered a health reading for him. At this time his mother also had a health reading. He thanks you for the help he has received from his reading. He now would like to know if his interpretation of his mother's reading is correct or not. Is there anything he can do to help her? Is what he's doing now wrong for her? He asks, please, could you please help him? His mother's name is S_____ M___."*
**We see of the same, and we should answer in this manner. Thy have brought forth unto the one known as soul Ray both for healing form. If treatment were continued in the present form, the help that was needed would be given. But we can say unto you unto this manner, we are not allowed to interfere with free choice. The free choice of your mother, thy have known.**

October 26, 1974: **Thy have other questions, ask.**
*"Thank you, Aka. Soul Mark [11-26-71-002-11] asks if she may help in some way her uncle, J_____ R_____... 'And if not, how may I help him to understand his physical condition?'"*
**We shall answer in this manner. Within himself he knows of his own physical condition. He has full awareness of this. But we say unto you, we have given you other tasks. We see of the need of the heart. Place this in our hands, and we shall place other things in your hands. Glory be the name of the Lord.**

October 26, 1974: **You have other questions, ask.**
*"Thank you, Aka. [10-26-74-001], he would like to know if his mother and dad will get back together?"*
**Yes, we see thy need. And we will answer in this manner. That that was meant in the beginning shall come forth in the ending. Have faith. We are not allowed to answer questions pertaining to the free will of another soul, but we have answered your question in a manner that only you, and you alone, shall see the full meaning of the same. Yet, we have answered your question.**

November 9, 1974: **Yes, we see thy need.**
**And we should answer in this manner. For each of you in your prayer should pray unto the Lord in such a manner as though you were**

talking unto yourself. But as you speak, remember that the Lord, God, should hear. But in your prayer make certain that your prayer does not defile another.

For many should pray for rain. And others should pray for the sun to shine. Yet the sun should shine and the rain shall fall upon the earth, each in a different way and in a different place. But should one pray for rain when the earth is not in need, then the prayer shall not be answered. And if one should pray for sunshine when the earth is in need of rain, then the prayer shall not be answered.

Do so in your own life. Do so in such a way that you do not offend thy brother or sister. But as the rain should fall, look not at just the rain and the cloudy skies, look, therefore, at the rainbow that should come after. Look at the earth, and say unto thy selves, "New life shall come forth, for the rain shall come and replenish the earth, and the sun shall come forth and bring forth the harvest."

November 9, 1974: Yet you say unto us, both in these times, "Why must the earth sleep?"

And we say unto you, that winter must come for the same reason that men must sleep. For the earth should replenish itself the same as man. It is a time for change. Nothing shall stand still, not your measure of time, nor your concept of time.

We have given you past-life readings to stir memories within yourselves of where you have been. But we say unto you, you are all parts of that that you have ever been. And all parts of that that you have been is what makes you what you are today. It is only good to know where you have been so you shall know where you are going.

Before you ask for a past-life reading, study your present plane reading. Look where you [have] been in this lifetime and you shall know where you shall go unto your next lifetime. But more important yet, you shall know the direction you are taking now. If there is a stone way in your path, you will remove this stone and not trip over it. But even the stone serves its purpose, for it is useful for the overcoming of karmic action into the same. Karma, as you would know it, is nothing more than knowing where you have been and changing the direction if it is not to your liking, for we say unto you, "if your right eye offend thee, cast it aside."

November 9, 1974: Soon upon your earth, your earth shall rapidly begin to change. You have seen changes in your lives that have multiplied.

We have told you of a coming famine, and the famine is at hand. We have told you the things to store. Yet if a man should work from dawn to dusk and only store in his warehouse a small proportion, give prayer upon that proportion you have stored, and the Lord shall replenish that proportion tenfold.

November 9, 1974: **Now we should say unto those who should be of the teachers in this work. First, we should say unto you, your directions should come from your ministers, and your ministers' direction should come from the prophet, but all should come from the same tree. Do not close the doorway to your minds, that new knowledge may not enter. Hold the doorway open and your growth shall continue beyond your wildest imagination.**

**And we should say unto the pupils, for none shall be greater than the teacher, or the pupil, or the master, for all shall come forth. But treat within each the respect you would want to be treated yourselves.**

**We say unto you, all of you, we have told you the parable of the Seven Spirits and the wheat field. We have brought forth unto you** *A Rose without Thorns.* **Soon it shall take flight upon the earth. We have told you of a new book to come, A** *Psychic Gift before the Dawn.* **We have told you of another book that should come forth at the same time. and it shall be your** *Workbook on Parapsychology.* **It should be named as such.**

**We shall open the doorways that many may enter. Close no doorways, that all may enter. Take no one from their faith, for remember, our Father has many mansions. Build upon what is there. Give unto those who should take of such, but let them take into the proportion of their needs.**

**It is true we shall expect more from the ministers, the teachers, and the pupils, for it is a binding thing that should come forth.**

November 23, 1974: **You have other questions, ask.**
*"Yes, Aka. There were two other questions, a couple of other questions that this subject had. [1-25-75-002]. One of them was, 'What could be done for a recurrent rash on her hands?' And what was the, why does she have severe headaches? 'What is the cause and cure of this?'"*
**We should answer in this manner. Come forth, therefore, unto soul Ray for healing, and the body, the soul, and the spirit, and the immortal body shall be healed of the same.**

November 23, 1974: **You have other questions, ask.**
*"Yes, Aka. [11-23-74-001] asks questions about her health....and she asks this. 'Considering my health problem would it be advisable for me to move to a higher altitude, like Prescott or Payson, and if so, where?' She would also like to know her time of birth."*
**We should answer in this manner. Thy time of birth was as the snow should fall, in the second day of February at 2 p.m. We are speaking of the time that the soul entered the body of the same, not of the time that you were emerged from your mother's womb.**

We would suggest that due to your health problem, you should take in consideration the altitudes of the same. From 4,000 to 3,500 feet above sea level would be most adequate. We would further suggest that thy should venture forth unto soul Ray for consultation of the same.

December 26, 1974: You have many questions, ask.

*"Yes, Aka. [12-26-74-001] asks a question...and she asks, 'How can I help my husband and help myself, and my family situation? Any advice you give would be appreciated.'"*

Yes, we see thy need. And first, we should say unto thee unto this manner. The answer unto your question lies within yourself. There is a time for all things upon the earth, a time for learning, a time for eating of the food of knowledge, a time when the mind, like the stomach, should become too full. You have doubts within your mind of your husband, and doubts within your mind of your children and their health. The health problem shall correct itself, within the children. The problem and the doubts of the husband shall also come forth in such a manner that fulfillment shall come forth. But we say unto you, because of thy worry thy are harming thy body.

# 1975 Health Readings

January 4, 1975: **You have questions, ask.**

*"Yes, Aka. I have a question regarding the health on* [1-25-74-001…Salem, Oregon]. *And the question his parents ask for him is, 'What is the cause of* [1-25-74-001]*'s recurrent illness, and is there any cure?'"*

Yes, we see thy need, and we have before us the body, the soul, the spirit, and the immortal body of the same. We shall say unto you, the cause of the reoccurring illness is that of pesticide poisoning, or defoliant poisoning, which is attacking the nervous system. It is also attacking the pancreas and the circulatory system; it is also attacking the respiratory system.

We shall answer in this way. The blood within the child itself cannot at this time fight off — the needed antibodies within the body to destroy the foreign substance — it has become weak. There are two manners unto which this could be remedied.

First, we would suggest the use of negative ion units, placed on a north-south axis. We would suggest that the child be placed with its head to the north and the feet to the south. The units should be placed five feet from the head and five feet from the feet. The child should be placed in this position, starting in five-minute intervals, five minutes the first hour, 10 minutes the second hour, 20 minutes the third hour, and 30 minutes the fourth hour. This should be repeated for a 30-day period. If this is done, this in itself will give the body chemistry time to correct itself and the necessary ions within the system to correct that within the same.

We would further suggest that these — the use of the sage tea should be used, drinking one cup on each hour intervals during the wakening hours of the child.

We would further suggest that that which is known as the mineral supplement unto which has been brought forth, the Negative Ion Mineral Supplement, could be used in this case. The necessary information is in soul Ray's mind.

It would further be suggested, if possible, that the child be brought forth for healing. If this is not possible, and the use of the above is used, then health shall be brought back unto the child.

You have further information.

Yes.

We would also suggest the use of the Jerusalem artichoke be used in the diet, that all sugar of any form be taken from the child and that of

the tupelo honey be used it its place.
Yes.

January 4, 1975: **Now, we should answer unto the question of the one known as [7-22-74-003]. And it is a private thing, yet the answer shall be given. They, both her husband and herself, have sought long for the conceivement of a child. And we answer unto you, do you not remember Elizabeth?** [See *Luke,* chapter 1.]
**Do you not remember Sarah?** [See *Genesis* 21:1-7.]
**That that you ask for shall be rewarded. Be patient, and that, the gift unto which you have asked the Lord, shall come in fulfillment.**
**But we have said unto you, the child into which you ask for shall be a special child. And therefore, the time and the preparation for its implantment will not be your own choosing, for it shall come of its own free will, for it should come upon the earth with a mission. You have asked, and so, the spirit that shall enter has asked — and the spirits of Aka have asked — and the Lord has seen that which would be placed upon the earth, but it shall be in the Lord's time. Further information on this subject shall be given at a different time.**

March 15, 1975: **You have many questions, ask.**
*"Yes, Aka. I have a request for a health reading from*
[3_15_75_001...of Faith, South Dakota]. *She says 'Please, I beg of you in Jesus' name, help me. I have been paralyzed from the waist down and unable to control my urine since a car accident July 3, 1965. At that time I received a blow, no cut, to the spinal cord in the first and second lumbar region.'"*
**Yes, we have before us the body, the soul, the spirit, and the immortal body of the same. Yes, we find, therefore, damage done unto the central nervous system. We find that certain nerves have been — a deterioration caused from the blow. We would suggest that this problem within itself could be corrected with the use of biotherapy. We would suggest that you should come forth unto soul Ray. There is no manipulation, only that of a nerve implant, that could be done. And this in itself must be done in the proper manner.**
**We say unto you, if this should be done by a neurosurgeon, take that of the sperm of the male, taking it, therefore, within 24 hours after it has been taken from the male; therefore, exposing the nerves, using that of the sperm to regenerate the nerves within themselves, and this way and in this manner, this could be corrected.**
**Soon you shall find within the sperm of the male new life-giving properties. This should be used in its proper source, for that that is brought from the seed shall grow unto the tree. We should also answer that the keys shall be both light and sound, used within its proper atmospheric conditions. As this sperm is used, it [must] be kept at an incubated temperature, in other words, at body temperature at all times.**

The key to [internal] life lies within the same. Also that that you should call cancer could be treated and cured with the same sperm, and an extract made from the same. The aging process of man could be reversed in the same manner, with using biotherapy in accordance with the same.

You have other questions, ask. One moment.

Yes, yes. Yes, Father.

Yes.

Permission has been given.

The healing that is needed to bring you unto this land shall be given and the means shall be set forth in motion. Ask in our Father's name, and you shall receive.

This is all on this subject.

March 15, 1975: **You have other questions, ask.**

*"Thank you Aka. I have another request for a health reading from [3_15_75_002...Phoenix]. The question they ask is, 'I would like a health reading, especially as to why my blood is anemic, and also is there anything I can do to keep from having any more outbreaks of cancer?'"*

Yes, we shall answer in this manner — with the use of the negative-ion unit placed on a north-south axis; that the subject matter should be placed on a mat that should be in height three foot above the floor level; that the ion unit[s] should be nine foot apart, and should be six foot above the body substance in height. This should be used in short intervals.

We would further suggest that the use of the new mineral substance that has been brought forth through soul Ray's mind be used in the treatment of the cancer substance.

There is yet another source that lies within soul Ray's mind that shall bring forth that that is known; the mineral substance within itself is chelated. Once ionized, and once [the] B-6 vitamin is placed within the same with that of the niacin or niacinamide in correct proportions, this should act as a purifier of the blood. The ingredients of B-12 should be added in accordance with the same. All of this and the knowledge of the same has already been implanted in soul Ray's mind.

New uses of that that you would call the chaparral has also been implanted in his mind.

New uses for the vitamins E, A, and D in accordance with other substances of the mineral compound, using that of myrrh and golden seal, and slippery elm in accordance with the same.

This is all on this subject at this time. Should further information be desired, ask.

March 15, 1975: **You have other questions, ask.**

*"Yes, Aka, I have a question or a request for a health — assistance,*

*from* [3_15_7 5_003…Phoenix]. *She asks for healing. 'Please help Ray and me to bring my high blood pressure down to normal, and also sugar. Thank you.'"*

That that has already been started shall be completed. The healing asked for shall be given in God's name. Continue with the therapy that soul Ray has brought forth. But come forth with faith, and faith shall breed love, and love shall bring healing.

April 5, 1975: **Soul Ray now grows weary. Yet we should answer in the mind the question of the one known as [8-27-73-001]. And we shall allow a message that is dear unto a departed one's heart to come forth. One moment.**
**Yes.**
**She asks but two things, that you go should forth in the work thy have chosen. Do so in the fullness of manner. And she says unto you, wed not but one who should walk by thy side in the manner that should prepare you for the greater work before you. But your days of loneliness should soon be over. She should thank you that you have released her. Yet she shall guide your footsteps into the new days of wedlock.**

April 5, 1975: **Yes, we see thy need.**
**Yes.**
**And we should say unto the one who has come from the land of the Coolidge, from this day forth, thy cup shall runneth over and fulfillment of thy life shall come forth, and that that thy have sought so long shall be fulfilled. And the healing that is sought shall be given in the name of the Lord, our God.**

May 15, 1975: **You have many questions, ask.**
*"Yes, Aka. [5-15-75-001…in Phoenix], and she asks, 'What should I do about my eyes?'"*
**We shall answer in this manner. Come forth into the land of the Eagle, the land of Globe, that the proper testing should be done by soul Ray. And we shall stand, and healing shall be given unto the same. But from the growth and from the journey you shall see from within as well as from without. Both are necessary. Glory be the name of the Lord.**

May 15, 1975: **Thy have other questions, ask.**
*"Thank you, Aka. [5-15-75-003] asks, 'I have been bothered by problems concerning a person named Garry and would like your advice as to how I can resolve them.'"*
**We shall answer your question in this manner. When a fisherman goes forth he should find a spot that he should cast his net. He should fish for but one kind of fish, that when he casts his net and brings it forth, he may bring forth nothing or fish of many kinds. Some he should care to**

keep, some he should care to cast back into the ocean. I should say unto you, you have caught a fish, yet you know not which is a fisherman, yourself or the other. Let the fish go back unto the ocean until you both make up your minds. Give yourself the freedom that is needed, and the time that is needed. And if that that you think is in your heart really dwells there, then it will be in truth. But there is much ocean, and many fish. Be as the fisherman who catches nothing; cast your net again.

May 15, 1975: **You have other questions, ask.**
*"Thank you, Aka, from [5-15-75-001], she is present here tonight and she asks, 'The doctors have diagnosed a serious health problem, which has resulted in being over-tired, which has affected my studies. What can you tell me on this? Thank you.'"*

We have told you before, come forth in truth unto soul Ray. Within his mind lies the answer of both *the health* and the correction of the same. We shall stand forth. But your spiritual development and your studies should be completed, for the time of the coming of the new Messiah upon the Earth is close at hand. The time of need upon the Earth of those with spiritual growth is now at hand. Cast these aside and you shall deny his coming.

May 15, 1975: **You have other questions, ask.**
*"Yes, Aka, from [5-15-75-008]...."*
**One moment.**
**Yes. Yes. Yes, Father.**
We have been instructed to say unto you these words. We shall take care of thy needs of thy physical body. As a new coveth comes forth unto the Earth, bring thyself into the same. Come forth unto soul Ray, and all things shall come, and all thy needs. Remember, thy wants and thy needs are two different things. We shall say unto thee, as the Parable of the Rose, and the book of *A Rose without Thorns*, the knowledge you seek lies within, for the greatest treasure within man should lie within himself. Think thee of the parable of the little girl who waited long by the healing well, while the others went forth before her. And when God looked down He did say unto her, "WHY DO YOU NOT HASTEN UNTO THE WELL?"

And she looked unto her Lord and said, "For my faith is my healing, Oh Lord. And my Lord's faith can never be used up, so why should I hasten?"

And the Lord did shed a tear, and the land was healed and the ocean roared, and all was blessed that day.

May 15, 1975: **You have other questions, ask.**

*"Thank you, Aka. From* [5-15-75-009…Phoenix], *she asks regarding herself, 'I would like to know what I am doing wrong, or not doing, to bring my high blood pressure down? Thank you?'"*

First we should say unto this one, we have before us the body, the soul, the spirit, and therefore, the immortal body. First we should answer unto you, thy biggest problem in the high blood pressure is emotional, and therefore, biotherapy should be sought out. The second problem is that of a problem of weight. Take forth the dietary substance soul Ray should give unto thee and the diet, and the high blood pressure problem shall vanish.

May 15, 1975: **You have other questions, ask.**
*"Aka, I have no further questions here tonight."*
Then we shall answer. Yes, we see thy need, and we shall give the healing that is needed into the one known as [5-15-75-010]. But we say unto you, we shall guide thy footsteps as long as thy remain our instrument. But beware that greed and need do not become confused. Healing shall be given in the name of the Lord and the [impart] therefore. Glory be the name of the Lord.

May 15, 1975: **And for those who should seek of the same, we say unto thee, we have placed an instrument at thy disposal. Use of the same, and the healing that is needed shall be provided. Glory be the name of the Lord.**

May 31, 1975: **You have many questions, ask.**
*"Yes, Aka. I have a question for a health reading from* [Mrs. S_____ M____ D_____, nicknamed Sandy,…Phoenix, Arizona]. *And she says she has trouble with her abdomen, throat, and frequent bruises on her legs. What can she do for this? And also any comments on childbearing?"*
Yes, we see thy need. And we shall answer your question in this manner, that the necessary herbs that are needed for the correction of the above situation lie at your fingertips. At the beginning we gave many, many health readings, as you would call them. But as we gave them, so should we prepare one that we would send within your midst as a healer with the knowledge to give healing into all, in equal proportions. Come forth unto soul Ray and he should bring forth unto the healing that is needed into the body, the soul, the spirit, and the immortal body of the same.

The bruising of the body is that of the, what you would call, of the thin skin, of the blood vessels being too close to the surface of the skin, and them being too brittle. The taking of the vitamin E substance in 2,000 units per day, with the taking of the mineral supplement, and the taking of 600 mg. per day, in the taking of the R.E. Lipo-C in the commodities of three, 3 times per day, in the taking of the niacinamide in the quantities of 300 mg. twice daily, of the taking of the Aloe Vera E Cream, moisturizing the whole body with the substance of the same, this in itself, the body would have a chance to rebuild the organisms within themselves, and your health problem would soon correct itself. But once again we would suggest that, come forth unto soul Ray, that the healing skills that we have implanted in his mind might speed up and increase the healing thy have asked for.

Of the child bearing, this is in past tense.

July 12, 1975: **You have many questions, ask.**

*"Yes, Aka. [7-12-75-001] asks, 'Will you please tell soul Ray how to cure my hands? They get sore to the bone, and get puss pockets between the fingers and on the palms.'"*

Yes, we see of thy need. And we have before us the body, the soul, the spirit, and the immortal body of the same, and therefore, we find within the body substance — yes — the imbalance of the pancreas, an imbalance in the blood substance of the same in the circulatory system of the same.

We should say unto this one, we have already placed, therefore, in soul Ray's mind that of a new formula, which will be taken both orally and placed on the outer skin, that should change the chemical balance of the body substance. We would also suggest that further bio-therapy be used in such a manner that the change might be complete. But we say unto this one, that that you have asked for shall be given in full.

Glory be the name of the Lord, our God.

July 12, 1975: **You have other questions, ask.**

*"Yes, Aka, [9-10-74-002] asks, why does she perspire so while working on some patients and not with others? 'Is this part of the healing process? I sincerely ask for God's healing help and guidance for the healing of patients' ills. I am also concerned with the continual ringing in my head, intensified at times — a rarity if it is not ringing. Is this common with humans? I would also like to know about the heat in my body. Is this also part of my healing work?'"*

We shall answer the question in this manner. We have before us the body, the soul, the spirit, and the immortal body of the same. First we should answer your question in this manner. We find, therefore, that of calcium deposits in the circulatory system, therefore, a restricting of the blood flow to the inner ear and inner eyes and restriction of blood flow to the brain. This, in itself, is damaging to the inner ear and to the bone structure of the same.

We would suggest the use of 400 mg. of niacinamide twice daily, and the use of the R. E. Lipo. These two substances — one would dilate the blood vessel, the other would aid greatly in the cleansing and the elasticity of the blood vessel within the same.

The perspiring — should a person labor in earnest they should perspire. It is a natural substance of cooling both the inner and outer body substance.

But we should answer further in this manner. That of a high cholesterol count in this system, this should also be corrected with the use of the mineral substance with B-6 and the use of the [lecithin]. A new formula has already come forth in soul Ray's mind, and a combination of such should soon be at your hand.

July 12, 1975: **You have other questions, ask.**

*"Yes, Aka, he has one another question. He asks, 'My twin brother, C_____ D. C_____, has some injured knees, and I was wondering what can be done to help. They bother him a great deal. He was born in Kingston, Pennsylvania, 1/1, January 1ˢᵗ, I guess,....'"*

**The information you have just fed us is incorrect, but we still see thy need and we shall answer the question. Take, therefore, of the Earth formula** [Note: Aloe Vera Earth formula Ray developed]. **Applied properly, the relief needed in the healing shall come forth, using the cream formula of the same.** [Editor's note: Aloe Vera E. Cream.]

July 12, 1975: **You have other questions, ask.**

*"Yes, Aka. I have a question from [7-12-75-004…Phoenix…]. She asks, 'When will I get well? And what line of work will I be best suited for, one that I can enjoy and be of service, and profitable.'"*

**We shall answer in this manner to your question. The time element in your healing lies within your mind. The healing can come at any time thy wish.**

**The second part of your question we shall answer in this manner. Seek out that in the line of the beautician or cosmetologist. There is that of the new facial substance which soul Ray has brought forth. With its proper use, and proper business management, this would give you a good livelihood.**

July 19, 1975: **Now soul Ray grows weary. But you have two questions about a person's health that should be answered. Ask of these.**

*"One moment. I am not aware of the questions, one moment…Here it is. I have a letter from a [7-19-75-002…in Tucson]. One moment…"*

**We shall answer of this.**

*"Yes."*

**And we shall say unto this person, soul Ray shall soon venture into thy land. Come forth, that he may administer the healing that is needed, both of the body, the soul, the spirit, and the immortal body of the same.**

**But the healing that thy have asked for shall be granted. And so it is done in the name of the Almighty God. Glory be the name of the Lord.**

[*Kay-ah, kay-ah.*]

August 23, 1975: **You have many questions, ask.**

*"Yes, Aka. I have a question for a health reading request for [7-314-1...Phoenix]. 'Aka, will you please tell soul Ray how to cure me. I am losing nerve control and muscle tone. I have degeneration in some muscles.'"*

**We see thy need, and we should answer in this manner. That that has been done shall continue to be done with the biotherapy treatments.**

**We should add further into this in this manner. If the ion units were placed on a north-south axis, placing the units nine feet precisely in distance one from the other, placing them exactly three feet above the surface of the earth — they must be precisely level, placing the head to the north, the feet to the south — the subject as such should be placed exactly three feet from the surface on exact level with the ion units. The therapy should start with 30-minute intervals each day, increasing unto the third hour, with the continued therapy of that of the swimming to restore the degenerated muscular tone. Further information on this subject shall be given from time to time.**

**Thirdly, we would suggest that the subject lose the fear within himself, for this, in itself, is the greatest destructive force, therefore, in the subject matter. As we have said before, the past is the past, the present is the present. You can make your own future. But that that should be the crippling disease should be manifested more greatly in the mind, and from the mind unto the body; therefore, with the light and tone changes within the mind substance, healing should continually be brought forth. But it must be done on a gradual basis. If this is brought forth too fastly, the degenerated nerve substance should become mutate, and therefore, not in control of the same.**

August 23, 1975: **You have other questions, ask.**

*"Yes, Aka. Soul Ruth [2-30-2] asks, 'When I was a small child I attended a masquerade ball where a young woman dressed as Salome carried on a platter a realistic wax reproduction of the severed head of John the Baptist. I have been haunted by this ever since, and it bothers me so much lately that I cannot sleep. Can you tell me a reason for this?'"*

**Yes, we see thy need and we should answer in this manner. As the garden is weeded, there are those who would rather eat the weeds than the fruit.**

August 23, 1975: **You have other questions, ask.**

*"Aka, [7-301-1] asks a number of questions. One, 'How can I finalize my healing?'"*

**We shall answer in this manner, the faith and knowledge within the mind — a cripple can only be a cripple as long as the mind allows it to be. The continued therapy, with full cooperation, which you have not**

The Health Readings - 1975

extended as yet, in biotherapy; you have been lazy, uncooperative, and therefore, the healing as such cannot be completed.

August 23, 1975: **You have other questions, ask.**
*"Yes, Aka, she asks, 'What would be the best career for me to pursue, and what is the quickest way for me to become financially independent.'"*
**Go to work, period.**
**You have other questions, ask.**
*"One final question from her, 'Also, should I pay Dr. J___ F__?'"*
**If labor is due, and the labor is honest, pay of the same.**

August 23, 1975: **You have other questions, ask.**
*"Aka, [7-314-2…Woodside, California] asks, 'Please give guidance and direction for me at this time. Should I go to California and go to medical assisting school? Thank you.'"*
**(Chuckle) Yes, we see thy need. You have gone forth for healing and have received the same, both mentally and physically. If the schooling was all thy desired, this would be a good thing, but you seek even that of the past. We say unto you, the past is the past. Walk on unto your future and let it become bountiful. If one should plant a tree, and seek the fruit the same day, they shall not receive it. But if they should plant the fruit tree, cultivate it, and tend it well, then the fruit shall be bountiful and sweet unto thy taste.**

**We say to you, you have made progress in the ability to make your own decisions. Soul Ray has implanted that in your mind with the use of biotherapy. He has taken nothing from your mind, only added to, the ability to make a decision, to carry it out, and to gather the fruit from the same tree. Continuing to run will accomplish nothing. Stand in one place, and let the tree grow.**

September 20, 1975: **You have many questions, ask.**
*"Yes, Aka. I have a request for a health reading tonight from [7-315-1…Scottsdale, Arizona…]. She asks, 'What is causing the constant buzzing and clicking noises in my ears, and is there any treatment that will cure this condition? This has existed for six years.'"*
**Yes, we have thy body, the soul, the spirit, and the immortal body of the same. We shall answer your question in this manner. If you should bring your problem unto soul Ray, the treatment of the same is a very simple treatment. The clicking or tone in the ears is a fusation [fusion?] of the bone structure of the same. It is brought about by the lack of circulation in the inner ear in the proportion of the bony structure that should provide that of tone and sound into the same. You shall find further that this condition is impairing the sight, and also the motor function of the brain, and shall soon bring on other complications of a radical nature.**

This could be treated by the use of that of the niacinamide, the vitamins of the Lipo-C, and the use of hot castor-oil packs placed behind the ears. We would further suggest that the mineral supplement be used in the treatment of the same. Further use of that of the ion, negative-ion units, would help to change the atmospheric conditions while the subject slept at night.

This is all on this subject.

September 20, 1975: **You have other questions, ask.**
*"Yes, Aka. I have a request for a health reading for* [7-315-2…Phoenix]. *The problem is headaches. But he asks for — the question is for a general health reading."*

Yes, we see thy need, and therefore, we have before us the body, the soul, the spirit, and the immortal body of the same. We find, therefore, that we have brought unto thy keeping that of the bio-therapy.

The headaches are due to two problems which should run parallel, one with the other. One is due to the fluctuation of the blood pressure. The other is due to that of stress. We find a third factor, that of a chemical substance within the bloodstream which, in turn, has caused that of the neutron [neuron] built between the two tissues of the brain in the upper left lobal area. Further we find, therefore, within the same, that of the sinus cavities, infection, therefore, within the same. We find, therefore — yes — the lack of mineral in the blood structure of the same, kidney, liver damage due to that of imbalance of vitamin substance.

We should say once again, bring this one forth unto soul Ray. The knowledge that is needed has been planted, therefore, in the mind, for both biotherapy and that that you would know as psychic surgery will be needed to impair and repair this and to bring about the full healing.

We would also suggest that the use, at this time, of that of the slippery elm, [myrrh?], that of the hops and mistletoe and sage, each in exact proportions of a balance of the same be used for the making of a tea substance. This should be drinke four times daily. [Note: drinke(n) is Middle English for drank.]**This would help in the cleansing of the system, and help to reduce the infection in the [bronchianing] areas.**

But without the necessary biotherapy, herbs and vitamins alone, or medication of any kind, would not fully restore this one to their health.

September 20, 1975: **You have other questions, ask.**
*"Thank you, Aka. I have a request for a health reading for* [7-315-3…Durango, Colorado]. *'Is there anything I can do to maintain the good health that Ray has gotten me in, other than I've already been instructed?'"*

Yes, we see the need, and therefore, we should provide the information. We have before us the body, the soul, the spirit, and the immortal body of the same, and we should answer in this manner. Continue the use of that of the Wonder Loss, in its exact proportions directed by soul Ray; continue [the] use of the other herbs and vitamins substances in their proper form; continue use of biotherapy at periodic periods of time.

You must realize that one part has been provided. Other parts shall come forth. At the present time we have implanted in soul Ray's mind many new formulas for the improvement of the health of all. He is slowly bringing these forth. We are providing that of the material needs. But you must realize also that due to his own health state we can only implant the knowledge. One thing at a time must be brought forth and a foundation built in the structure of the same.

New machinery, that that shall be needed, will take time in the provision of the same. In this time of recession, the hearts of many have grown cold to his efforts. But we shall continue to prevail and provide, that all may receive from his healing, both by herb and by the energy substance we have provided within him, and the knowledge of the same, taking of the knowledge, using it well.

We have said before, we may knock upon the door, only you may bid us enter. Take forth, therefore, that that we have provided, and let it spread into your land. Take forth of the vitamin and herb substance, and let it spread, therefore, upon your land, as well as the knowledge. A healthy mind and a healthy body will function better together.

September 20, 1975: **You have other questions, ask.**
*"Yes, Aka. I have a request for a health reading from* [6-274-3…Dallas, Texas]. *She asks, 'What is behind my daughter, A____ L_____ B_____'s learning disabilities and how can we best correct this? Please be specific.'"*

We shall answer your question in this manner. Soul Ray has given you full information in specific terms. Listen therefore.

Of your own health needs, and that that you have asked for, the necessary surgery has been provided. We have restored your health, that of your husband, and that of your daughter. The learning difficulty is that of a bored child, nothing more. We shall say unto you that further biotherapy would improve this.

September 20, 1975: **You have other questions, ask.**
*"Thank you, Aka. I have a request for a health reading from* [7-315-4…Grants Pass, Oregon…]. *Her question is for help with her arthritis and muscle cramps of the skin, three kinds of arthritis, also trouble with her heart and lungs."*

Yes, we shall answer in this manner. A new substance shall soon be provided unto soul Ray, that of the chelate-orotate method used in the mineral supplements. It shall be provided and isolated very soon. Be patient.

We have placed before you that of the Aloe Vera Earth formula, and cream formula. Use of these. Use of the mineral supplement, therefore, at hand at the time. Use, therefore, of the hops, a tea seeped [steeped] of the same before bedtime. Use, therefore, of the sage three times a day, a cup of the same.

Of the heart problem, we shall answer in this manner. This we shall maintain, for the healing that is asked for shall be given. But we shall answer you also in this manner. A place has been prepared.

September 20, 1975: **You have other questions, ask.**
*"Thank you, Aka. I have a request for a health reading for* [7-325-5…Alta Vista, Virginia]. *She asks for a health reading; she has a hearing problem, leg and stomach and weight problems. Also would like to know if she will marry again?"*

Yes, we see thy need. We have before us the body, the soul, the spirit, and therefore, the immortal body of the same.

Yes.

We should answer your question in this manner. Of the stomach problem, we should suggest that of the Aloe Vera Gel, two ounces three times per day.

Of the weight problem, we would suggest that of the Wonder Loss formula of the same, three teaspoons three times per day.

As for the marriage problem, we shall answer in this manner. If a gardener should plant his garden and tend it well, then it shall reap a bountiful harvest.

September 27, 1975 [in Philosophy]: **You have other questions, ask.**
*"Yes, Aka. I have a question from* [7-316-1] *who now lives in Yuma, Arizona, and asks, 'What can we take to nullify the poison cotton and lettuce sprays that we have to breathe? Also, Aka, please tell me about my health conditions.'"*

First, we should answer in this manner. We have brought forth the substance that is known as the "Goldenseal with B-6" formula. This in itself is constructed in such a manner to cleanse the system and maintain the toxic level of the same.

Of your health conditions, this in itself is a general question. Your main health condition at the present time is condition of the liver, and a toxic condition within the same, a blockage. Using of the substance we have just suggested, this problem could be readily dissolved.

As we have said before, we have brought forth that that is needed for your needs. We have seen the need. Therefore, we have implanted the knowledge, and the substance is before you.

September 27, 1975: **Now we should say unto you, due to the condition of soul Ray's health and the overtaxing of his body substance, your reading shall be short. We have given unto you that that is needed.**

The Fifth Angel walks upon your earth.
Now is the time of the Cherubim.

October 11, 1975 [in Philosophy]: **You have other questions, ask.***
*"Yes, [7-317-2] has another question: 'What is your opinion of diet and refined foods as a cause of sickness?' She has asked in the past especially about white sugar."*

**We shall answer your question in this manner. The white sugar, in refining, in itself, does little but take, therefore, from the substance of the same.**

**In this particular question you are asking both for that of hypoglycemic patients and diabetic patients. We would suggest the use, therefore, of the tupelo honey that should come from the region of the Florida land. This should contain within the substance three different types of glucose. This substance will feed slowly into the system, and therefore, can be handled by the system much easier than your other sugar forms.**

**Of diet within its same, and roughage, roughage must be needed within the system, therefore, that the system may digest its food more readily. Cooked food quite often, if prepared in a wrong manner, could take, therefore, of the vitamin substance within the same. But in this day and time, I would look closer into the mineral lacking in the food substance.**

**The oritate method and chelating method, and the combining of the mineral substance, both with the use of the ionization and the use of the B substance, or your B$_6$ substance, within this would, therefore, help very much in the repair of the lower colon and the damage, therefore, into the same, as surgical techniques seldom may help these regions because the diseased area only will become diseased again. Correction can be made without surgery in this fashion.**

**Your question should cover a great latitude, and therefore, we shall add more unto it from time to time.**

*Editor's note: Also see what was said just before on this date.

November 8, 1975: **You have many questions, ask.**
*"Yes, Aka. I have a question tonight from [1-1-5]. He asks, 'Aka, I would like a health reading; is there anything I can do to improve my hearing?'"*

**Yes, we should say unto you unto this manner. We have before us the body, the soul, the spirit, and the immortal body of the same. Therefore, we find in this subject the lack of the substance, as you would know it, as B-2 and B-1. This, in itself, has caused hardening of the arteries, shutting off the blood supply to the inner ear and the bone structure of the ear substance of the same. This is also affecting the eyes, and is also affecting the memory pattern of the brain. We would suggest**

that come forth unto soul Ray that the necessary adjustments of the vitamin substance and herbs come forth that this may be restored.

We also find within this body substance within the liver area, kidney, we find, therefore, large quantities of pesticide. This is creating a blockage of the liver. Less and less of the liver is being used. This also could be corrected in the same manner.

We find also within this subject that of a heart problem. The arteries between the lung and the heart have been weakened due to the lack of circulation throughout the body. In essence, this has caused, as you would say, back pressure upon the heart valves themselves. We would suggest that the above mentioned be corrected, and therefore, the heart function would correct itself.

November 8, 1975 [in Philosophy]: **You have other questions, ask.**

*"Yes, Aka, I have a question from [6-281-1]. She says, 'Dear Aka, recently I have been reading a book entitled,* Everywhere the Light, The Story of Zitelle. *It is written by Neil Bishop. I have some questions regarding this work. Please comment. "There is an essence in almonds unknown to mankind. The same applies to raisins and dates and figs." Can you tell us more about which nutrients are vital for special kinds of illnesses, and which nutrients more emphasis should be placed upon?'"*

Yes, we shall answer your question in this manner. But first we shall say unto you, what should be good for the biochemical structure of one humanoid should not, therefore, be good for another. Therefore, many tools are needed. You speak of the almond substance within the same. We should say unto you, you have now a drug called Laetrille that has been brought forth from the apricot-pit substance. In its present form it is dangerous to man. The almond, an extract made from the almond, added to the Laetrille in its pure form, and taking that of the chaparral and adding to, in the correct proportions desired, and that of the calcium-magnesium base, would change the structure, therefore, and be useful in the fighting of the virus-type cancer. Yet, it would be fairly useless in other types of cancer without the use of large doses of 50,000 units of A, the vitamin A.

What we have tried to show you in nutrients, once a substance is placed within the body structure, the body, therefore, shall change its form. The biochemical structure of the body substance shall change the form of one substance in one person in one way, and another in another way.

It is quite often you have seen in a subject the yearning or the desiring of a certain substance. This is the mind itself speaking out from the body of a food substance it needs. Yet sometimes that that it reaches for is not that that should be put through the stomach, for nothing should be placed in the mouth that the stomach cannot digest, and nothing should be placed in the mouth that the circulatory system cannot purify and find useful. Food substance, this in itself you shall find, through genetic breeding the cell structure shall be changed to meet the required needs, much as man adapts to his environment. If you lived in a land where all you had to eat was fish and vegetables, you would soon find through genetic breeding and time the body substance would produce fully all that was needed. Yet, even in that environmental condition there would be certain vitamin-mineral substances that should be added.

We would not suggest that a vegetarian become a meat-eater or a meat-eater become a vegetarian. It may be done, but it must be done in a gradual manner. This is why we have suggested that certain proportions of that that you have stored for future use be used now, that the body may gradually adapt to this substance.

You have many different types of medical substance. The size, the weight, the height, must all be considered in the administering of these, as such. The amount of protein *per se* must be calculated very carefully, and the amount of carbohydrates should be calculated very carefully, and so on, in such a manner that a very balanced, nutritional diet for the subject at hand may be brought forth. But always take in consideration that not even one snowflake upon your earth is identical, nor no part of the same snowflake may be identical. Each cell is different and apart, and the cell structure of each human, fish, fowl, or animal is different.

December 14, 1975: **Yes, we see thy need, and we should answer in this manner in this way, for love is giving without expecting anything in return, for love is hope, and hope is love. It comes to the very young and to the very old, and without it man would perish from the earth, and God would perish from within.**

December 14, 1975: **Therefore, we should answer of your question. We say unto you, the one thy seek is safe, yet frightened. We see of her, therefore, in the Phoenix area. We find her, therefore, at this time alone and seeking.**

**We should say unto you, her pride is what keeps her from returning.**

**Yes.**

**We say unto you, go forth [and to] your police and place a missing persons report. This, and their finding of the same, will bring her back into safety. But it will tell unto her that she is wanted by all of her children.**

**We should say unto the child who has known of this, and yet, not spoken out, remember the Ten Commandments, to honor thy father and mother, [that] love begot love. And love comes unto each in a different manner. So who are you to judge what love must be?**

# 1976 Health Readings

January 26, 1976: **You have other questions, ask.**

*"Thank you, Aka. [8-326-4] asks, 'Is there any reason for my fear of being with people. Is it karmic or must I just be with people more? I can't seem to relax with more than one person.'"*

**We shall answer your question in this manner. First we should say, we have before us the body, the soul, the spirit, and the immortal body, and therefore, the records contained within the same. We shall answer your question that this does not come from a past-life experience, but from a present life experience.**

**We would suggest that two forms of therapy should be sought out, one of two forms, either that of biotherapy, or that of hypnotic therapy. Or, a third alternative, come unto soul Ray that this question can be answered in privacy, for it contains and should only be aired in the privacy between two minds.**

January 26, 1976: **You have other questions, ask.**

*"Thank you, Aka. [8-326-5…Green Valley, Arizona] who is here tonight…asks, 'I want to know what I can do to better the health of my two youngest children, who are with me, and to save my marriage. I also wonder if there is anything I can do for my two children, that is, sons in Chile, and my parents?'"*

**Yes, we see thy need, and we shall answer in this manner. The health question should be brought forth unto soul Ray. That that is needed shall be implanted in the mind of the same in a wakening state.**

**That of the marriage is of a delicate nature and should not be aired in public or made for public record. That also should be brought unto soul Ray that private counseling might be given.**

**Of the last question, we shall answer in this manner. You can go back to nothing. You have walked forth and away from that that lies behind you. There shall be a time and a place when the past [shall] come forth and beckon you, but leave that of the past alone until that day arrives. There is a time to do something; there is a time to do nothing. Now is the time to do nothing.**

**As we have said, we cannot interfere with the free choice of another. This is the God-given right of every soul upon your Earth and all others. Quite often men try to play God. This is a foolish thing to do.**

January 26, 1976: **You have other questions, ask.**
*"Thank you, Aka.* [8-326-7, of Tucson…] *asks, 'Do I need surgery?'"*
**We shall answer in this manner and say, yes. The decision of how this may come about must come from within.**

January 26, 1976: **You have other questions, ask.**
*"Thank you, Aka.* [8-326-8…Canada…] *asks, 'Do I have cancer?'"*
**We find not of this substance.**

**You may confuse our answer; therefore, we shall clarify of the same. It is not of a true cancer substance, no. We find a virus, therefore, in the body substance, but of a different nature. This could be readily eliminated with proper treatment.**

February 14, 1976 [in Philosophy]: **You have other questions, ask.**
*"Yes, Aka, soul Ray has a question. 'What is the next step to do about my blood disorder, and is chemotherapy recommended or what?'"*
**Yes we see thy need, and we should say unto you these words. Two programs must be initiated. One is within the diet substance of the same. More of the seafood substance must come into the diet. Second, we should say unto you that as blood is extracted, a blood exchange should be made in such a manner that the new antibodies of the blood placed in the system would have a chance to combat the situation. A form of chemotherapy, as you would know it, should be used. This should be used in the form of the use of antibiotics — if treated in intervals, not in heavy, stringent manner; in other words, a series of antibiotics should be used in one-week intervals once a month. This would allow the system to correct itself.**

**We have said before, we will maintain the body substance and give forth the healing that is needed.**

**We say unto you, to answer your question within your minds, "Why then should he suffer, when we could heal the body?"**

**We say unto you, that part of the biological change of the blood structure is due to that of the energy force he chooses to use in his form of healing. Under different atmospheric conditions there would be no problem, such as placing him closer to the ocean substance or lower altitude. Yet, this again would not [seek, suit] his need within himself. We would suggest more frequent trips to the ocean.**

**But, we should say unto you, his choice is to find a cure, not for himself, but for the many others upon the land who carry this disease substance in their bodies also.** [Editor's note: He had polycythemia and later was diagnoses with systemic lupus erythematosus. Many people who had lived in south Tucson in the 1950s-60s when Hughes Aircraft used trichloroethane to clean aircraft engines, as Ray did, later developed Lupus (SLE), brain cancer (which Ray later did), ovarian tumors from these chemicals in the ground well water.]

We would also say unto you that if you could learn from him the use of the bio-therapy, this could be used to alter the chemical, biochemical process of the blood substance.

But we say also, he should bring forth and use more of the exercise of the swimming. He is spending far too many hours working, both in the bio-laboratory, in the healing, and in the laboratory to produce the substances to heal your bodies.

Yet, as we have said before, he is a stubborn lot. His greatest joy comes from seeing others healed and the bringing forth of the substances that will heal the body, the soul, the spirit and the immortal body of man. We cannot change nor take from him his free choice, for this is his will, his free will. His love of life extends beyond that of his own life. For his love of life is seeing life renewed. Much as his roses come into bloom, his greatest joy is seeing the blossom within another human being. To understand the healing, you must understand the man. Yet his quest for knowledge shall never end.

You have many other questions in your mind this night. But all have wondered long about this one, and so, we shall finish what we have started. From the beginning, as we have said before, he came unto your Earth as the sons of the God did come forth, and therefore, he did bring karma unto the Earth. Through his own free choice, and his desire to remove this from the Earth, we say unto you, the Eagle in is flight and nothing we can do can stop it, for he shall expend his last breath preparing the way for the coming of the Messiah. It is his choice.

He shall continue bringing forth that of the bio-therapy, and the means of treating your diseases, [and] the means of seeing them in their truer form. Deny him that and he would die. Deny him the right to heal the sick and he would die. Deny him the right to seek forth and bring forth knowledge that will stand long after he is gone from your Earth, and he would waste away. For building, whether it be of stone or man, he shall do to his last breath. [Editor's note: See his last reading in 1989.]

February 25, 1976: **You have other questions, ask.**

*"Yes, Aka. From [8-330-1], 'Will I remarry my first husband? Will he be able to make a change? I would appreciate any further information you could give me.'"*

We should say unto this one, we have before us the body, the soul, the spirit, and therefore, the immortal body of the same. And we should say unto you, the two of you have bore this karma together. Each have faults. Each should correct these faults. Each should learn to overlook the other's faults. Your marriage and your reunion can only come when you can love one enough to free them.

In this case, there are certain things that should be removed and cast aside. We shall say unto you, it is written in the book of Moses that should a man and a woman divorce one another, they must, therefore, go before their God and ask forgiveness before remarriage into each other. If this is not done, then they have sinned against God and they have sinned against man and they have sinned against themselves. They must go unto each other and ask forgiveness.

But we should say unto you, you could seek out others who should be and look for the characteristics of the one you have left. And should you meet this new person, they would have those same faults as the other person, and so would you. Would it not be wise to rebuild the house and start with the foundation that you already have?

Build the foundation well, and the marriage shall stand, and it shall bear fruit and the fruit shall be good. And the fruit's fruit shall bear fruit. We say unto you, for you, as the descendants of Abraham, are the children and the seed of God.

February 25, 1976: **You have other questions, ask.**

*"Yes, Aka. From* [6-275-1…in Alameda, California], *'Thank you, Aka, for what you have done for me. What can I do for others to help myself and them stay that way?'"*

We shall say unto this one, we have before us the body, the soul, the spirit, and the immortal body of the same. And we should say unto you, a promise unkept, whether that promise be to yourself or to another, is a lie unto yourself and a lie unto the other. We say unto you, a way shall be made that you should be brought back forth unto the land and united with your wife, in the land of the Eagle. And a way shall be provided that you shall make your livelihood in this land. Prepare for this and prepare for the reunion.

But we say unto you, learn to look unto all things and see the beauty within. To love is to love enough to let that that you love have freedom of choice. But this must go together; she in turn must learn the same. There is much for both of you to learn. Give it time, and that that you desire and the knowledge you desire shall be laid before you.

But we say unto you, we have placed into thy hands *A Rose without Thorns*; pick it up. Read it once, and as you read each chapter write down what you feel the meaning is. And then reread it again, and again, at the end of each chapter write down what you feel the meaning, what you have gained from the chapter, is to you. And then, read it unto the third time, and then this time write down once again what you have found within the whole book, and you shall find a peace and a truth within yourselves. Can you understand of which we speak?

Yes, we see thy understanding, but not in full. Listen carefully. Reread this transcript and you shall understand in full what we have said.

February 25, 1976: **You have other questions, ask.**

*"Yes, Aka, from [6-281-1] and she asks about, 'Would it be advisable for her husband to seek help from Dr. McGarey? And also could you give any information about her health?'"*

We should say unto you, our time should grow short.

The help that Dr. McGarey would give would be good. We should say unto you, the help that soul Ray might give might be good. Use of your free choice to make this decision, for both would give honest service.

February 28, 1976: **Thy have many questions, ask.**

*"Aka, the parents of [8-331-1] request a health reading.... And the mother asks, specifically, 'How we can help her overcome her allergy to milk and susceptibility to all manner of infections, and how to build up her resistance and aid her digestion?'"*

Yes, we see thy need. We would say unto thee to take that of goat's milk, taking, to one pint of goat's milk to one-fourth part of Wonder-Loss Formula. This would allow the system a chance to gain the biochemical balance needed in the system. It would also allow the assimilation of the glucose needed from the protein substance of the same. It would also be suggested that that of the tupelo honey be used in small proportion, only enough to slightly sweeten this substance and make it better to the taste of the child. If this were done, the child would soon — the child's own biochemical substance then would have a chance to balance itself and the problem would end.

We would further suggest that that of the night-blooming cereus plant, the root proportion of the same, or tubular proportion, be used and fed to the child. This must be crushed — only quarter-by-quarter-inch pieces at a time be used, and no more than three parts of this in the course of a day — crushed into a fine pulp. Do not lose the juice form, using all of the substance. This would allow the [antibodes, antibodies] in the body to build. The plant itself contains that of the [antibodes] necessary to ward off diseases within your system. This must be done very carefully and very precisely, for too much of this could make the soul sick and it would have a violent reaction to this substance.

We would further suggest that the child be fitted at this time for corrective lens substance. This is hard, we know, for you to understand. It is because of the imbalance of the eyesight. The equilibrium of the motor area of the brain is affected, as such.

Small amounts, as no more than 50 international units, of vitamin A should be added to this substance.

This is all on this subject at this time. Should further information be needed, ask.

February 28, 1976: **You have other questions.**

*"Yes, Aka, from [8-231-2] and he asks about his neuralgia and lumbago troubles present in lower back, [and] the intense pain and arthritis manifestations in both of his hands."*

Yes, we see of thy need. First we should say unto you unto these words. We have before us the body, the soul, and the spirit, and the immortal body of the same. The location is incorrect at this time. One moment please.

Yes. Yes, yes.

Yes, we find this, this soul in the land of the Phoenix.

Yes.

Now the information may be given.

We should say unto this one, number one: the problem of the back is due to the overweight or gluttonous of this one. The back structure was not meant to carry this amount of weight. Therefore, the use of the Wonder-Loss substance to reduce this and bring it under control — dietary should be used. The use of any sugar form should not be used in this diet. The use of the tupelo honey only — *no* sugar substance of any type should be used, for this subject is that of a borderline diabetic. The use of the cheeses or heavy spices should be taken from the diet. The use at the present time, every third day, of 1 ounce of castor oil to 1/4 ounce of that of the lemon juice to 1/4 teaspoon of the baking soda, mixed well and taken internally — this would clear the blockage of the bowels and take the pressure from the lower back as such.

The controlling of your eating habits — more of the saltwater sea-life protein substance should be used in your diet. This should be in the diet at least four meals in the course of one week. Beef, that raw as possible, should be consumed in one form or the other, two meals of each week. Of the seventh day, that of the gizzard of the chicken should be used. As much raw vegetable as possible should be placed in the diet. This may come in many types. That of the papaya should be used as a digestive enzyme with each meal.

With the present course of treatment that soul Ray has brought forth unto you, full recovery would come forth at this time.

But we would say unto you that that of your own experimentation shall destroy the heart substance should you continue at its present course. It is very dangerously close to doing of such. Quit experimenting with your body. Quit experimenting with that of your wife.

The vitamin B-12 is a good vitamin if it is used in its correct proportions. Overused it can destroy the liver, kidney substance.

February 28, 1976: **You have other questions, ask.**

*"Aka, should I continue with health questions or general questions at this time?"*

It should make little difference.

*"I've got a request from...[7-316-2...he lives about 1/4 mile south of* [B____], *California...].*"

**One moment, please. We should say unto you unto this manner, the full data must be given.**

*"Aka, [2-50-2]'s doctor requested that she ask for a health reading, particularly in relation to the problem of repeated gum infection."*

**Yes, we see thy need, and we have before us the body, the soul, the spirit, and the immortal body of the same. Therefore, we should say unto you, the infection brought forth, first unto the land by that of the spray substance upon the land, did infest the animal substance and the land substance. The repeated handling of the animals without better sanitary conditions should only prolong this in the animals and yourself.**

**We should say unto you at this time that the use of the antibiotics suggested are correct, but we would say unto you, finding that of a very light-bristled toothbrush, use that of the vitamin E after the mouth has been washed thoroughly with normal toothpaste, working this into the gum substance. First, before this should be done, a cleaning of the teeth and the corrosion from that from the water and that of the — that are in the teeth should be done. Then, after this has been done and the anti-biotic been used, then using the A, vitamin A, as we have suggested, then using that of the Aloe Vera in rinsing the mouth. We suggest that it should be used in this proportion — taking 1/4th pint of Aloe Vera and adding 3 teaspoons of dehydrated sea salt into the Aloe Vera. This should be used as a mouthwash, making certain that it penetrates throughout the whole mouth, and gargling with the same. This in itself should clean away the problem.**

**We should say unto you, should you continue to wish to control this problem, the use of the sage tea, at least 6 cups a day, must be consumed in the body substance — and the continued use of the Wonder-Loss formula with the Lipo Formula. These would bring your health, and hold the health substance. We would further suggest the use of 60 micrograms per day, twice per day, of B-12 be used by this. This could be taken orally.**

March 6, 1976: **You have other questions, ask.**

*"Yes, Aka, I have a request for health assistance from [6-281-1]. She asks, 'May I have a health reading, please, specifically dealing with the constant pain radiating down the left side of my back, with a weakness of both arms, and numbness in left leg.'"*

**Yes, we have before us the body, the soul, the spirit, and the immortal body of the same. And therefore, we have before us the body. First, we should explain into this subject, because of the extra matter substance in the spine, this is a problem within itself. Soul Ray could remove this. But his suggested therapy would be by far the wiser course.**

We shall first explain to you that the motivation, or the problem within the same, is that of what you would know as your flu, brought on further by your own anxieties. You have feared two things. First, we shall explain unto you, we have come here to harm no one. We have come to prepare the way for the coming of the Messiah. We have weeded the garden at times, as the need, or as a good farmer should tend his field, for the growth and maturity of all concerned. But we have said that nothing shall stand in the way of this work on either side. We did not mean this as a threat; we meant this as a statement of fact.

Your own anxieties have brought forth the greatest problem in the back region. Therefore, bio-therapy would be suggested in the treatment of the same.

We would further suggest that no radical course of action be taken. The healing that you have asked for shall be given. It shall be whole and complete. Each time in your life when this anxiety has risen, the problem has removed itself. Soul Ray has brought about the dissolution of the problem before. He may do so again.

We would suggest more rest. We would further suggest the use of the Wonderloss. We would further suggest, one moment.

Yes.

Accept in your own mind that that is here and the love that is given [is for] you. If you could accept these things — let the dead bury the dead; let the past be the past. Do not destroy that which is before you and which cares for you. We have placed flowers at your feet, not thorns. You came unto soul [1-1-1] unto wedlock. You knew of his work then, and you accepted it as such. But there is a time for all things. There is a time when a man and a woman should be as a man and a woman. We have given unto you this time. We shall continue to watch after and continue to place the healing and bring it forth. Fear our hands not, for they are placed with love.

March 6, 1976: **You have other questions, ask.**

*"Yes, Aka. [7-317-2] would like your suggestions for their medical future and any movements. Also, she ask, does she have any radical health problems requiring treatment?"*

We shall answer the last first. The only radical health problems at hand should be none more than soul Ray can treat adequately and take care of.

We say unto you, you have reached with truthful hands. We shall see unto thy needs.

But we should say unto you that you should prepare a way for [of] your own private practice. This could be done with the guidance of both your husband and that of soul Ray. You shall be much needed. You have been a healer beyond that of your medical knowledge for a long time. We shall say unto you, think thee of thy youth as a child. Your hands could heal then. Your hands can heal now.

You do not have to remove yourself from the orthodox healing to build a private practice in this community. We say unto you, the building blocks are now being handed into your hands. We shall say unto you, [with] that of the Euclid property substance, both land and a building could be constructed upon the same and a good clinic be established. This should be brought forth into your own mind. We shall implant that into soul Ray's mind that is needed to fulfill the knowledge, the substance of the same and the building needs of the same that you may bring forth in privacy and further planning may come into reality.

As we have said before, your physical needs shall be continually maintained by soul Ray and ourselves, for where he touches, we shall touch. But we have known for some time that his energy substance could not continue to sustain *all* of those who should need of healing. This is why we have brought you forth.

March 6, 1976: **We shall say unto [6-281-1], our plan has but budded. Fear not, for that in thy doubts shall be removed.**

April 3, 1976: **You have questions, ask.**
*"Yes, Aka. I have a request for a life reading for [5-213-1]. He asks specifically, 'To better understand my present reincarnation.'"*
We should say unto you, we have before us the body, the soul, and the spiritual [body] of the same; we have before us the immortal body. We shall say unto this one, you [should] ask us, "Why should I be placed in the position of a cripple?"

We say unto you, you made [of] the choice unto yourself, but not for karmic reasons. You made the choice that you might become part of the preparation for the coming of the Messiah. But only in this way would you have reached unto the one who could heal, who could [bring unto some] that [of] the light and sound that could heal the body. Only in this way could you understand that the body is like a perfectly tuned instrument. Out of balance it would play a sour tune. Therefore, [it would take] this ability, as such.

You have contemplated the love, and [become afraid]. We spoke unto you, we have brought unto you and shown unto you this love that we have given. Yet, it has taken a long time for you to reach forth to find the [true] meaning, yet there is more to come. When you have found the true meaning then you shall find that the affliction shall [be there] no more.

You are reaching. We say unto you, reach farther. Each day, say unto yourself, "That is [reaching distance]." But the same way, [the healing] will come.

We say unto you, this is not the way of all, but it is your way, and your choice, for this time, for this place, for this purpose. Look long unto the Eagle's eyes. [Editor's note: one microphone blew out.] **And there you shall find the pathway.**

April 29, 1976: **You have questions, ask.**
*"Yes, Aka, from [8-333-1], and he asks, 'Can you give me any information about the improvement of my breathing, and heart difficulties?'"*
**Yes, we see thy need, and we shall answer in this manner. We have before us the body, the soul, the spirit, and the immortal body of the same. Part of the improvement is due to that of your reaching for within yourself and bringing forth the spiritual self. The other part is due to that of the gift we have given unto soul Ray that he might give unto you. We shall further say unto this one, further improvement shall be given.**
**We shall ask that you give us, with the rest of your questions, all of the data.**

April 29, 1976: **You have other questions, ask.**
*"Yes, from [8-333-6], she asks, 'Will my liver be healed?'"*
**We have said, "Ask and you shall receive," and so it shall be. For all those who should ask for healing, let them do so, and let the deliverance of healing come forth. Glory be the name of the Lord. Glory be the name of His people.**
**Praise be given unto the name of the Lord. Praise be given unto the name of His people, for they are the people of the Earth.**
*[Arkan yahnah, seay, seay].*
**And healing shall come forth unto thee.**

April 29, 1976: **You have other questions, ask.**
*"Thank you, Aka. From [8-333-9], and he asks, 'How and when is it possible that I will stop stuttering and stammering once and for all?'"*
**We shall answer your question in this manner. Come forth unto soul Ray for bio-therapy treatment, and your problem shall end. And the knowledge that you gain shall help others.**

May 8, 1976: **You have further questions, ask.**
*"Yes, Aka. [7-317-1] asks, 'Should I sell the car that nearly killed me?'"*
**(Chuckle.) If thy had a horse that kicked you in the head and you should lose of an eye, should you wait until you lose the other?**

May 8, 1976: **You have other questions, ask.**
*"Yes, Aka. Soul Mark [3-115-2] asks, 'There are many interpretations, through many channels about where we are at this time in the series of prophecies of the book of Revelations. Please help us.'"*
**One moment, please. We should further answer unto soul [7-317-1]'s question.**

First, we should say unto you, you came to us in doubt. When we gave of you the three days, you saw them not. Yet, when other situations were asked for, the informations were given, and you did not come truthfully before those involved with you. As it would be said, you took them down the gate, and then let the trust they had placed in you fall aside.

You asked us for many things. Then you did come to soul Ray and ask again. We gave you but one small of a proportion of the proof that we may lay at your hand, of our being. We said unto you, if you should write, you should write in a righteous manner, and truthful. In your bargaining, if a word is given, the word must stand. It is sometimes necessary that a board may be applied at the backside of a mule that they may move. We have given you ample proof. Ask for more and we shall accommodate in the same manner.

June 5, 1976: **You have other questions, ask.**
*"Yes, Aka. [8-338-3] who is here tonight asks, 'What caused the swelling and itching and discoloration in my feet and legs? Two weeks later I broke out with big bumps; I still have them and it had been eight weeks ago.'"*
We should say unto thee, the condition was caused by the heart, and the circulatory system of the same. But we should also say that it is a condition brought forth from the contact of insecticide and defoliant substance. This affects the heart in such a manner that the body need to extract the poison — but it also affects the heart in such a manner that could be, and given in a prolonged basis, could become fatal. Therefore, we would suggest the use of biotherapy on a continued basis. We would also suggest that the returning back to the vitamin substance that was suggested, that the body may have a chance to rebuild itself. But healing shall come. Do not be afraid.

We also should say unto this one, thy have a diabetic condition, which has been told to you before. It would not be favorable, the use of either honey or any sweetening source, only that of the Tupelo honey should be used. We should further elaborate upon the use of honey as a food substance. It *does* contain many vitamin and mineral substances. It is a good source of three types of glucose — the Tupelo we speak of. Normal honey contains but one type of glucose, which should turn into a pure sugar form. This to your system is poison. Take not that into the system that could destroy it.

June 12, 1976 [in Philosophy]: **You have other questions, ask.**
*"Yes, Aka, Dr. [3-116-4] who is here tonight asks, 'How can I effectively treat cancer with present knowledge? Is cobalt therapy effective?'"*
**Cobalt therapy is not effective. The cobalt should bring forth the destruction of healthy cells that cannot be replenished in the system. It shall also bring about a total biochemistry change in the system, which**

will slowly destroy the system, the body. If you should treat it, treat it first as a preventative measure with the use of vitamin A.

If you should go into the removal of the first stages of different types of cancer, this should be answered at a different time, for the various stages of cancer in its related state comes in many form[s]. But we should say unto you, these come in the form of virus. Bring this question forth at a different time that we may *fully* answer this question.

July 9, 1976: **You have other questions, ask.**
*"Thank you, Aka. [8-341-2] who is here tonight, asks, 'I am going to have to visit my mother; I would like to know her reaction to my visit, and if it would be best to wait until I am 18 years of age.'"*

Yes, we shall answer your question in this manner. Because of the past karmic path of the mother, the reaction would not be favorable at this time. It would be by far better that this subject should wait until her 18th birthday.

We further see unto thy need and the questions that have lingered in thy mind. Both we and soul Ray did see into that of the one known as [6-285-1]. For much as Thomas, the doubter, the faith to see, to feel, to know — it was sadness that we gave unto such a message. Yet knowing of the direction unto which he would travel, it was necessary to give him the knowledge. Yet he shirked our words.

It is true, that we could have prevented some of his destructive nature. But as we have said before, we should allow nothing from either side to interfere with this work. We come but for one purpose, and that is the preparation for the coming of the Messiah, and the thousand years of peace upon the earth and the universe. We come to bring forth the promise of a new heaven and a new earth. We have come not to change the prophesies of Isaiah. We have come not to change the laws brought forth in the Ten Commandments by Moses. Nor have we come to change the coveth [covenant] brought forth by the one known as Jesus Christ. But we have come forth for this time, in a time of need and desperation of our Father's children, to bring them into the fulfillment of the awareness of themselves. [See *The Revelation* chapters 21-22.]

You have often asked unto yourself what talent you have. And we shall say unto you, you have many talents. One of such you have inherited from your father. You have inherited more from your father than you realize.

If a flower is in bloom you do not push it to blossom, to mature. It is a beautiful thing to watch these things come forth, and so it is within yourself. You have just began. You have much beauty that you are afraid to share. Throw away these fears. Bring them forth. Let others share in that that lays beneath, and it shall *all* become a beautiful thing.

You have many of the talents that your Aunt [2-19-2] had within her, yet they are yet to mature. We say unto you, she stands beside you, to guide you. You shall feel her gentle touch.

You have many other questions in your mind. All things shall be brought forth within time. Be patient. We shall fill thy idle hands soon, and fulfillment shall come within yourself.

We know of the feelings and the mixed feelings that lay dormant, yet alive within you. But it was not by chance that a way was prepared for you to come unto the Eagle's Nest.** We say unto you, pick up the *Rose without Thorns* and read it very carefully. You shall find much knowledge within for self-guidance.

July 9, 1976 [in Philosophy]: **You have other questions, ask.**

*"Yes, Aka. I have two questions that I feel are very important tonight. One of them is, we are running out of water at my home and want to tap a good source for present and future needs. Should we, one: continue drilling where we are, or deepen the big well, or dig at the northerly end of the dam, or deepen the shaft in the pasture, or is there a better solution?"*

**We should say unto thee, heighten the dam and deepen the big well. One shall supply the other.**

*"Thank you Aka. I have one other question: This is that our trial attorney in the herbicide case says that the other attorneys have used up all of the funds and there is nothing left to work with. Should we let him represent us in a malpractice action against them, or how can we best proceed to wind up the entire matter for final settlement; is there a better solution to this?"'*

**We would suggest that he should represent you for the return of the monetary value. What was done was both illegal and [yet] immoral. Yet it was not unexpected. Questions should be brought forth and answers should come forth in the same manner. We have said unto you, if you are struck upon the right cheek, turn the other; but if you are struck on the other cheek, then the mighty hand of God shall strike.**

**Too long has falsehood sought to bring fame unto those who should suffer misery. We should say unto thee, that "an eye for an eye, and a tooth for a tooth," and so it has been; they did seek forth their own karmic punishment.**

**We would suggest that a quick settlement be brought forth as soon as possible. A way shall be provided for all.**

**The first step should be that this should be turned over to the bar — state bar association — and should be brought forth by your attorney unto the bar association, that such criminal charges should be levied against the attorneys who acted in theft. A hearing, therefore, should first come forth before the state bar association, and then should be followed by such action as you should deem necessary. The monetary value should be returned.**

We say unto you, we have given you riches far beyond that of money. All of the others did have permanent inflictions [afflictions]. We gave unto you grandchildren of good health. We gave unto you children of good health. We gave unto you yourselves in good health. Your riches have been plentiful.

Their riches, even though they have been monetary, have not been plentiful, for they have carried an edge of sadness. We are sad, for we came to prepare that of the healing of the body substance unto all who would ask for it, but we cannot give it where it is not asked for. It is said, "Ask, and you shall receive; knock at the door and it shall open." Bid us enter, and we come with the glory of God.

September 3, 1976: **You have questions, ask.**
*"Yes. Aka. I have a request from* [7-32-1] *for* [8-345-1...Salem, Oregon]. *His mother asks, 'What is this person's purpose in life, and how can the mother help in that goal? What is the cause of bedwetting and how to stop it?'"*

Yes, we have before us the body, the soul, the spirit, and the immortal body of the same. First, we should answer in this manner. Before this question should be placed before us, permission should come from that of the child, so that an honest answer and the sincerity of the truth may be placed before him.

The problem of the bedwetting is both of the psychological and the physical of the same. We shall explain in this manner; if he should wet the bed he should get attention. We see a small bladder capacity, but this, in itself, should not be of the real reason. There are certain sectors or proportions of the brain which trigger certain muscles that say, you shall go to the bathroom, as you would say it, urinate, and when you shall urinate. These may be triggered in the sleeping state, but part of the awaking state is there also and present at the time. We would suggest that biotherapy be used as a corrective measure, both as a psychological means and that of a physical nature.

We would further say unto this one, thy wish to know unto where he has been so you may know where he is going. We have placed this in the first of this reading.

As far [as] an occupation is concerned, this one would serve well in that of an electrical engineering; this should be his strong point, for this is from which he came, and it would come natural as an occupation.

We would also suggest that further development of the psychic gift born within the child should be developed, and soon. But it should not be pampered. It should be brought forth in a true and just manner. Nor can it be forced. He must know the difference between make-believe and truth. But as he should practice, do not continue this subject on this at a prolonged time. Take a small proportion of each day in the development of this region. This also could be further developed with the use of biotherapy.

This is all on this subject at this time.

September 3, 1976: **You have other questions, ask.**
*"Yes, Aka, [6-284-4] who is here tonight asks, 'I would like to know the exact time I was born? I was born in....'"*
**9:52 a.m.**
*"Thank you, Aka."*

September 3, 1976: **You have questions, ask.**
*"Yes, Aka, I have a question from [7-316-1....Yuma, Arizona], and he asks, 'Please Aka, would you comment about my left lung?' He would like to know about his left lung."*
Yes, we have before us the body, the soul, the spirit, and the immortal body of the same. Yes, not only of the left lung, we see also emphysema of the right lung, also. We find traces of tuberculosis in the earlier ages, in a dormant state at the present time. We would suggest unto you, that come forth unto soul Ray that healing may be administered in such a manner for healing of the same. We find other physical imperfections in the body substance of the same.

That is all on this subject.

September 3, 1976: **You have other questions, ask.**
*"Yes, Aka, I have a request for a health reading from [4-123-1], who is here tonight. He'd like general health reading and his time of birth."*
Yes, we have before us the body, the soul, the spirit, and the immortal body of the same. Yes, we see thy need.

Yes.

First we should mention that of the imbalance in the antibodies within the body substance of the same. This is being readily corrected with the use of biotherapy and that of the herb substance of the same's. We also find that of — yes — of that that would be known as trace cancer, or that of a component's left over of pigment cancer in the area where the incision was made. We find error in surgery, therefore, of the nerve, several nerves, and the searing of the same. We find a separation of the tissue in the muscular substance in this arm. We also find, therefore, a degeneration of the bone marrow; this in itself may also be corrected with further biotherapy and that of psychic surgery done into this region.

Further work should be done in the pancreas region, and a balancing of the same, that a full release should come forth of that of the pesticide defoliant substance in the blood in the same.

We find other impurities in the system, one of which is that of arsenic poisoning. This has come about by the use of that of apricot, or that of the apricot pit, which contains dosages beyond human tolerance.

We shall answer your question in this manner. The seed was meant for planting. The pit was meant for maturing, to bring forth fruit for the body substance. There is many herbs and many roots and many particles of the same which were brought forth for the use of your medications and cures to your disease substance. If this substance was brought forth in its proper — and in a proper formulating substance — it would work, but not on all cancer substance and *not* on the form of cancer which you possess.

You have long feared that word. We say unto you, cast it out of your vocabulary. We shall assist in the healing of the same. We see no cancer in its active form at this time. We see further surgery that will be needed.

We also find that this of the Laetrile substance is also affecting that of the eyesight and certain parts of the brain substance in itself causing deeper and deeper proportions of depression and depression state.

This is all on this subject at this time.

September 3, 1976: **You have other questions.**
*"Yes, Aka, one moment. I have a question from* [7-321-1]. *She says, 'I have trouble with my right leg from the hip down. The sole of my right foot is very painful.' She asks for help."*
Yes, we see thy need. The help that you have asked for has been given. Blessed be the name of the Lord.

September 24, 1976: **There is one here who has asked for healing, not for herself, but for others. We shall give of the healing that is asked. But we say unto you, bring of this unto soul Ray in an awakening state that those things that are needed in the healing process may be given also.**

October 1, 1976: **You have other questions, ask.**
*"Thank you, Aka.* [8-349-1…Reno, Nevada] *asks how to cure the thin walls of her capillaries that seem to be hemorrhaging in various parts of her body? Medical science says it's hereditary and incurable."*
Yes. We would say unto these words, taking three substances that are specially designed in the Lipo-Flavonoid form, bringing the dosage of the same into four times the normal dosage, this in itself could restore the blood vessels, and therefore, allow them to become the main carriers, and also restore the capillaries which are coming to the surface and bursting. Come forth — we say unto thee — that these things may come about. We should say unto thee, when this substance is brought forth, take that of

the *Yucca bacatta*, and add to of the same. Add therefore, this substance, and the results you desire, shall come forth in the manner you desire.

October 1, 1976: **You have questions, ask.**
*"Yes, Aka, I have a question from [8-50-1] who is here tonight. He says, 'For about a year I have been having severe neck, upper spine, and shoulder pain. It has now worsened to glandular swelling on both sides of the neck, and I have been having migraines lately. What is causing the difficulties, and what might be done to correct the situation?'"*

**Yes, we have before us the body, the soul, the spirit, and the immortal body of the same.**

**Yes, we would suggest the biotherapy be used, for there could be a completeness. But we would also suggest that look into the front part of the reading and the fulfillment shall come forth.** [Editor's note: See the Parable of the Merchant Who Met the Healer.]

**We would also suggest that within soul Ray's mind, the combining of certain compounds with the new substance you call *Yucca bacatta* extract, this in itself would bring forth a deadening and a killing of the virus substance in thy body. First, you have had an arthritic disorder. This was compounded with a man-made virus, which is now being used or called Swine Flu. It has many sides. Within soul Ray's mind, in the combination of the herb substance and the use of the Liquid C Cough Syrup shall be the answer, also the use of the "surgery" which is being performed and has not yet been complete.**

**But listen unto what we should say. When the horse is brought, at the merchant's auction, you do not buy it by the piece, you buy the whole horse. The same thing should apply for the use and the ability of the healer that you seek out. You have asked for healing. This has been the first step. The healing you have asked for shall be given in full.**

**By kindling the spark within yourself, now you shall reach outward and inward. We would also suggest, in your own habit form, upon awakening in the morning, eat protein as soon as you arise. You have that of hypoglycemia; therefore, eating of protein as soon as you awaken, do this before you drink the coffee, or any smoking. Balance your diet in such a manner that the protein substance should be the predominant factor in your diet. In such, you shall find that this in itself, the worst part of the migraines shall disappear.**

October 1, 1976: **You have other questions, ask.**
*"Yes, Aka, I have a request for a health reading from [8-30-2...Litchfield Park, Arizona]. She says 'Aka, would you please give me my exact birth date and also a health reading?'"*

**(Pause.) The information which is given is incomplete. Data does not compute.**

October 15, 1976: **You have questions, ask.**

*"Yes, Aka. I have a question for* [8-350-2...Sun City]. *And she asks, 'Could you please give me my exact birth date?' And also she requests a health reading."*

Yes, we see thy need. **The birth time was 8:46 — or at the time the date would be, in the Year of the Cow, in the Century of the Dragon, in the Day of the Horse, in the Hour of the Moon, in the Second of Scorpio.**

**You ask for a health reading. First we would say unto this one, that of the hardening of the arteries is the predominant factor, which is causing the loss of both the hearing and the eyesight. The lack of vitamin substance in the system is also causing the aging process to be excelled. The intake of pollution substance has caused scar tissue of both lungs, and slight asthmatic condition. We find that of a yeast infection, or staph infection, the vaginal region. We find very poor circulation, impairment of the respiratory parts of the organism. We find that of the growth of fatty tissue in both the left hip and right breast. These in themselves could cover further complications.**

**We would suggest the use of the sage tea in substance. We would further suggest, because of the arthritic condition within the substance, the use of that of the** *Yucca bacatta* **in the right use which has been brought forth under our direction. We would further suggest the use of other vitamin substances; these substances [in] exact substances could be brought forth from soul Ray in the awakening state.**

**This is all on this subject at this time. One moment.**

**Yes.**

**We further find a thyroid, on the left side, an over — a small growth tissue in this substance, not malignant.**

**You have other questions, ask.**

*"Yes, Aka.* [7-320-1] *—"*

**One moment. There is other information on this subject** [8-350-2] **of a confidential nature. We would suggest that this subject come forth unto soul Ray that this could be discussed.**

**Yes.**

**Now you may continue.**

*"All right."*

October 15, 1976: **You have other questions, ask.**

*"Yes, Aka.* [8-351-1...Icehouse Canyon] *asks, 'Will my husband find work on land so he can be home instead of at sea, and also will I lose all of the excess weight I have gained in the past seven years?'"*

**To the first question we shall answer in this manner, he shall find that that he seeks, but not in the abundance that he seeks for. In the second part of your question, follow the directions soul Ray has given unto you, and you shall receive that that you ask for.**

October 15, 1976: **You have other questions, ask.**

*"Yes, Aka. [6-290-5…Litchfield Park, Arizona] asks, 'I would appreciate any message the Father would have for me. Thank you.'"*

**First we should say unto thee, the healing thy seek shall come. Of a physical nature, we are facing two problems — one, that of approaching of menopause; the second, of that of a man-made virus which still hangs into thy body substance. We would suggest that soul Ray bring forth unto the Aloe Vera laxative form, and using of this in two-ounce substances in that, that the elimination system may be cleansed; the using of the Wonder Loss substance to stabilize the blood and losing of the weight; the use of the Vitamin C Cough [Syrup] substance, that as this be brought up, the body in its biochemical condition should be excelled into such a way that the destruction of the disease may be come about.**

**Third, we should answer unto thy question unto this manner. The Lord, God, looks upon thy need, for you have come in faith, as you have asked in faith. Fear not, for you are not forgotten. Blessed be the name of the Lord; blessed be the name of His children.**

November 5, 1976: **Now we should say unto the one known as Ruth [2-30-2], healing shall be given; have faith. Glory be the name of the Lord.**

November 5, 1976: **You have other questions, ask.**

*"Yes, Aka. I have a question from [8-352-2], and is here tonight. She asks, 'I have been advised by persons I trust and admire to give up my job and write professionally. I am not in great health and stress is causing me many problems. Is this the time to quit teaching and begin writing?'"*

**We would suggest the taking of the sick leave that is at hand, that the restoring of your health might come about. But a teacher you are, and a teacher you shall remain, whether through writing or standing before a class and teaching. At the present time, your health is the most important factor. We shall assist in the resurrection of the body substance and the healing of the same.**

**We say unto you, as Jesus said once before, "Destroy this body, and we shall rebuild it in three days." We say unto you, the body is the temple of God. Respect it in such a manner and it shall serve you well.**

# 1977 Health Readings

January 21, 1977: **You have other questions, ask.**

*"Thank you, Aka. Aka, I have a request for a health reading from [9-357-1...Phoenix]. She asks, 'Dear Aka, I would like to have a general health reading, and what suggestion you can make so that I can prevent any health problems. My concerns at this time are varicose veins, eyes, and ache in my right arm. Thank you.'"*

Yes, we see your need. We have before us the body, the soul, the spirit, and the immortal body of the same. Most of your problems have already been taken care of by soul Ray. That that you call varicose veins are not of that of such. This condition is caused by hardening of the arteries, which will not allow the blood flow to return back unto the usual manner. The suggestions that have been given to you at this time are now beginning to work.

The condition of the heart has been corrected.

The suggestion of the elevation of the feet while you sleep has greatly [enhanced] your condition. Further therapy in this line should be continued. The therapy has been good.

We would further suggest that within a short period of time, a full scan of the system be done in the laboratory here in Globe. This would ease your mind, and at the same time would help soul Ray in determining farther therapy.

This is all on this subject at this time.

February 25, 1977: **You have other questions, ask.**

*"Yes, Aka. Thank you. [ 9-360-1] asks for assistance for her son, [9-360-2]. She asks, 'I wonder if Aka can help my son with the problem he has had with his breathing? If it is allergies, please specify, so that we can try to control it. I am asking this for my son who is age three years.'"*

Yes, we see thy need. That that you ask for shall be given. Bring the child back unto soul Ray. The knowledge that is needed we will implant there. And the cure shall come, and the healing shall come, as you have asked.

February 25, 1977: **You have other questions.**

*"Yes, Aka. [9-360-4] asks, 'I want to know if my husband has a heart problem and is for his reason for drinking so much.'"*

This we cannot answer. We cannot interfere with the free will of another soul.

February 25, 1977: **You have other questions, ask.**
*"Yes Aka. Thank you. [9-360-6…Las Cruces, New Mexico] asks, 'How can I overcome my almost obsessive fear of interacting with people and lack of self-confidence? Can I get rid of these hang-ups once and for all, and be free to love my life to the fullest and be productive?'"*

Yes, we say unto you, go on into the biotherapy. These things shall come one step at a time. The love of life can be only enjoyed in its fullest by knowing that one day on this earth you can learn more than you can in a hundred years on the other side because you experience life. There you observe life.

Yet death is nothing to fear. It is that which man chose, and of his own free choice. It was only through death and rebirth could he grow back to his Father's mansions.

Those things that you ask for are already at your fingertips.

September 21, 1977: **Now you have many questions, ask.**
*"Yes, Aka, from [_____ …Phoenix], and she says, 'I am very mixed-up about a relationship. I don't know which direction to run. I don't even know why. Could you help me make the right move in the right direction, because there is a lot of strain right now?'"*

Yes, we have before us the body, the soul, the spirit, and the immortal body of the same, and we see thy need. We say unto you, have faith. Do not lose the faith, and the guidance you seek shall be given. And wedding bells shall ring. We have placed these in words in a manner that only you shall understand. Continue to come forth unto soul Ray that he may give you full spiritual and mental therapy, and the physical of the same. There is nothing to fear but fear itself. You have laid your hands and your faith in God. Fear not. For we do not sleep; we are with you all of the time.

September 21, 1977: **You have other questions, ask.**
*"Thank you, Aka. From [L_____ G____'s son…in Miami]: 'I am thinking of purchasing land. Where would be a good place for me? Will children come in the next five years? Is happiness eternal?'"*

(Chuckle) Yes, we have before us the body, the spirit, and the immortal body of the same. Happiness is that which you make. Without tears, how would you know when you were happy? Life has come unto you as the seasons come unto the earth. Yet the Lord, God, made man that it took less work for him to laugh that for him to cry. Yet crying is a necessary release of emotions, and a healthy one. Anger, rightly directed, is a healthy release of emotion. But the happiness that you seek, the eternal happiness that you seek, shall come within your love for man and your love for God. But it must come in a truthful manner, from the heart and the soul and the spiritual substance, therefore, within the same.

You speak of purchasing land. The Globe area would be a wise purchase at this time, for it shall multiply in its financial value in a three-year period.

But you have a greater question within your mind. And we shall answer it in a manner that shall be private unto yourself. If you deny yourself, then you have denied God. When you stand before God and say, "I take this to be my love," God hears you. But if you really love this other person, say it where man can hear you. Do not be ashamed of it.

September 30, 1977: **We shall say unto you, because soul Ray is very tired, our time is very short. Therefore, we shall not give unto life readings this night, but you have other questions, ask.**

*"Thank you Aka. We have a request for an emergency health reading from [10-372-1...Tucson, Arizona]. He is very weak and is not improving."*

**This data does not compute.**

*"The name is spelled [N_____...]"*

Yes, we have before us the body, the soul, the spirit, and the immortal body of the same. We say unto you these words. Healing shall be given.

November 25, 1977: **And we shall say unto soul Ray these words. The house that you were called to was the house of your grandmother, the soul of your grandmother. Upon the death of your grandmother you gave forth her name unto a child, but they are not one of the same.**

The houses that you sought protection in were those among you who you have looked for and counted on to protect you against the evil ones. Yet, in your heart you have never thoroughly counted on anyone, for your desire, to do it yourself, as you would say. Since you were hurt, this has become an obsession with you, to prove to the world that you could stand as a man, even though your body was left in a limited condition. We have done that to restore as much of your body as possible, but we are not God; we cannot create. God has placed His hand upon you, and He has brought His disciples of the Old and of the New unto you, to show you that the fields you would harvest from shall come from many places. [Editor's note: Testaments?]

We say, fear not, but use your own discretion in self-preservation, for you have turn both cheeks.

November 25, 1977: **You have other questions, ask.**

*"Yes, Aka. You have spoken about soul Ray's [1-1-1]'s dream. Is there anything in my dream that would amplify it, or is it some other subject?"*

**Both are one of the same.**

*"Thank you, Aka."*

November 25, 1977: *"We have a health-reading request from [9-373-1…Idaho]. His first question is, "What was the cause of my recent stomach and intestinal problem?"*

We should answer the question in this manner. We have before us the body, the soul, the spirit, and the immortal body of the same. We find, therefore, the upper hyatic [hiatal?] hernia, a twist of the intestine of the lower colon, ulcer in the large intestine two inches from the mouth of the stomach. Most of the cause of your problem is that of an emotional problem, and it shall continue — and the fact of not eating properly. This is all on this subject.

*"He has further questions. Do you wish to take those questions at this time?"*

Yes.

*"He asks, 'Is there any damage from my smoking?'"*

Yes.

*"He asks, 'What is the cause of my bursitis and what to do for it?'"*

We suggest thy consult soul Ray, and therefore, follow his suggestions.

*"He asks, 'What are the two small red spots on my right leg?'"*

(Chuckle) Lack of circulation.

*"Thank you, Aka."*

November 25, 1977 [Also in Philosophy document]: You have other questions, ask.

*"Yes, Aka, we have a question from [9-373-4]. She asks, 'In the July 1976 issue of* Rays of Philosophy *in a question asked of you regarding cancer and the cure, you asked that the question be repeated at a later date. The question was, "How can I effectively treat cancer with present knowledge." Is this a time you can fully answer this question, and will you?'"*

Yes, we will answer this question. Now that soul Ray has brought forth the yucca extract, cancer can be fully treated. He should further go on with the research and the development of the new extract that he has in mind. This new extract would work more rapidly, and work upon all phases of the cancer virus. This includes leukemia.

It would also be advisable that the new extract he has in mind should be used as a preventative toward cancer. And with the further development of the new protein supplement he has in mind, cancer could be a forgotten disease. For as we have said before that arthritis, cancer, diabetes, and the most predominant disease of your nation, that which you would call of low blood sugar, could also be treated and cured. Heart, different heart diseases could be treated. Diseases of both the respiratory and the circulatory system could be treated now with great success.

November 25, 1977: **You have other questions, ask.**

*"Will this new formula be suitable for the treatment of* [9-373-4] *'s cancer?"*

**Yes.**

*"Thank you, Aka."*

# 1978 Health Readings

January 20, 1978: **You have many questions, ask.**
*"Yes, Aka, [2-30-2] asks for your assistance in healing."*
**We see thy need, and healing shall be given.**

January 20, 1978: *"I have a question, Aka, from [10-374-1...El Paso, Texas]. She says, 'I am having a struggle with a relationship. In four months my friend leaves for Korea for a year, and there is a lot of strain now because of what has happened to each of us in past marriage. I am confused and scared, as I don't want the relationship to end.'"*

**We shall answer in this manner. If you were riding a horse across the desert and you came to an oasis, and the horse desired to stay in the oasis, and there was another horse there that you could go on your journey on, it would be advisable to get on the other horse and ride on.**

**But fear breeds more fear. And jealousy can become as a monster to evil and devour and consume. We say unto you, place your hope and faith in God. And do not bear false witness, either in yourself or in the other.**

**Take forth these things we have said unto you unto the other, and let a choice be made. But do so in such a manner that regardless of the decision reached, that you shall walk forth in such a manner that love may be carried on in your life, for love is the greatest gift God has given man — and laughter, and joy. But remember, love may enter as a winter storm, fierce and cold and deadly. But remember, there is also the spring.**

March 17, 1978: **You have other words, ask.**
*"Yes, Aka, I have a question from [10-378-2...Albuquerque, New Mexico]. She asks, 'What is the cause of the recurring dull pain in and over the left eye, and how am I to prevent it? Also can you give me my exact hour of birth?'"*

**The exact hour of birth was 2:64 — correction, the exact hour of birth, your time, would be 3:04 a.m.**

**The recurring of pain, as you would call it, we would say is caused from an asthmatic condition.**

April 21, 1978: **You have questions, ask.**
*"Yes, Aka. I have a question for some health assistance for [6-23-72-001...Oakland, California]. And what he's asking is, he normally is very*

*energetic, but for the last little while, he has been coming home and falling asleep at 6 p.m. and sleeping until 7 a.m. the next morning, and no one can wake him. He wants to know what is causing his loss of energy and this problem?"*

Yes, we see your need, and we shall answer unto your need, your question in this manner. The loss of energy is a cellular problem in the blood within the same. We would suggest that you should seek out the counsel of soul Ray and he shall advise you in full detail of that and the answer unto which you need. But healing shall be given unto your body, and soul, and the spirit of the same. And healing shall come into thy as a light.

June 23, 1978: *"Aka,* [8-326-9…Tucson, Arizona] *asks, 'Please give me some advice, because ultraviolet rays have made so many sunspots on my face. If these are keratoses, they will change into skin cancers. Also I do have a hidden cancer started elsewhere. I never stop thanking you for sending my husband's message to me on July 5, 1976.'"*

We shall say unto you these questions. Soul Ray did bring you the answer in his last visit, but we should also say unto you that further work should be done in this area. Upon soul Ray's mind now should come forth the answer for your cure of cancers. Come unto him and speak, for the answer is near at hand in his research.

June 30, 1978: We know that each of you here have come with questions in your minds. We have answered most of these. If each of you will look carefully in the parable we have given you shall find an answer to your questions.

That that you shall receive is the last into which you have asked, and that is the healing. You have entered at the Eagle's nest, and therefore, that which you ask for shall flow as an endless well — for remember, soul Ray is I and I am soul Ray. Once again we have given you a riddle.

Now is the time of the Cherubim.

July 28, 1978: You have other questions, ask.
*"Thank you, Aka.* [6-284-4] *asks, 'I would like to know if there are any problems physically with my husband and I at this time that is preventing me from conceiving our second child?'"*

We should answer your question in this manner; that of your complete physical histories is within soul Ray's mind. Once again, if conceivement of the same should come forth, it would be suggested that both you and he should come forth unto soul Ray that he may prepare the way for this one who should arrive.

July 28, 1978: You have other questions.

*"Yes, Aka. [9-373-4…Washington] asks, (1): 'Please advise Ray Elkins of something that will regenerate new hair on the heads of mankind.' That's her question."*

**(Chuckle.) This has already been done.**

August 25, 1978 [in Philosophy]: *"[10-387-3…Huntington Beach, California] says, 'Aka, will you please give me a health reading and any advice you can give me on marijuana smoking pertaining to me.'"'*

**First, we should answer your question in this manner. That that is done in moderation would not hurt thy body. That that is done in above moderation shall damage the brain, the circulatory system, the spleen, the heart, the liver, the kidneys, the respiratory system.**

**The health reading you wish we shall give at a different time.**
*"Thank you, Aka."*
**One moment, please.**
**Yes. Yes.**
**We should also say unto these words. As it has been said before, a little wine is good for the stomach, a lot should damage the whole body. We should say unto you on the marijuana subject, that each time you bring forth unto your body this substance, it is not just man's law you have broken, but God's, who says, "THY SHALL BRING NOTHING INTO THY BODY THAT SHOULD BE HARMFUL UNTO IT."**

**But you should also take into consideration the vultures that you are feeding by buying this substance at this time, the vultures which leech upon mankind. The time shall come when this of the marijuana shall be legalized. There shall always be those who shall abuse the use of this and pay for it, not only themselves, but their families; their children, their mothers, their fathers, their brothers, their sisters, and their friends shall pay the highest price.**

**At this time we shall say unto you, there are many who should use this money to farther build your Communist empires, where they are not allowed the worship of God. In this manner you shall feed the hand of the Anti-Christ.**

August 25, 1978: **You have other questions, ask.**
*"She asks, 'I have terrible tumors or cyst-like lesions all over my face that are painful and ugly. Why do I have these?'"*
**We would say, one, a disease of the lymphatic system, two, as the lymphatic system feeds into the circulatory system, both must be corrected that this could be ended. We would say unto you, come unto soul Ray and he shall give you the necessary information to end this, both karmas.**

September 8, 1978: **We shall bring the light and we shall bring healing into the one known as [6-274-2].**

September 8, 1978: **You have questions, ask.**

*"Yes, Aka. [6-281-1] asks, 'My husband insists on having the house sporadically sprayed with Chlordane.' She says that this is causing her a great deal of illness, and she doesn't know what to do unless she moves out of the house because it makes her so ill, and she doesn't want to do that; she's asking for help. And, what can you suggest?"*

**We shall place in the mind of soul Ray a form, to build a pesticide that shall control these things. It shall be of a natural source that shall not be harmful to the human body. Worry not, it shall be no more.**

September 8, 1978: **You have other questions, ask.**

*"Yes, Aka, would you tell me if the course I am pursuing in making my foot well is adequate, or if there is something I should do?"*

**We should do that that is needed to bring this about. Soul Ray brought unto your mind the sign of the pentacle that no longer could you be attacked. For all that once placed and walked through the sign of the pentacle, no harm may come to them, yet all evil that should enter should never leave. We shall implant in his mind a new method of doing this that should not — that shall be done at the four corners of your property, that none may pass through from this day forth.**

**One moment.**

**Yes.**

**It shall be done.**

**Soul Ray must make the signs, and it shall be complete. Each of you in turn shall make the signs, and it shall be complete. Blessed be the name of the Lord.**

September 8, 1978 [in Philosophy]: **You have other questions, ask.**

*"Yes, Aka. [7-317-1] asks, 'Do you have any advice for me? Thank you.'"*

**As we have said before, you have looked for the buildings and the places of knowledge, yet we told you they were beneath your feet. We say so now. Soul Ray did show unto you that of the processing of the prickly pear, that the fruit, a pure fruit, uncontaminated, could be brought to the Earth. A way must be prepared for this.**

**And now we shall also tell unto all of you, that by the drinking of this fruit you shall have a cleansing of the body, of the kidneys, [of] the liver, and the removal of poisons, therefore, within your system. We shall give further information at another time.**

**We will also say unto you, come unto soul Ray for consultation.**

November 3, 1978: **You have other questions, ask.**

*"Thank you, Aka...One moment, Aka...Do you have any advice on the health of [10-287-3], Aka?"*

We do not have of this information. We do not find the request by himself. The request was made by his mother and grandmother.

*"Thank you, Aka."*

November 10, 1978 [in Philosophy]: **You have other questions, ask.**

*"Thank you, Aka. I have a question from* [10-380-2…El Paso, Texas]. *He asks, 'Will you advise me how to get out of my emotional and financial troubles as soon as possible?'"*

**Yes, we shall advise you, in this manner. Look at your needs and not your wants. We have given back unto you the life that you desired, and yet you ask for more. Soul Ray has placed into your hands the necessary means to help you financially, and it shall soon come into fulfillment.**

**It is good to ask and good to receive. But if God sent you into the desert and gave you water and food and you left it behind, would you stand in the desert and blame God because He did not give you another, and another, and another? Would you do the same with your children? Do you want God to become your crutch? "The Lord is our shepherd, thy shall not want." He has said nothing about being your crutch.**

**It is not important what a man has done, it is what he *shall* do.**

November 10, 1978: **You have other questions, ask.**

*"Yes, Aka,* [10-391-3…New Mexico] *asks, 'How can I best overcome nervousness?'"*

**The data is incomplete. One moment, please.**

**Yes, yes.**

**We would answer your question in this manner. One moment.**

**It is still incomplete. Give — the birth date is not correct. Request further data on this subject, and information then may be given.**

*"Thank you, Aka."*

December 1, 1978: **You have questions, ask.**

*"Yes, Aka. I have a question for* [10-392-1…Quartzsite, Arizona]. *The question is, 'Is there another course of treatment for my condition other than the one that has been prescribed by the doctors under whose care I am now? I have either a neurological or muscular disorder of a chronic wasting nature and now weigh 65 lb. I am 5'5" tall. I also have some kind of bugs in my urine that are visible to the naked eye. Please help me.'"*

**Yes, we see thy need.**

**And we shall say unto you, the Lord is with you. Glory be the name of the Lord.**

December 29, 1978: **You have other questions, ask.**

*"Thank you. Aka.* [10-391-3…New Mexico] *asks, 'I have been highly nervous most of my life, and would like to know how to overcome this state.'"*

With the use of bio-therapy. Come unto soul Ray, and these things that you ask for shall be brought into completeness.

# 1979 Health Readings

March 9, 1979: **You have other questions, ask.**

*"Thank you, Aka. I have a request from* [11-398-2…Tennessee], *and he asks, 'Sir, the distance is great for me to travel and reach soul Ray; is it permissible for you to use distant healing to heal my eyes, please?'"*

**Yes, we see thy need. We shall give you that which you wish. And healing of the body, the soul, the spirit, and the immortal body shall come forth. But we say unto you, go into meditation, and distance shall not be a barrier, but we shall give you the sight to reach this land, if you wish.**

March 16, 1979: **You have questions, ask.**

*"Yes, Aka. I have a question from* [6-274-3…who is here tonight], *and she asks, 'All things considered, physiologically and physically, can I wisely have this predicted child now? Please explain in detail the ramifications pro and con.'"*

**At a different time the child could have been born unto you and your husband in a graceful manner. Now it [would] be much more difficult, both psychological and physical. But the choice is yours to make. In the next three-year period, the life as you know it, financial, shall greatly change. It shall become a necessity that small communities come forth and bind together. This will change your way of living up to this point. It shall change the child you have now, and this one that you shall ask for. Times shall almost reverse themselves.**

June 22, 1979: **You have many questions, ask.**

*"Yes, Aka.* [ 6-281-1] *asks, 'Is there anything else I can do to help my daughter?'"*

**Yes, we see thy need. We have answered that question in the first of this reading. We shall explain further. In truly loving her, turn her loose. She shall fall many times before she shall rise. Let her get up by herself. But you shall not continue to not love her, but love her enough to know she shall go her own way at the expense of you or anyone else, for she loves with the right hand and destroys with the left. But yet, within time, this shall mould away. But do not be surprised or angry at the decisions that she is making now. They are her own. You have placed *all* that you can. But you must remember, she is also her father's daughter.**

June 22, 1979: **You have other questions, ask.**

*"Thank you, Aka. I ask for healing for* [3-115-2] *in Scottsdale Memorial Hospital."*

We say these words unto you, as we said in the beginning of the reading[s], if they should ask — that we may not violate their right, their freedom of choice — therefore, we may enter. But in this case, they have closed the door unto us. But love them, for it is their choice. We promise you unto this much unto these things, that she shall not have pain. This much we may intervene to do. Yet, there is still hope, should they come unto soul Ray.

June 22, 1979: **You have other questions, ask.**
*"Yes, Aka. I have a request for healing for* [6-290-3...in Union City, California]*; his eyes have been injured."*
**Yes, we see thy need, and healing shall be given.**

July 20, 1979: **You have questions, ask.**
*"Yes, Aka. I have a request for health assistance for* [11-404-1...New York]*, and she says she has had two unsuccessful stapedectomies in the ears and she has been encouraged to go have another one in Pennsylvania, and she is wondering if this would be successful, or how can she save her hearing?"*
**Yes, we see thy need, and we shall answer in this manner. Without the necessary circulatory system first being repaired, the operation you speak of would not be successful. We should answer in this manner. We have placed great knowledge into that you would know of soul Ray's mind, and we work through him in his healing efforts, and as we say, we, from whatever need of the information at the time, we place. Come unto soul Ray and let him give unto you that that is needed. We shall provide the healing if you shall provide the faith.**

August 3, 1979: **Thy have other questions, ask.**
*"Thank you, Aka.* [11-405-3...Roswell, New Mexico] *asks, 'Will the pain I am now having leave soon?'"*
**Yes. Yes, this shall be done. We shall also answer your question in this manner. If thy climbed to the top of the mountain and stood there, and thy food bearer did bring thee food and laid it upon the mountain, and thy walked back down partway of the mountain, and they left that upon the mountain that had been given, who should be blamed, the food bearer or yourself? If you should desire that which you seek, take the gifts that are given, one at a time, and carry them with you. If you want a total release of the pain that you speak of, soul Ray shall give it. But to totally release it, go unto ten people and speak, therefore, of the wisdom that you might have gained here, and tell each ten that they shall approach ten, and unto each of these ten perform one deed of good**

standing, and so it shall grow, and they shall be relieved of their pains also.

September 19, 1979: **Thy have other questions, ask.**
*"Thank you. 'What will clear up the ringing in my ears?'"* [11-406-4].

We shall answer in this manner. The ringing of the ears is caused by damage to the nerve. The damage was caused by lack of circulation in the inner ear. If you wish to cure yourself, we would suggest that the following formula be used, in connection with proportions therefore of in this manner, that that should have been created into the Alpearon, two tablespoons twice daily, and that of the niacinamide, at first 500 mg. and then in three weeks' time increasing therefore into 1500 mg., and then therefore increasing into 2000 mg., and three tablespoons of the Alpearon, taking in this manner. But there is more....[Editor's note: Inaudible.]

September 19, 1979: *"Thank you, Aka. 'Why have I been unsuccessful in carrying the child? Will I be successful in delivering a healthy, living child in the future? Please give me advice on this and proper obstetrician.'"* [6-274-3].

We see thy need. We shall answer in this manner. All that is to be done that you may carry a child has been done. We would suggest coming unto soul Ray for private consultation, but we advise you in this manner: Time is a fleeting thing. It is like a river that you would say, "It looks like it is the same river," but it is always changing, every second of every moment.

We say unto thee of these words, that which was important before, [inaudible] a child, has already been given unto another....[Inaudible.] Now we shall say unto thee, come forth, therefore, as a godfather unto this child, and put thy efforts in teaching this knowledge and the fulfillment of the same.

And you say unto us, "Where is this child?" And we shall say unto you, the child was born at the same moment as the fleeting of the child in thy womb. And it was born at what is known as The Top of the World near Globe, Arizona. And the child's name shall be as the rays, or the king, and the meaning shall be of the same. And the last name shall be known as keep this child and its parents, and your fulfillment shall come unto fulfillment, and therefore, as Jude did come and teach unto Jesus at a time, so you shall teach unto this child.

September 19, 1979: **You have other questions, ask.**
*"We have, Aka. 'Will my cardiac condition improve? Should we invest our time in our new business? Will it be a success?' There is no name to this."*

Cardiac condition shall improve.

We would say unto you, come unto soul Ray on this subject, on both subjects, that that that thy wish to know should be said in private. The answer we would answer in the form of a riddle, but we do not feel that you would understand this riddle.

September 19, 1979: **You have other questions, ask.**
*"We have, Aka.* [11-397-2]. *'Should I move to Tempe, or nearer, and will I be cured?'"*

The cure thy seek shall come forth, and the move thy seek shall come forth. We say unto you, that which we said just before shall go unto all of you, and each of you shall take of it in your own way.

September 28, 1979: **You have other questions, ask.**
*"Yes, Aka.* [11-407-2...El Paso] *asks for help in regard to circulation, headache, blood pressure, and dizziness."*

Yes, we see thy need, and the help you need lays before your feet. As we have said before, that those who seek healing, a way shall be laid before them.

October 12, 1979 [in Philosophy]: **You have other questions, ask.**
*"Yes, Aka. I have a question from* [11-408-2...Ingram, Texas]. *It says, 'For many years I have been trying to be a vegetarian. Is man supposed to kill animals and eat their flesh, or will he ultimately become a vegetarian? Shall I pursue vegetarian diet or not?'"*

We shall say unto thee, the words of thy own Bible, "Into the fifth generation." If thy mother and thy father are carnivorous, and their grandfather and their grandmother were carnivorous, you may change your diet, but it shall take time for your body's metabolism. And one of the greatest sources of strength unto the same is of protein, and the source that it has adjusted itself to extracting the same from. When drastic diet changes are made, it can be harmful to thy health. This is why we have suggested that a slow, gradual adjustment be made.

At the present time, your body has *not* adjusted to this. The wanton killing of animal — nay, this is not good. For it has been said that the Lord, God, did place in man's dominion the fowl of the air, the fish of the sea, and those animal[s] that are [of adjust] placed forth and placed under his dominion, and for his use. You shall find that a balance of the earth at the present time into all life form is made in this manner, whether it be the lion or man.

In some places upon your Earth, man, generation from generation, has eaten nothing but that of the vegetarian diet. If you've tried to place before them that that you would know as meat, of any kind, it could be very destructive to the system. The same thing applies to a bi-carnivorous man. This can also be. But the bi-carnivorous man can adjust more easily to the vegetarian diet than the vegetarian can adjust to the carnivorous.

We see that you do not fully understand, and we shall answer in this manner. The chromosome structure, in other words, the life pattern set forth at birth, should serve man throughout his life. If it should be bent, it should be bent very slowly.

November 9, 1979: *"Thank you, Aka. I have a question from* [11-409-1...El Paso, Texas]. *He'd asked that, 'Am I going to get rid of my pains?'"*
Yes. The healing that is asked for shall be given.

# 1980 Health Readings

January 4, 1980: **And we shall say unto [1-1-5] and [1-1-3], glory be the name of the Lord. And glory be those who have faith in the Lord, our God. But we say unto you, we shall give healing where it is needed, as you have asked, and it has been asked. But smile.**

January 4, 1980: **You have other questions, ask.**
*"Thank you, Aka. [12-413-3…El Paso] asks, 'Will I regain my full health, my heart problem; will it be healed?'"*
**Yes. The healing you have sought shall be given.**

January 4, 1980: **You have other questions, ask.**
*"Aka, [12-412-4…Whitewater, California] asks, 'In Jesus' name, I pray you for good health, to be able to be useful and helpful as long as I live. I would like also to know what planet I am originally from. Thank you.'"*
**Earth. The mother of all planets.**
January 4, 1980 [in Philosophy]: **Yes, we see thy need, and we shall answer in this manner. All that God places before you He places for a time, to fill your need, to take you one step closer to your own, made destinies. There are those who think they have been cast down, when the truth is they've only been cast upward.**

January 11, 1980: **You have other questions, ask.**
*"Yes, Aka, thank you. I have a question from [12-413-2…Long Beach, California]. The question is, 'What can I expect in regard to my brother, W_____'s, disability?'"*
**We shall answer your question in this manner. We may answer questions that do not conflict with another's free will. Since you do not have the permission of your brother, we may not answer this question.**

January 11, 1980: **You have other questions, ask.**
*"Thank you. [12-412-3…Albuquerque] asks, 'What career or situation is within God's will for E_ and myself? Will E_ recover fully from his chest ailment?'"*
**We shall answer once again, we may only answer for yourself. And we shall say unto you unto this manner, that you shall follow the route of the artist. But there is much hard work before you.**

March 7, 1980: **You have a question, ask.**

*"Yes, Aka. I have a question that D\_\_\_\_\_ W\_\_\_\_\_ brought in from* [7-316-1]. *He asks, 'Dear Aka, what should I do to get this health problem solved? Do I need an angiography?'"*

**Yes, we see the need. And we should say unto thee, so that the physicians who are studying you might understand your case better, this might be needed at the present time. But we should say unto thee, we shall give unto thee that of the health that is needed, and then come unto soul Ray for further healing. That that is needed shall be furnished to you and to your physicians that this might come about.**

March 14, 1980: **You have questions, ask.**

*"Yes, Aka, I have a question from* [12-417-1]. *She asks, 'I need to make a decision regarding where I am to live. Should I remain in Tucson, or consider living in Globe? Also, what other methods should I consider that would be beneficial to my health? Advice will be appreciated.'"*

**We shall answer in this manner. The time shall come when your journey to Globe shall be a necessity, both for your moral and physical support.**

**But that of the pursuit of your health lies in these things that soul Ray has asked you to take. Taken in its proper proportion, the circulatory system may be restored. You were born with a heart murmur, or that of a small passageway in the heart itself. It has long healed over. It may be detected as a problem when it really is not.**

**We say unto you other things, and as we say them, take them as we give them to you, and in the manner we give them to you.**

**As long as you stand and worry where you are, then you shall be alone. Your faith, that you have been taught, tells you that life is the most precious commodity upon your Earth, that the body you contain is a temple of God, and therefore, the temple must be contained in its most perfect form. We should also suggest that soul Ray go into the bio-therapy farther with you, and that of hypnosis therapy, to stop that of the intake of the nicotine itself, which is harming the arteries and valves of the heart. It should be done, though, in such a way that the tapering off of the same should not affect the respiratory part of the system. The final choice in all of these things shall be yours.**

March 14, 1980: **You have other questions, ask.**

*"Yes, Aka,* [12-417-4...Deming, New Mexico] *asks, 'Will the operation that was performed on my son be successful?'"*

**Partially, yes. Help shall be given.**

March 28, 1980: **You have other questions, ask.**

*"Yes, Aka. I would like to ask for comfort for* [9-360-1] *on the death of her brother, and also ask our, give our prayers for his soul and spirit and his development. Do you have anything to say for her?"*

Yes, we see this. And we shall send those that are needed to help this soul across. And the next time when you see him, his return we shall make come forth as fast as possible, for he shall be needed on the Earth, stripped away of his profanity and brought forth into the lesson he shall learn. If this can be done, and he shall be receptive, then wait, and one day you shall see him again. At this time he sleeps in torment, and there are those who are about to awaken him. So fear not, for we see the love that you have sent him, and it shall be the weapon we shall use to awaken him with, for it is the only weapon that he will allow us to penetrate through with.

Glory be the name of the Lord; glory be the name of His children, forever and ever.

May 9, 1980: **You have other questions, ask.**

*"Yes, Aka.* [8-338-2] *also asks — she would like to have some help with the allergies that she has, knowing what she is allergic to? She says, 'Thank you, very much.'"*

Yes, we see thy need. And we shall answer you in this manner. The animals that you love the best are those that you are the most allergic to. So we would suggest that these things in this quantity be placed forth and taken in a daily basis — that of the local honey of your area, of the pollen of the same, and that of the vinegar made of the prickly pear, be put together in equal parts and taken as a tonic twice a day. This shall bring forth and allow for your allergies to adjust.

May 9, 1980: **You have other questions, ask.**

*"Yes, Aka, thank you. Do you have any words which might be of comfort to* [2-30-27]*? Thank you."*

Yes, we see thy need. And we should say unto thee, that that was in the beginning has been in the past and shall be in the future. All things that are to be prepared and laid before the table must be done in a loving manner. As the fields are left for the widows, so should love be given unto all mankind. Full fulfillment of these things you have asked for have come forth. And the healing of [2-30-3] shall be the same.

May 9, 1980: **You have other questions, ask.**

*"Yes, Aka, thank you. What is the source of the reoccurrence of herbicide contamination that seems to be affecting us? How should we deal with it?"*

We shall answer you in this manner, in the pollen — that that that should come from the root that should come into your plants and come forth at this time of year. We should suggest that that of the

Alpearon be used. And we would suggest that that of the sage tea be used, and that of the prickly pear be used. And it should come forth, and tea should be placed, taking 1/4 of the water of the Dripping Springs, to 1/4 of the prickly pear; therefore, the Yerba Santa be placed and the sage be placed in the same to make a tea. And the honey of the local area be used. That, with what you would call, for the male, which you have named the M.E. 10, and for the female, that you call, the Femina 6, or the — yes — with the new formulas that have come into completeness, with the necessary vitamins placed forth into them, these also should be used.

June 7, 1980: **You have other questions, ask.**
*"Thank you, Aka. [10-381-2] asks for her daughter [12-423-2…Albuquerque, New Mexico], 'The doctors have wanted to do tests on [12-423-2]. She is small, and they consider her weight and height curve abnormal. Is there a reason to be concerned? She has a small appetite, recently increasing. She has had diarrhea almost constantly for a month; what is the cause? And what can I do to promote a natural, normal healthy body?'"*

We see thy need, and we shall answer in this manner. First, the size of the child is perfectly normal. Who is to say whether a child is to be six-foot tall or five-foot tall? These things could be altered and changed quite simply by stimulating the pineal gland. But don't you think that it should be the free choice of the child? The diarrhea comes from that that you feed the child. We would suggest that warm goat's milk be used in sequence with its regular formula. And you will soon see that the problem shall end. Part of the problem is that that you would know of as a virus, which is passing. The healing that is needed shall be given. For remember, these children that came at this time came for a special purpose.

July 18, 1980: **You have many questions, ask.**
*"Yes, Aka. I have a question from [12-425-1…Littleton, Colorado]. He's here. He asks, 'Will I be healed or cured of the leukemia I suffer presently?'"*

We see your need, and we shall answer in this manner. You have lived in a righteous manner before your God. Ask and you shall receive.

But it is your choice. If you choose to pass beyond, you choose only through rebirth that you might come again and walk with the Messiah. If you choose to stay, you choose because you wish to prepare the way for the Messiah. In your heart, the Lord sees both of these. He shall not take your life; it shall be your choice. Soul Ray shall administer unto your body, but he cannot take away your free choice, for it is not his given way. You shall make the choice. And whichever it is, soul Ray shall respect your choice, and so will the Lord, God, your Father, who art in heaven and within you.

Glory be the name of the Lord; glory be the name of His children.

July 18, 1980: **You have other questions, ask.**

*"Yes, Aka, thank you. Is there anything more we can do or should do to assist the transition of* [11-407-1]*?"*

**We shall answer your question in this manner. This one chose of his own free choice, that he might bring forth and place his love into you and unto soul Ray and all those around him, that this disease that he died of, that you might find the cure for the same.**

**We shall place in soul Ray's mind further knowledge. And we shall place into all of your minds that should work in this, further knowledge. For he walked upon your Earth, and gave you love, and he did so, as you would say, in death.**

**Yet he is not dead. He lives. For as one a long time ago asked, "Where is heaven, and where do you come from?" — he now walks upon the universe and the stars, and his love is bountiful, yet without limit.**

[Editor's note: See Aka's words of November 16, 1970.]

**He will soon be born again, for it is his choice to walk with the Messiah. He came to you in love and he left you with love. For those who shall prepare the way for the coming of the Messiah, it was his gift to you. Glory be the name of the Lord.**

July 18, 1980: **Now we should say unto you, for [12-425-3], healing shall be given. For it has been asked for.**

**And we should say unto you, for all those who seek healing, let them place their faith in the Lord, God, and it shall be given.**

August 1, 1980: **You have many questions, ask.**

*"Yes, Aka. I have a question from* [10-390-1] *who is here. He asks, 'Our backs seem to be very weak. The vertebrae won't stay in. Is there something causing this that we don't know about? Is there anything that we can do other than what is already being done to help our problem?'"*

**Yes, we see thy need. We shall answer in this way. There is tension in your house, and a house divided cannot come together. And healing that is given cannot stay, for it is driven out by the dissention. We say unto both of you, lay this aside. Become as one of the strangers in the parable. For the answer to your question lies within this parable. "If thy right eye offend thee cast it aside." But remember, do not become so busy casting aside things that you cast the better part of yourselves aside. Love one another, as you would wish others to love you.**

October 17, 1980: **You have other questions, ask.**

*"Thank you, Aka. I have a question from* [12-428-2…Albuquerque]. *'Is my whole family suffering from witchcraft?'"*

**Yes, we see thy need. And we should say unto you in this manner. Much as we have said in the parable before this, those who would practice black arts have nothing more to do, and shall gain nothing more**

[in] knowledge, for they know not where to look. They think they have all the knowledge locked in a little bag before them.

But we shall also answer your question in this manner. You have asked and you have received. And through the blessings given unto soul Ray unto you, all harm has been taken from your family. So what you say, now does not exist.

October 17, 1980: **You have other questions, ask.**
*"Thank you, Aka. [5-206-2 and 2-33-1...Flagstaff], both suffer from severe allergies for about one and one-half years. 'What causes these, and what is the remedy,' they ask?"*
**Yes, we see thy need. And we shall answer your question in this manner. The cause is the conflict within yourselves. The remedy is to extract the conflict.**

November 28, 1980 [in Philosophy]: *"Yes, Aka. I have a question from [12-419-7...Corrales, New Mexico]. He asks, 'Could you tell me how long I can expect to continue my partnership with the One Hundred Ranch, Inc.? If the government takes over the present ranch will we continue at another location?'"*
**Yes, we shall answer your question, and we answer in this manner. The partnership shall continue, as long as you shall desire it. When the government does take over your ranch you shall continue at another location. But there are many things in the making at this time which shall change and alter the pathways unto which you have taken. Part of those pathways you have already taken. You shall find that unisis within yourself, and those around you, shall bring gladness into your heart, and the great depression which has been within you shall be lifted as a shroud. And in its place shall be placed before you the wonders of the earth, and the gladness of God. From it, like a great horn of plenty, shall come forth into your life. Fear not, lest you breed fear. Cast it from your side. Replace it with the first part of the reading, the cardinal, and all things shall come into fulfillment at an abundant way of the Lord, our God.**

November 28, 1980: **You have other questions in your mind and we shall answer them at this time. And, "This is a real heart problem? And what happened?"**
**And we shall answer in this manner. Because you do not allow the weight to be lifted from within you, it is a re-creation of the same problem that brought you here in the beginning. But we say unto you, soul Ray now has answers that he did not have before. The problem shall be dissolved, and you shall be allowed to go forth and fulfill those things that are needed for you to fulfill. There are other blessings ahead in the months to come which you have not yet even dreamed of.**

# 1981 Health Readings

January 30, 1981: **You have other questions, ask.**
*"Thank you, Aka. [3-63-1] asks, 'What is the cause of my dizziness and what should I do for it?'"*

We shall say unto you, you have that of hardening of the arteries, but you also have that of arthrosclerosis, which should lead into other complications, and *has* led into other complications. We should suggest that you come unto soul Ray for counseling, that these problems may be taken care of. Healing you ask for, and healing shall be given.

February 16, 1981: **You have other questions, ask.**
*"Thank you, Aka. [13-433-5…Phoenix] asks, 'What should I do to improve my physical health and energy level?'"*

Yes, we see thy need, and we shall answer into this manner. One of the first things that you should do is to adapt to a good exercise program. And do it as it is supposed to be done. The second you should do is adapt unto your diet into a good balanced diet. As you exercise, your appetite shall increase, but you should be maintained — your weight should be maintained, for you shall burn this off. The third that you wish, we would say unto you, has and is being given unto you.

February 20, 1981: **You have other questions, ask.**
*"Yes, Aka, he also asks for a health reading for himself and any other information he can use for his spiritual development."*

The health reading he has already received. The spiritual development and guidance that he has asked for has been given. The direction he has asked for has been given. We do not interfere with freedom of choice. This is your choice. *You* should make it yourself.

February 20, 1981: **You have other questions, ask.**
*"Aka, [11-408-1…Texas] asks, 'Does my brother, T___ W_____, have M.S., and if so, can he be helped? Thank you.'"*

We shall answer your question in this manner. It is not a true multiple sclerosis, no. It would be more a pre-stress letdown, or a pre-stress syndrome, and he could be helped, yes.

February 20, 1981: **You have other questions.**
*"Thank you. [13-434-2] asks, 'What will give me peace of mind?'"*

The acceptance of the Lord, God, as the one and the only God, and the knowledge of knowing that He is always with you — and also, that you should make labor unto Him. You do not understand that which we speak. And we say unto you, all that we say shall be made clear into you before a fortnight.

February 20, 1981: **We say unto you, [6-281-1], that that you have wished for has been accomplished. Your uncle now walks in the light of the Lord, and he has passed through without great difficulty, for your father waited for him. And soon, you shall feel both presences near you once again.**

April 24, 1981: **You have other questions, ask.**
*"Thank you, Aka. In our preparation of the issue on holistic healing, we realized we have asked only about the health of sick persons, when perhaps we should have been asking about well people. For example, why does Soul Ruth [2-30-2] burn out the flu in three-and-one-half hours when it takes others around her three weeks to get over it? And why does Soul Paul [2-30-3] never get intestinal flu? How can our resistance help others?"*
**We shall answer your question in this manner. Both of you are manufacturing herbs, with vitamins. These enter through the tissue and into the system, and therefore, you'd feel better protection than the average person has. But in the healing process, there is a saying that "time waits for no one." But there is also a saying, that few wait for time.**

April 24, 1981 [in Philosophy]: **We shall answer your question in this manner. You mentioned this flu, which is a man-made deferment [detriment?]. First, it contained 12 initial viruses. Now it has mutated into 48 viruses, any and all capable of making the human being immobile. There is a second side of this which has not been seen. Your Government released the 12-sided virus in the beginning. Your Russian government issued a 12-sided virus, and the two have combined. Therefore, it is double, the 48 sides at this time. You have two great powers now seeking to destroy that that they brought forth — and it is destroying them. It was warned many times that if you pollute the land, you may die in a wasted land. Now we shall say unto you, in these, the summer months, there shall be a cleansing upon the earth, and not in a way that either your Government or the Russian government shall understand. And not to please either government. For the Lord has looked upon the suffering of His people, and says, "THIS IS ENOUGH." Therefore, it shall be lifted.**
**Soul Ray has brought forth in many ways, ways of counteracting these things. Continue the use of that that you call the "Flu Special," all of you, until the cleansing is complete.**
**You have other questions, ask.**

*"Yes, Aka, I have one more question on this. In what form will the cleansing come?"*

**From God.**

*"Thank you, Aka."*

May 1, 1981: **You have questions, ask.**

*"I have a question from [13-437-1.] She called from Tucson this afternoon, and she says the doctors believe that she may have stones in her bile duct. They are giving her disodium phosphate and choline tablets. She asks, 'What is really wrong with me, and how may my health be improved?'"*

Yes, we see thy need. And to the first question we shall answer in this manner. We have before us the body, the soul, the spirit, and we find, therefore, not stones as such, but nothing more than plaque. These are not in the bile duct itself, but in the artery, therefore, that enters the same, and therefore, we have an inflammation of the blood vessel or the artery, as you would know it, swelling, and therefore, restricting the bile duct.

There are different manners of taking care of this. The first, if you wish it, would be with [the] "normal surgery," and a bypass or artificial blood vessels being placed in the place of the same.

The second would be that that you [would] know as chelation therapy.

The third would be as soul Ray would do it, with the use of the Alpearon, the Golden Seal, that of the Nia-C in correct proportions, much fluids, the use, therefore, of the sage tea in large quantities, and last, that you would know as Gerovital.

May 1, 1981: **You have other questions, ask.**

*"Thank you, Aka. [13-437-2] asks, 'Why am I having all this illness? Is this past-life? And how do I go about getting well?'"*

We have just explained the why and the how. It has been said before, respect that and know of that of the way others believe, but respect that unto which you believe and know of, yet with the doorways open.

You live as a person who is afraid to pass through a doorway. You live with the Roman Catholic belief within you, and you feel a conflict of the knowledge that has come from soul Ray. You believe within yourself that you are violating your faith in your church by believing in what soul Ray is able to give you. This is not true. [For was it] not once has he told you to leave your faith? He has only added to that you already have. When you can accept these things and create a balance within yourself, a total healing shall come forth.

May 1, 1981: **You have other questions, ask.**

*"Yes, Aka. Thank you. [12-413-3] asks, 'Will my brother recover from his mental illness, and where is he now?'"*

We would say unto you, come unto soul Ray in private. This is not a question that should be answered in public.

May 22, 1981: And now we say unto all of you, yet we shall say unto one of you, the Lord sees your affliction. Had it not been for your affliction, you would not have taken the time out to show the love that was needed. You would not have sought this place in which you are now. You would not have found the knowledge within yourself to use the compassion you have used this day. So we say unto you, this small affliction of the body, has it not been worth this for the growth of your soul, your spirit and your immortal body?

You are wondering if we are speaking to you. That is the thought that has gone through your mind. So you might know it's so, we will speak your thoughts. You are almost ready to jump with joy with the realization that you think it is true. Is not our words true?

The call which you made this day, you grew more than you have in a long time. It shall not stop now, but shall continue as a butterfly. You have been as a butterfly in the cocoon. You are coming out of the cocoon to spread your wings and be beautiful, before all men, and before your God.

May 22, 1981: Yea, and we say unto you and to all of you, who have ears to hear, and eyes to see, hear our words. Take them from this place this night. Put them to work for you, that your souls may grow. And through the [soul's growth], so grows the spirit, and so grows the immortal body, the temple of God.

May 22, 1981: Now is the time of the Cherubim.

June 8, 1981: You have other questions, ask.
*"Yes, Aka. From [13-441-6], 'What is the state of my health? Will I get my house built?'"*

Yes, We see thy need, and we have before us the body, the soul, the spirit, and the immortal body of the same. At first, we shall answer your question in this manner. You shall have your health restored, you have already taken the steps needed for this to come about.

June 8, 1981: You have other questions, ask.
*"Thank you. From [13-441-7], 'What is the state of my health, particularly the abdominal area?'"*

Yes, we see thy need, and we shall answer in this manner. In that of this, the short intestine, there is a puffin out, a blistering out of the same. This is causing a disease of the colon. You have take certain steps for the correction of this at this time, and we say unto you, come therefore unto soul Ray and you shall find the answer for the same.

June 26, 1981: **You have many questions, ask.**
*"Yes, Aka. I have a question from [9-360-1], and she asks, 'In the reading of June 13, 1973, you referred to a soul who left his body due to a mental disease. Upon leaving the body, a lost soul possessed it. Is there any connection with this problem and the problem of my uncle? Is there anything we can do to help these people?'"*

Yes — the person, and we shall explain. The mental disease which possesses a body is like a death. When the soul and the spirit can no longer function within the body, it leaves to join the immortal body. Therefore, it has no use for it. The spirit, who has lost his soul and his immortal body, which comes into this body, gains nothing, and can do no harm except those who would allow it, and would leave it by simply, if you ignored it. [Give prayer] into the Lord of thy intent. And know that nothing falls on this earth, leste the Lord should know of it.

And fear not. Do you think that the Lord should allow one of His children to wander lost without making an attempt to bring it home? We say unto you, nay. The Lord has gathered His flock, and your uncle among them.

July 17, 1981: **You have other questions, ask.**
*"Thank you, Aka. I have a health question from [6-290-5...Litchfield, Arizona], and she asks, 'Aka, would you please give me a health reading and any advice concerning my health. Bless your, dear ones, and light and much love to you and our Father.'"*

We see thy need, but your health reading has already been given this day from soul Ray. It is complete. Fear not, for we have said before, for soul Ray is I, and I am soul Ray. Where one dwells, so does the other.

July 17, 1981: **You have other questions, ask.**
*"Thank you, Aka. I have a question from [13-443-1...Casper, Wyoming]. It asks, 'How come I'm allergic to cats? What can I do for my nose?'"*

(Chuckle.) We shall explain to you in this manner. That of the cat fur is much like the wool of a sheep. It is like a fishhook before it allows the cause of many, many things that it touches to lay dormant in it. The easiest way is to wash your cat. And do so with a fragrance which you like.

August 21, 1981: **Now we say unto you, you have questions, ask.**
*"Yes, Aka. I have a question from [7-316-1...Winterhaven, California]. He asks, 'What herbs, minerals and food should I eat more of?'"*
We see thy need, and we shall say unto you, soul Ray has already

answered these questions for you. If you have not heard him correctly, come forth and he shall give you this information.

October 2, 1981: **You have many questions, ask.**
*"Yes, Aka. I have a question from* [13-446-1...Payson, Arizona]. *'Will the full straightening and healing of my eyes be given through Mr. Elkins?'"*
**Yes, we see thy need. And that that you have asked for shall be given through the instrument you asked for. As it has already begun, so it shall be done.**

**We shall answer another question within your mind. The love is a fleeting thing. In youth, it travels sometimes with heartbreak. but time is a healer and a renewer. For that that you think at the moment is the most important of all shall just be as part-time, a learning time, for the day when your fulfillment shall come.**

October 2, 1981: **You have other questions, ask.**
*"Thank you, Aka. I have a question from* [13-446-3...Clovis, New Mexico]. *'Will my son, Eddie's, eyesight return, or will he seek the help of Ray?'"*
**We shall answer your question in this manner. Freedom of choice is one of the most precious gifts God has given. It has also been said, "Ask and you shall receive." And it [was] also said unto you, "God helps those who help themselves." But ask in my Father's name, and all things are possible. If that is what you wish, and he wishes, then that that is necessary shall be given unto soul Ray that this may be possible.**

October 2, 1981: **You have other questions, ask.**
*"I have a question from* [13-446-4...El Paso, Texas]; *'Can I do anything about my hypertension?'"*
**Yes, we see thy need. We shall answer in this manner. The steps that you are taking are the correct steps. But remember, that even unto the healing of God, or man, could only last when you yourself become a party to the healing process, a commitment upon your part. All that can be done can be destroyed in the twinkling of an eye with negative thought, and yet, be restored in the same manner with a positive thought.**

**There are those things upon your Earth that are useless, and stupid, cruel and vicious, all without logic, all without compassion or knowledge.**

**We have seen many times, throughout the centuries, when men have stood up and said unto other men, "Look at me, for I am great, for I and I only have the ears to hear and the eyes to see the Lord, God," that "He speaks only to me, and from me to you." You know, deep in your heart, that no matter where you are, in heaven or earth, if you prayed unto the Lord, God, He is with you. If you cast Him from you, He is not with you. It is your choice, your time, and your place. Choose wisely.**

November 6, 1981: **You have questions, ask.**

*"Thank you, Aka. I have a question from R___ E____. 'What can be done to improve my liver function?'"*

Yes, we see thy need. We have before us the body, the soul, the spirit, and the immortal body. And we shall explain in this manner. And we shall try to do so that your physical problem shall be still a private thing.

First we should say, that as we came unto you we promised not that we would repair your whole body. You have done a good job in that which you have done so far. But first, you must take more time for that which is physical exercise.

The second, as we have said before, that which is known as the dialysis machine, or a machine which you use to clean the blood.

If these things are not available, the third; because of the thickness of the blood itself, [in] the removal of blood in 500 c.c. lots in the time only necessary to replace the volume, and then, testing of the liver function until it cleanses itself, this will work as well as the other. But as the removal of the blood and the inability to fight off germs because – then the use of that of gamma globulin to help build up the immune system would be necessary.

You know your own condition. You know that rest is necessary as well as the exercise. But last, you know that the more pressure, emotional pressure placed upon you, the faster the disease will progress. Utilize the ranch in such a manner as your father has told you, "The outside of a horse is the best thing for the insides of a man." You know this as well as any. Put that time forward.

November 6, 1981: **You have other questions, ask.**

*"Thank you, Aka. I have a question from* [10-387-3…Litchfield Park, Arizona]. *And he asks, 'I would like to have a health reading and advice on my investments.'"*

We have given you both.

We say unto you, our time now grows short, and soul Ray now tires.

November 13, 1981: **You have other questions, ask.**

*"Thank you, he has one other question. He asks, 'What can be done to help the negative situation that seems to be increasing between my daughter-in-law and her mother towards my wife especially. Our son seems to be caught in the middle and we want to set things right. Should we ignore the problems, or talk it over with our son?'"*

We shall answer your question in this manner. Sometimes a squeaky door needs oil. [To] find this in your door and oil it without words, without conversation, you shall find that when the squeak is gone, the problem[s] shall disappear. And it shall not take, as you would know it, verbal communication upon your part.

November 13, 1981 [in Philosophy]: **You have other questions, ask.**
*"Thank you, Aka. [13-449-4…El Paso, Texas] asks – he would like a physical exam and requests a health program pertaining to diet and exercise."*
**Yes, we see thy need. And we answer in this manner. *All* these things have already been given unto you. We shall give you one other question in this manner. Feed your soul. For it is only when the body, the soul, the spirit and the immortal body bind as one should things that you seek be complete.**

**You wish to give a gift, and we ask you this questions. If you should give a gift wishing nothing in return and asking nothing in return, then it is truly a gift that you have given. When you have not given it in this manner, then it is not a gift you have given, but a barter. Therefore, do not lie to yourself. Look at it as it is, and know it for what it is. And accept it or change it, whichever is your desire. When this happens, the true question that you ask us will be answered in full, for then, and only then, shall the happiness which you seek become fulfilled.**

November 13, 1981: **You have other questions, ask.**
*"Thank you, Aka. [13-449-5…Donna Ana, New Mexico] asks, 'why myself and immediate family, my husband, two sons and daughter, have kidney stones?'"*
**Because of the water you drink – second, because of your diet; third, because of the lack of intake into your systems of the necessary vitamins which would restore the blood vessels, destroy the plaque that forms the kidney stones, and let it be released from your system, the dilation of the blood vessels in the right amounts. If you wish these things, you know where this help can be given. This is all on this subject.**

November 13, 1981 [in Philosophy]: **You have other questions, ask.**
*"Thank you, Aka. [11-409-1] asks, 'Aka, will I get my GS-5, and will I get loose and buy the old house and be happy?'"*
**Part of the things that you asked for have already happened. The happiness must come from within, as you already know. We have said before, ask in thy Father's name and those things that are needed shall be given. But when you ask, make certain that those things you wish for and ask for are what you want.**

**Speak unto your Father as you would unto yourself. Therefore, if you do so, God shall hear, and listen, and act. If you stand and repeat what someone else has told you, which means nothing to you, how can you expect it to mean anything to God? Talk is a very cheap commodity. Acting is a very rich commodity. Take the action that is needed, so that**

that you wish for shall be yours.

November 13, 1981: **You have other questions, ask.**
*"Thank you, Aka.* [13-499-6…El Paso, Texas] *asks, 'What specific guilt complex am I holding to prevent myself from completion?'"*
(Chuckle.) **The thought that you hold a guilt complex − that is all, just the thought. Release the thought, and the other thing shall leave you. The beginning and ending of a karma may happen within the second, or within the blinking of an eye. What do you have to be guilty for? Do you not know that our Father has seen all things?**

**Our Father has not judged you. Why should you judge yourself in this manner? Are you ashamed of the temple that our Father has given you? There is no other vehicle like it in the whole universes or galaxies. It is a good vehicle. Quit using yourself as a whipping boy. Stand up, and know that you are the creation of God, Almighty. And with your uniqueness comes the unique gifts that lie within you. Put them to work and forget this guilt.**

November 20, 1981: **You have other questions, ask.**
*"Thank you, Aka. I have a question from* [7-304-8]*, and she asks, "This entity wishes to ask for guidance at this point and any information that will be beneficial for the future, related to past lives.'"*
**We shall say unto you, we have watched you run in many directions, for we have before us the body, the soul, the spirit, and the immortal body. You have tried your utmost to destroy this, for no one else may harm you but yourself. You have tried to destroy all things that we have given you and all things that you brought forth from other lifetimes. The only help that you need is the help that you already know in your heart and your soul. Place yourself, your heart, your soul, your body, as the temple of God; open the door that He may enter.**

**You have acted at times after time to destroy this temple, yet you have not succeeded. But if that is your fullest wish it shall be given. But knowing that you seek within you the spirit of God, which already dwells there, let it blossom forth. All the tools you need are inside of you. All the knowledge you need lies before you. Ask and you shall receive. Give unto the Lord one-tenth of the love which He has given you; give unto your fellow man the same amount, and give unto yourself the love the Lord wishes for you, and in all ways you shall be serving God.**

November 20, 1981: **You have other questions, ask.**
*"Thank you, Aka.* [11-450-1...El Paso, Texas]*, she asks, 'What specific fear keeps me from achieving my goal of recalling childhood memories?'"*
**Yes, we have before us the body, the soul, the spirit, and the immoral body. [And] therefore, we shall say unto you, your fear of**

recalling childhood memories is that of a delicate nature, one into which you were basically raped. The person [who] raped you, you know of this, and your love for the person who did this. To block this out, you have blocked out all the good and wonderful things of your childhood. You have forgiven this person in your heart, but not in your mind. Forgive them, and the memories shall return, but first forgive yourself.

November 20, 1981: **You have other questions, ask.**
*"Yes, Aka, thank you.* [11-450-2...El Paso, Texas] *asks a question, 'What specific guilt am I using to block myself from regaining custody of my son, V_____ A___ R____, age 4?'"*
Yes, we see thy need, and we have before us the body, the soul, and the spirit there of the same. There is no guilt. There is fear within yourself that you might not do the best job of raising this child to its full potential. When that is removed, then the things you desire shall come into fulfillment.

Remember, the beginning and the ending of a karma can happen within the very moment that you realize that there is no problem, no karma at all. But if you continue to use yourself in the manner of continued persecution of yourself, it shall destroy you. Be transformed − turn around, and you shall know of yourself, and like yourself, and respect yourself. But be not [in] such a hurry to cast things out that you cast the better part of yourself away, for you *are* that that you are.

Remember the story of Jesus and Mary Magdalene, when they brought her before him? And they said unto him, "Rabbi, you know the law. This person is to be stoned."

He reached down and picked up a stone and said, "Let he who has no guilt in his heart cast the first stone. Let he who has not sought, or thought or lusted in his mind cast the first stone." They all turned and departed. He threw the stone away.

And she said, "But Master, strike me, for surely you have not sinned against your Father."

Jesus smiled and laughed, and said, "Little but do you know. We are none so perfect as our Father. Rise, my daughter, and live."

And she did.

December 11, 1981: **You have many questions, ask.**
*"Thank you, Aka. A* [13-452-1...Dripping Springs, Arizona] *asks, 'What is the cause of my headaches, and what can be done to correct this problem?'"*
Yes, we see thy need. First we should explain in this manner. The inflammation of the nerve in itself is the direct cause of thy headaches. A great deal of this inflammation is the lack of the blood supply in these. To go without this system [re-staying? retains?] in pain substance. The nerves in the back of the neck have become inflamed to the arthritic

state, and yet, the body keeps continuing to cry out, "Warning! Warning, for see, I am not well! Repair me."

These to the parts necessary to repair the body is locked up within the birth. They allow the doors to be opened; they allow us to enter, allow us to convey messages. Many shall think that the answer we have just given you is not so. Whatever you give unto the Lord, He shall give you tenfold, be it love, or money, or yourself.

# 1982 Health Readings

January 8, 1982: **You have other questions, ask.**

*"Yes, Aka. [14-453-4...Houston, Texas] asks, 'How can I rid myself of mental pain, depression, and anxiety? Any information on obtaining peace of mind and spiritual development?'"*

**Yes, we see thy need. Peace of mind, we have spoke of in the beginning of the reading. Spiritual development, we spoke of that also. Yet, we see a physical problem; [it] impairs your from functioning at your fullest. We say unto you, come, therefore, unto soul Ray that this obstacle, or should we call it, [a] many-sided hexagon, be removed.**

January 29, 1982: **We shall say unto you, the words that were said unto the healer, and from the one who said them, for [R____] said unto Ray, "Why me; why must I die, when you have saved so many?" And soul Ray looked into his eyes, and said, "I have not the answer for you. Only the Lord and yourself have that answer."**

**And now [R____] says unto you, he has that answer, for he went, therefore, to prepare a way for many, and he went, therefore, to renew the wine of life.**

February 12, 1982: **You have questions, ask.**

*"Yes, Aka, thank you. I have a question from [7-316-1]. He asks, 'At what number does my blood residue stand at? What should I take for my lung trouble? Thank you.'"*

**We have told you before, and we shall tell you again, we have placed a healer before you. If the healer does not suit you, go elsewhere.**

February 12, 1982 [in Philosophy]: **You have other questions, ask.**

*"Yes, Aka. Thank you. I have a question from [14-455-2...Albuquerque, New Mexico], 'What is the importance of selenium to humans?'"*

**Selenium, in itself, is an ingredient that should change forms once into the system. It becomes a nutrient to the brain. It is a guiding light, as you might know it, to the reproduction of cell structure. The brain cells, as you know, are not connected. They produce electrical charge which sends a signal from one cell to the other. It is like a great organ being played. The selenium in itself aids in turning on the electricity necessary to light the organ and keep it in harmony.**

We have placed it in a way which you will understand which we speak of. There are other things that must be added to it that it may enter the bloodstream as it should, because in [the] one which you are thinking about, it cannot enter the bloodstream by itself. It needs the vitamins, as you would know them, as B-12, B-6, and B-3. These would act as a catalyst agent. We would also suggest that by placing the DNA factor of that of the mesquite with this, it would then work as a nutrient, not only to the brain, but it would also work in such a manner to prevent disease of many different types. It allows your own defense mechanism to be triggered, and built, therefore, into a complete substance.

If you have further questions on this subject, come unto soul Ray, for he has done thorough research in this field, and [has thought] to build a product accordingly.

March 5, 1982 [in Philosophy]: **You have many questions, ask.**
*"Yes, Aka. I have a question from* [14-456-1…Litchfield Park], *'Please give me a health reading and any other advice.'"*

(Chuckle) **We see thy need. But the health reading you do not need, for you know, therefore; all those things that lie within you, you have brought unto soul Ray. You also know the advice that we would give you is a very simple thing — be happy.**

**Love is a wonderful and beautiful thing. Do not allow it to bring hardship or burden into your life, for there is not need for that. The freedom of love is the kindness of all things; yet man makes it so complicated. If you see a flower and it is beautiful to your eyes, and [to] smell the fragrance brings total satisfaction to your nose, and when you reach and pick it up it is smooth and delicate in your hands, you do not have to think of its wilting. You do not have to think of it dying. It is a thing to appreciate at the time when you hold it in your hands.**

**Love is like the wind, tame but untamed, cooling and refreshing, yet it carries the storms. Yet the storm shall pass and in its place a bright new day shall arrive, and maybe a new love with this day.**

**Love is a word you use so often, yet know not the meaning of. Yet the moment given from one to another is worth a lifetime of all other emotions. In some ways it may be stored in the memories of your mind for all of eternity, for once it has been there, and you hold it in a delicate manner, nothing can change it. Though time may dim the memories of the emotion, yet even time has a way of sweetening the taste.**

**Do not become confused, for the love that soul Ray has given you is eternal. It is a love that a father would give to his daughter, as God would give to His child. It has not changed nor altered.**

**Do not become confused with the paths that lay before you. Touch them with love. But there is one thing that can destroy love — if you smother it, if you take the flower and crush it in your hands.**

March 5, 1982 [in Philosophy]: **You have other questions, ask.**

*"Thank you, Aka. I have a question from* [14-456-2…Litchfield Park, Arizona]. *'Please give me any health reading and any advice.'"*

**We see thy need also. And we shall answer *your* question for your health the same as we have before. Soul Ray knows your health and your problems, and that that has been needed has been placed in his heart, his hand, and his mind.**

**We have answered the second part of your question with that of your sister's, and with the first part of the reading. Therefore —** [long pause].

March 5, 1982: **You have other questions, ask.**

*"Thank you, Aka. I have a question from* [14-456-4]. *She asks, 'What is the main cause of recurring pain in the left chest and back?'"*

**Yes, we see thy need. And we have before us the body, the soul, and the spirit of the**

**same. And we shall answer your question in this manner. The circulation within your body is not complete. This of the new virus, or the old virus, whichever you care to call it, is the main source of the pain. Soon that shall be gone, and even that which carries it shall be gone, [and] defaced of your earth.**

March 5, 1982: **You have other questions, ask.**

*"Yes, Aka. Regarding that statement, I just wondered if the bacteria that was developed to eat Agent Orange is the same bacteria that will attack these viruses?"*

**It and others, for the meanest, [or] the greatest, shall come forth to destroy these bacterias, for it shall become, in the form in which you would know as, the wind of God. And soon your land shall feel it. Fear it not. Some shall.**

March 5, 1982: **You have questions, ask.**

*"Thank you, Aka. I have a question from* [14-456-6]. *He asks for 'the cause of right leg circulation and right hip joint problems.'"*

**We see your need. These questions have already been answered by soul Ray.**

August 13, 1982: **You have other questions, ask.**

*"Yes, Aka. I have a request for* [12-419-5] *who is in childbirth, has been in labor for about 31 or 32 hours. And she has asked for assistance."*

**It has been given and shall be given. Fear not.**

August 13, 1982: **You have other questions, ask.**

*"Yes, Aka, thank you. [8-350-2, born…1905…Litchfield Park, Arizona] asks, 'Would you please give me a health reading, also healing? I love you.'"*

**We see thy need, and we shall say unto thee unto these words. The reading is not necessary. The help that you shall need shall be given. Glory be the name of the Lord. Glory be the name of His children, forever and ever.**

*[NOTE: AUGUST 13, 1982 WAS THE LAST READING IN 1982.]*

# 1983 Health Readings

June 3, 1983: **You have many questions, ask.**
*"I have no questions except life readings tonight, Aka."*
**Soul Ray's health cannot do those at this time. And we shall
answer the questions within your minds.**

**First, we shall say unto the one known as [15-461-1], as the stars
should sit in the Orion Belt, so shall the truth that thy seek come into
fulfillment. We say unto you, we have placed the knowledge of thy health
problems in the hands of soul Ray. It shall become and made as complete
as possible. Of the other questions you have in your mind, we say unto
you, we did *not* leave you unprotected.**

August 5, 1983: **You have other questions, ask.**
*"Thank you, Aka. I have a question from [3-69-2], and she asks, [3-
69-2] and [2-30-2] would like to know the meaning of 'Marsha.'"*
**Yes, we see thy need, and we shall say unto thee, it is a babe yet
not born, but the seed has been sprinkled. You shall know it, and it shall
know you. It shall be a joyous time. But its journey into this world shall
be a hard time. It is within your powers to make that journey easier, if
you wish.**

August 12, 1983: **You have other questions, ask.**
*"Yes. Aka. [1-1-1] would like to know how he can lose weight. He's
tried everything and seems to be putting on more."*
**(Chuckle.) First, we would say, with more exercise, both morning
and evening, the utilization of his pool – and he should do so now in such
a way that it can be prepared to use in the wintertime.**

**Next would be that that he may prepare himself by diet. There
are many substitutes for sugar. Eat the fruit that is in season, and as you
can it, utilize that. Pastry should be limited to one or two days a week
only, and a minimum amount of that – a balanced diet, more of the green
vegetables, yet more of the solid beef, or red meat[s] for him, because of
his metabolism.**

**We would also mention the fact that because of a thyroid
condition, longstanding, the retention of fluids within his body, the new
tablet which has been suggested to be made, when complete, shall greatly
assist in this.**

We would also suggest that he has with him several forms and ways of exercise — one of these is to go back to riding as soon as possible; next, unto the boating exercises which he had in mind.

We will give further information on this from time to time as questions should arise.

August 12, 1983: **You have other questions, ask.**

*"Aka, [3-69-2] and [2-30-2] say, 'We need more information on Marsha — who Marsha was in the past, and how we connected to her?'"*

We shall say unto you, it is a babe yet unborn. It is a babe that is important. Translate the word of Marsha, and where it comes from, its originality. It will show you its origin. And it shall show you how it ties together for the babe that is yet born, and the importance that it should be born. It shall need your assistance. It shall also need the assistance of its mother, and [in] her cooperation. This will come within time. It will also need the assistance of its grandmother. She knows of herself. It is vitally important, for there shall be a struggle in the womb for possession of the soul of this one.

August 26, 1983 [in Philosophy]: **You have other questions, ask.**

*"Thank you, Aka. [12-423-1] asks, 'Aka, thank you for our readings. At this time would you please give me the time of my birth? Also what will heal my leg?'"*

The last shall come first, and the first shall come last. We say unto you, the water of the healing springs, when it is complete. And when it is complete, and soul Ray shall call on the Kiva of the springs, and when the Madonna is placed upon the mountain, then all shall be in readiness.

**9:45 a.m.**

September 2, 1983: **You have other questions, ask.**

*"Thank you, Aka. [9-371-5…Peoria, Arizona] asks, 'Please give any advice or guidance regarding our property or personal affairs. Should we relocate? If so, when and where? Thank you.'"*

We shall say unto you unto this question unto this way, unto this manner. At the present time, due to a physical impairment, things have become confused unto you, and you have become dissatisfied of that that you dwell, and where you dwell in. And we say unto you that where you dwell has brought you happiness and prosperity. If you seek beyond this point, then there is only to look around you, and that shall be given also.

September 9, 1983: **You have other questions, ask.**

*"Thank you, Aka. I have a question from [15-470-2…El Paso], asks for help with overweight problems, to solve husband-wife problems at home; she desires peaceful harmonies, a loving home. She's asking for suggestions*

*for her to better help others who ask her to help them heal themselves, and also how can she liquidate debts and prosper?"*

We shall answer your question in this manner. Prayer is the greatest answer to most, and all of your problems. But prayer alone, without intent, shall solve nothing. Therefore, bring [full] prayer, and bring [full] intent, and that that you seek shall be fulfilled.

September 16, 1983 [in Philosophy]: *"Aka, I have a question from R___. 'What is causing the GH-12 and the GH-22 to sting? At times the complaints are greater than others. Is it something done while mixing the formula?'"*

We will explain in this manner, that the formula must be sustained at an even temperature. That that stings should be of the B substance of the B-3 substance. We would suggest that, in smaller quantities that in the place of the B, of the niacinamide, that niacin be substituted. This should be measured by one-half. You shall find a greater result, but also it shall do away with the stinging properties that go into the buffering of the niacinamide.

September 16, 1983: **You have other questions, ask.**
*"Thank you, Aka. [2-30-2] asks for help on her present health problem."*

Yes, we see thy need. Soul Ray has already answered your question, that of the GH-22 should be used.

November 11, 1983: **You have other questions, ask.**
*"Yes, Aka. [14-456-3] asks for guidance for her oldest grandson who seems to be having trouble lately."*

We see thy need. And the guidance you seek shall be given.

# 1984 Health Readings

January 13, 1984: **You have other questions, ask.**
*"Yes, Aka. Could you please help us find out what is causing soul* [1-1-1]*'s weight problem?"*

**Yes. We have a thyroid condition, which could be easily corrected. We also have a water problem, or fluid retention. The body is not releasing the fluids from the body; therefore, it is retaining them. We also have a blood disorder which is causing the spleen to swell and become bigger. The imbalance of the glandular substance is causing him to retain fluids and build more blood than normal, and more irregular cells than normal. At the present time, if the physician at hand does not recognize these, then we would suggest that he seek out a different physician, because the quickest way for him to stop this problem is with certain drugs that are prescribed medications. We would suggest that the physician at hand be asked, that if he cannot handle the job at hand, for him to be sent into a specialist.**

**We have also seen growths in the abdominal area, which is causing a malfunction [of] the pineal gland, which is causing the biochemistry of the [molecular] system to be off to an extent that the rapid amount of weight gain can be controlled.**

January 13, 1984: **You have other questions, ask.**
*"Thank You, Aka."*

**One moment. It must be fully understood, it's because of [soul Ray's]'s high energy that his [molecular] structure is quite different than yours. Therefore, what would be normal for you would kill him. If you check his temperature, you will find that it is not the same. You shall also find a high raise in the red cell count. We would suggest that further questions be brought up on this subject until a total recovery.**

January 20, 1984: **You have other questions, ask.**
*"Thank you, Aka. I have a question from* [3-69-2]*; firstly, a health question. She has had a drive to write from right to left and write words backwards. And she wonders if you could give her some explanation for this."*

**First, we would say that it is a form of [dyslexia] which is involved. This urge should be greatly resisted, and help should be sought out from soul Ray for the reason. It is not something that should come natural, or not something from the past, but a problem that exists in this**

time, in this space, of this day.

January 20, 1984: **You have other questions, ask.**
*"Yes, Aka. I have a question from* [13-446-1…Payson]. *She said that, 'In 1981, you said that Mr. Elkins would straighten and heal my eyes. May I ask why this has not been accomplished? Please give guidance in soon reaching this goal.'"*

Yes, we will answer your question in this manner. The work that was needed to be done has been done, not once, but three times. Each time you did not give the eyesight and that of the eyes time to heal because you were too busy doing your *own* thing. If you wish this to happen, then do as you are asked to do, and healing may take place. If you do not wish this to happen, then continue as you are now. But remember, a dog who bites his own tail learns nothing and goes nowhere.

January 27, 1984: **You have other questions, ask.**
*"Yes, Aka. He [16-479-1] also asks, 'What is the cause of my skin disease, and how long will it take to cure it?'"*

The cause of your skin disease is the substance which you readily call, Agent Orange, [which] you were exposed to. It is a chemical, or we shall say many chemicals, that was placed together by men who thought they would do the earth a service. Instead, they have done God and man a great unjustice. You have come unto soul Ray for healing; listen to him. That which he is offering you shall bring forth healing. When he tells you to go, therefore, to the valley of the healing waters, do so. [Editor's note: Dripping Springs on Dripping Spring Road, Arizona.]

January 27, 1984: **You have other questions, ask.**
*"Yes, thank you, Aka. I have a question from* [16-479-4]; *he asks, 'Are you going to fix my eye tomorrow?'"*
**We say unto you, ask soul Ray.**

March 30, 1984: **You have another questions, ask.**
*"Thank you, Aka.* [15-461-1…Globe] *asks, 'Do I need to take anything else to rid my system of [this] foreign substance? Could you be specific?'"*

Yes, we shall be specific. So far, those things that are needed, soul Ray has brought unto you. He is now building another substance which shall complete the cycle. But you have had the blessings you asked for, swiftly and surely. Each of the things you have asked for has been given. Do not be impatient.

**You have other questions, ask.**
*"Thank you, Aka. You may have answered this, but I will read it to you also. He asks regarding his asthmatic condition and infectious condition."*

Yes, we have answered that.

**August 24, 1984: Yes. You have other questions, ask.**
*"Thank you, Aka. A question for Aka from* [11-398-2], *asks, 'Sir, will you please tell me what to do to correct what is wrong with this body, especially with the [lynching] plantars and the places on the legs? Thank you.'"*

We have answered this question. For we should say unto you, the [waking] mind of soul Ray so is our mind. For the knowledge that is needed for the healing of the body, in the beginning, we did [the] health readings; we did them as we developed his mind and his skills. Now that is completed from the time and new knowledge shall continue to come into his mind. As we have said before, if you are sent into the desert, and God has given you the food and water, and you do not take them [when] able, what should we do?

**September 14, 1984: You have other questions, ask.**
*"Thank you, Aka.* [12-424-2] *asks, 'How can I improve my memory, particularly name retention and mathematic functions? Is there any harmful levels of mercury or lead in my system that is causing memory or other problems?'"*

Let the last be first, and we shall say unto you, no. These things are not there.

We would suggest that the present form that you have taken should keep your mind alert and active. But something that would act even better as a stimulant would be for you and your wife now to plan ahead to that time of retirement when you might go into a business. You have several hobbies which could become good businesses, should you care to use them.

**September 28, 1984: You have other questions, ask.**
*"Thank you, Aka.* [10-392-1…Quartzite, Arizona] *asks, 'Aka, would you please tell me what is wrong with my health and what can be done about it?'"*

Yes, we see thy need. And we say unto you, we have placed a healer before you. Before, we gave long health readings. The purpose for this was to help mankind at the time. Since that time we have placed the knowledge into the one known as soul Ray. Come unto him, and seek his counsel. If it is not that which you wish, then go elsewhere. Find that which satisfies you, for that is food for the body.

**September 28, 1984 [in Philosophy]: You have other questions, ask.**
*"Thank you, Aka. I have a question from* [16-490-5], *and the question is, 'Medical doctors have told my husband he has muscle disease. Will this get better?'"*

Yes.

September 28, 1984 [in Philosophy]: **Once again we shall say this unto you, our time is short.**

**For those who would wonder of the chemical that was brought forth into this land — the chemical that destroyed babies, and brought mutates into birth, and killed adults — you say unto us, "When you said it was gone from the land, and the land would be safe, during the long rains, is this true now?" And we say unto you, this is true now, but remember, nothing is ever gone. You may live on all lands with caution, for that that was in the land went into the seed and into the root, and into the seed of seeds, and so it is in human and plant and animal. When those who were exposed to it realize this, to the full measure, [for] the land that they live on, and take the necessary precautions, they will be safe.**
[Editor's note: In the late 1960's, the U.S. Forest Service had sprayed "Agent Orange" on mountainsides near Globe, Arizona, as a defoliant to lessen undergrowth and cause more water runoff.]

October 5, 1984: **You have other questions, ask.**
*"Thank you, Aka. [16-491-1] asks, 'Where do I go to get my health?'"*
**We do not see this. We find not of this.**

October 5, 1984: **Ask another question.**
*"Thank you, Aka. [16-491-2…Tucson], 'I would like to know more about my daughter, S\_\_\_\_\_, who she is, and about her relationship with myself and R\_\_\_\_\_….'"*
**Yes, we see thy need and that which you ask for. (Sigh.) You asked for information which does not concern you. You violate the freedom of choice of another; this we will not assist you with.**

**We say unto you, if you ask the Lord, God, for guidance, you shall receive that from both sides to guide you. If you have lost your arm, and you ask for help in using one arm in the place of two, do you think that He would send someone who has never lost their arm, and not learned to use one in the place of two? This is how these guides are chosen. You choose them. You ask for them.**

October 5, 1984: **You have other questions, ask.**
*"Thank you, Aka. [16-491-3] asks, 'Will my wife recover completely?'"*
**Once again you ask a question [for] another, but we shall answer in this manner. She will recover according to her choice.**

# 1985 Health Readings

January 4, 1985 [in Philosophy]:**You have other questions, ask.**
*"Thank you, Aka. [17-497-1…in Nevada] asks, 'Can a disease or an illness be helped by mind control by the person who has the problem?'"*
**Long ago, soul Ray brought forth knowledge of the type of mind control that can not only help [to] cure diseases — have him share these thoughts with you.**

February 22, 1985: **You have other questions, ask.**
*"Thank you, Aka. [17-500-1...Texas] born on March the 4th, 1984, and he asks, 'Our son, R_____, was killed about four years ago. Is there any message that he wants to give us?'"*
**We shall answer your question by saying this. There is new birth within your family. Look unto the eyes of the child, and you shall find your son.**

February 22, 1985 [in Philosophy]: **Now we should say unto you unto these questions. Should soul Ray continue into his line of thought into a new serum, which he has in his mind to build, he shall find an answer for two things, that which he calls the flu, and that which is called, AIDS.**

February 22, 1985: **Now soul Ray tires, and we should say, remember, this is the time of the Cherubim.**

# 1986 Health Readings

January 23, 1986: **You have other questions, ask.**

*"Thank you, Aka.* [18-512-4…Dallas, Texas], *and she asks, 'Can you tell me a way to correct the malfunction in my pituitary gland which has caused abnormal water retention in my system for years?'"*

**Yes we see thy need. We shall answer your question in this manner. It is the pituitary gland which controls the nervous system, sending messages back and forth to the different portions of the body. The pineal gland controls the biochemistry of the body. The water retention that you have can be controlled quite simply by the use of the product known as "Wonderloss," taken in quantities of three, four times a day. But we see other needs.**

January 31, 1986: **You have other words, and other questions, ask.**

*"Thank you Aka.* [13-442-2] *asks, 'Under the circumstances of the robbery of my parents, _____, what avenue should we take? I need to benefit of their wisdom."*

**We should answer your question in this manner. Take no action at this time, but watch. And let those who know that you are watching be ever aware that they are under observation. And they shall take no action. For as all concerned, we should ask you to rise above what you have seen. Your father has departed; he rests well; he has passed through well. He is now visiting, and enjoying himself well, with many good friends and many good relatives who passed before him, for he was well received on the other side, as you would call it. These things you yourself shall know. When you seek wisdom, we have placed he with you who knows of avenues and ways. You can always have relatives, but it is nice to choose your friends.**

February 14, 1986: **You have other questions, ask.**

*"Thank you, Aka.* [18-514-2…Texas], *and asks, 'How can I be healed of this severe allergy cracks in my hand[s] and feet so my energies can be used completely for my channel resource?'"*

**The information that you need is being placed into soul Ray's mind. It shall be conveyed from one to the other.**

May 16, 1986: "[12-423-1] *asks, 'To please tell us what is the problem with the horses − Pegasus, Cat Magic, and now the latest one. What treatment should they be given?'"*

The horse, Pegasus, was poisoned. The horse, Cat Magic, had a twofold problem − one of poisoning, the other of parasites. There *is* treatment for this. The ground must be kept clean. Horses are curious, and when they are bored they will take their curiosity out on what they find and try to eat it. The colt, which soul Ray calls, Trouble, has a twofold problem at this point, and one is with parasites and the other is that which he has eaten. If you will think, all three horses became ill in the same area where the old barn was. This area should be plowed very, very deeply, and then picked from the earth all substance there in the same which might be harmful. We have seen your need.

May 16, 1986: **You have other questions, ask.**
"*Thank you, Aka. [2-30-2] asks, 'Please assist [J___ C_____] in her passing.'"*
**We see this.**
"*Thank you, Aka.*"

May 16, 1986: "[4-125-2] *asks for − number 1, 'I ask for spiritual guidance, growth, and healing.'"*

The spiritual guidance is but at hand. The healing is also but at hand. The greatest healing is the healing of the mind.

There is a parable, a parable of the healing well. Each day a young girl went to the healing well. And she took from it and drank from it. And each day she drank more and more, for she believed that the more she took, the more she would heal. It is not in the amount needed to take, it is not in how much you can consume, but the quality of what you are given.

May 16, 1986: **You have other questions, ask.**
"*Thank you. Aka, she asks, 'Will you give me guidance about G_____ S. B_____ in relation to me?'"*
Friendship is a wonderful thing. It must be given. It also must be taken care of, and cherished.

June 6, 1986: **You have other questions, ask.**
"*Thank you, Aka. [18-518-3…Taos, New Mexico], who is here tonight...asks, 'How will Green's back be healed?'"*
Soul Ray has answered that question. It may happen one of two ways. By what you call conventional medicine, the L-4 vertebrae shall be repaired, and can be fused, with the L4 in what is called performing a laminectomy, and that also of the S-1 or sacroiliac of the lower sector of the spine with the same method. Or, he may seek out, as he has done, the

help of soul Ray, and by the use of the substance of the same it shall become whole. The choice shall be his. You must realize, due to the breaking of the spinal column, it shall be difficult, but the help that soul Ray has asked for shall be given unto him.

June 13, 1986: **You have questions, ask.**
*"Thank you, Aka. [18-519-1…Grand Junction, Colorado] asks, 'Because of my health, how can I make a living for myself and my family? Whom do I contact to get my good health back?'"*
We shall answer your question in this manner. You have come to the source of the well; drink from it and drink from its knowledge. If you took the retirement, it would take a little time, but you would live to see it all. And you would also live to see the children grow. You would also live to see other occupations that would allow you to do that which you wish in a monetary manner. The choice is up to you. Soul Ray will do those things that are necessary. But you must listen. If you do not wish to listen, then do that which you must.

December 19, 1986: **You have other questions, ask.**
*"Thank you, Aka. [E_____ P_____] asks, 'What is my sickness?'"*
Yes, we see your need; we shall answer your question in this manner. It is that of a spastic colon brought about by your surgery. This shall be brought about into a cure. Soul Ray has now brought you into a realm of wholeness. Allow this healing to happen, and it shall be so.

# 1987 Health Readings

January 2, 1987: **You have other words, other questions, ask.**
*"Thank you, Aka. [M_____ M_____...Tucson, Arizona] asks, 'I suffer in my stomach; this affects my mind. How can I get ok permanently?'"*

**(Chuckle) yes, we see thy need. First we should answer your question in this manner. We have before us the body, the soul, the spirit and immortal body of the same. The mind causes the over-secretion of acid into the stomach. There is a substance known as Tagamet. If it should be used as your physician should prescribe it, it should function and solve your problem. The second part is a problem with your sugar. Eliminate this from your diet, and that of chocolates and heavy, other spices. Also eliminate your cheeses or alcohol from your diet. If these things are done, your problem shall end.**

January 2, 1987: **You have other questions, ask.**
*"Thank you Aka. [J___B____ Jr.] asks, who is here tonight, asks, 'Dear Aka, please relate to my grandmother, _____, born _____, left from this plane _____. I love her and I want her to know this and that I feel sorrow for not spending more time with her. Please advise if she has anything to relate to me. Thank you, with love.'"*

**We should answer your question in this manner. Even upon the other side, freedom of choice is respected into the highest. One moment, and we shall ask.**
**Yes.**
**You should know this, that the one you speak of has passed through, and rebirth upon the Earth has already taken place. It will not be long until you know this person. Be glad, for it is their choice.**

January 23, 1987: **You have other questions ask.**
*"Thank you, Aka. [E_____ P_____] who is here tonight, asks, 'Why do my kids turn against me now in the time of my sickness?'"*

**We say unto you that as you stand, and bore your children in truth before the Lord, it is not always with understanding that a child can see. You will notice there are some among you who when they see blood will faint; there is others among you, when they see faint and pain, they will run. Yet, because they do not know how to, as you would say, "handle" this in their own system, they do not know how to face pain;**

they do not know how to face illness. But your illness is short lived, and you shall go on to do many things.

January 23, 1987: **You have other questions ask.**
*"Thank you, Aka. [L_____ B_____] lost her left hearing aid on December 31st. 'Can you please help me find it?'"*
**Yes.** [Surprised chuckle.]**We would say look on the bedroom, where you sleep. And we would tell you that you have a chest of drawers, a place where you keep your clothing. And in the top drawer on the left hand side you shall find it.**

January 23, 1987: **You have other questions ask.**
*"Thank you Aka. [M___ H___ R_____...Albuquerque, New Mexico] who is here tonight, asks, 'Will my health improve? Will I find love and peace of mind?'"*
**We shall answer, yes, unto all of these things. But remember, a gift that is given – if you were given the greatest of jewels and you put them before swine, [and the] swine did devour them, you would have nothing. Cast not your pearls before swine. It is hard, we know, to understand that what we have spoken. But think upon it and you shall understand.**

January 23, 1987: **You have other questions.**
*"No, Aka."*
**Yes. We shall say unto this one who has traveled far to be here and who is very afraid, the healing you seek shall come unto you. Fear not. It shall come one step at a time. As the healing[s] come, there shall be a healing of the body, the soul, the mind, and the spirit. Fear not, for you are not alone. It is said, "Seek and you shall find." And so it shall be true. The love of the Father is for all. Let it flow through your veins; let it be and vibrate through your very being, and know the Lord, God, is God.**

February 20, 1987: **You have many questions, ask.**
*"Yes Aka, thank you. I ask, Aka, for help to a lady named [J__ R_____...Houston, Texas] in which her husband passed away in January, and is finding – 'Needing much peace of mind.' Can you help her? Thank you."*
**Yes, we see thy need. And we have before us the body, the soul, the spirit, and the immortal body.**
**There has been much deliberation of the "yeas" and "nays" of this situation. But we shall say unto you, blessed be the house of the Lord, thy God, and blessed be His child who should enter. This one is awake and well. He is concerned greatly for your welfare, and he sends his love. Know these things that he said unto you.**

You feel that the communications between himself and soul Ray might be over, yet they are not. You feel, because you are still receiving literature from the Universal Philosophy, that it was only for your friend, your beloved. And we say unto you, it was meant for both; now it is meant for you.

See these things clearly and know that nothing passes from the Earth that our Father does not know. Nothing passes without a reason. The day shall come when you will see that smile again, yet in another. Blessed be the name of the Lord, thy God; blessed be the name of His children forever and ever.

February 20, 1987: **You have other questions, ask.**
*"Yes, Aka. Do you have a few words of wisdom for [K____ H_____] who seems to be having much trouble at this time? Thank you."*
Yes, we see thy need, and we shall answer your question in this manner. The Lord has seen the conceivement, the reality, within a child. He would not allow its removal. We know, at this time, you do not understand. But understand these things. That that was given shall not be taken away. That that seems impossible at times, when you look at your burden, know that the Lord is with you always. **"Ask and you shall receive."**

February 27, 1987: **You have other questions, ask.**
*"Thank you, Aka. W_____ L_ H_____ who is here tonight asks, 'Will _____ make it and what is wrong with him?'"*
We see thy need. And what you really ask for is healing. But let the healing be asked for for themselves.

We say unto you, there comes a time in animal or in man, or in fowl or fish, when those things between God and themselves become one knowledge, one thought, and one image. Allow that to be that is, and you shall allow all things to serve God and themselves as they wish. Ask for healing and it shall be received, and [be] granted. But remember, there are many types of healing.

May 1, 1987: **You have other questions, ask.**
*"Yes Aka, soul Ray asks, 'In J____ R_____'s recent trip to Washington D.C., could he have come into contact with something that may have [caused] him to have a relapse?'"*
Yes, we see thy need and we shall answer in this manner. Because of these things that he was taking, in their exposure to a colder climate, they did react upon him in a more abundant manner. But you must realize that there is a greater amount of pollution and a different type of pollution, almost into the form of what is known as acid rain, that is now within the atmospheric conditions of the Washington D.C. area. We say unto you, because of type of medication that you would take, when you

came in contact with these chemicals they would cause a completely different reaction within your body, body substance.

May 1, 1987: **You have other questions, ask.**
*"Thank you Aka, at this time I misplaced a question from W_____ S_____. Would you have a message for him?"*
Yes, we see thy need, and we shall answer your question in this manner. You have come forth this day unto soul Ray for counseling. And he has given you the counsel that is needed. We say unto you, you grow in despair because of your separation from your family. We say to you, let us reach out and carry your burden. It shall be yet a time more before your job shall change. But we say unto you, be patient, for that which you reach for is at your fingertips. But look, as you have said, unto the Universal Philosophy. Open the door that you may enter. We shall fill your cup.

May 1, 1987: **You have other questions, ask.**
*"Yes Aka, at this time could you tell us how soul Ray's body is now?"*
The body needs time to repair. We find additional growths in the sacroiliac. These will need attention. They are allowing spinal fluid to leave the body. They are also causing the nervous system, and pressure to be applied into the spinal cord, which is causing the nerves to be, as you would call them, cross-circuited.

We would suggest that due to an increasing pressure from a blood disease known as polycythemia [verigo] [vera?], this is also creating a greater problem within him.

We can help him to help himself. Know these things, that there was great damage to the brainstem area and to the whole spinal column. We do not create, only our Father creates, and God in His wisdom has allowed a regeneration of certain tissue within his body. But there is other tissue, because of the work he seeks out, because of his desire, now more than ever, to bring healings into a completeness. In his frustration, because he knows within his mind that that has been given him to create new medications that could be used for the curing of the substance you know as AIDS. But his frustration grows because he reaches into the upmost realms of the universe. Yet, he is a doer, a dreamer and a doer. These are not commonly put together. He knows that his body will burn out one day, and he wishes to leave with you a legacy of the knowledge. He wishes to reach forth and bring forth an end to disease and famine.

There are many things that we could say, yet we would violate his freedom of will if we said more.

May 1, 1987: **You have other questions, ask.**
*"Thank you, Aka. S__ B___, who is also here tonight....and he asks, 'How is my health in general?'"*

We see your need. We say unto you, you have an arthritic condition, which is causing you to lose your hearing. You also have a condition, you are borderline diabetic. It is also affecting the eyesight. We say unto you, allow yourself to have these things [which] are needed to restore your body.

And we also say unto you, do not seek out a higher altitude than you already live in, because you have a problem called secondary polycythemia. You are not receiving adequate amounts of oxygen into your system, as it is. These things can be corrected. We could go into elaborate detail of this reading, and should you request one a second time, we shall do so. But bring these things before soul Ray and he shall give you answers and solution[s] to answers.

May 15, 1987: **You have other questions, ask.**

*"Thank you Aka. J __ R____ asks, 'Dear Aka, please advise me any useful or predominate information regarding the passing of my father J__ R____, date 6-2-10, in Washington D.C. Please also advise if there is anything that he would like to tell me, or any member of his family.'"*

We should answer your question in this manner. Know of these things that we say − for we are not allowed to interfere or violate the freedom of choice of any person, and therefore, we must have the permission of the soul himself. One moment.

Yes.

He should say unto you these words.

"For behold, my son, say these words unto your mother, 'For I am not dead; I live on. I shall live on to another day that we should see each other.' And say to your sisters, 'Behold, for I am with you.' It has been my choice at the present time to remain on this side and be, as you would know it, a teacher. Do not despair, my son. In life, many times I did not tell you I love you, but know it to be true, these things I have said."

June 6, 1987: **You have other questions, ask.**

*"Thank you, Aka. 'Dear Aka,' J__ R____ ...asks for 'any advice on speeding his recovery, to include vitamin supplements, diet, medication, etc. Please feel free to offer this advice at any time. With love.'"*

We understand your need. And we would answer your question in this way. When the emotional stress has left your house then the rest of you shall get well. We would answer by one other question. Soul Ray has a new substance in his mind that you shall soon use to speed your recovery, and those and many others with similar problems.

June 26, 1987: **Now we say unto you, soul Ray grows weary; yet we see other questions, and even with their emergencies. We look unto the land of California and we see a child, and the child has the disease of** cancer. And we see your concern. And we see soul Ray's agony, and we should give him that that he desires for the child.

Glory be the name of the Lord, thy God; glory be the name, of the name of His children, forever and ever.

July 10, 1987: **You have many other questions, ask.**

*"Thank you, Aka. L____ K_____ who is here tonight, and also resides in Houston, Texas, asks, 'Could you please advise me what to do to improve the condition of my back and spine?'"*

Yes, we see thy need. The time is needed that soul Ray may give continuous treatment to this. There is also additional knowledge that we shall place unto his brain that shall bring about a total healing. Be patient. That which you ask for shall come first; you have asked for a deliverance of the spirit. You shall have both.

July 31, 1987: **You have other questions, ask.**

*"Yes. Thank you, Aka. M____ _____ who is here tonight asks, '[Could] the contamination from mining in this area be the reason that I and most of the people [are not breathing] so well. If so, how is it affecting my body?'"*

We would answer your question in this manner, we see your need. And we would say, under normal conditions the mining does not affect you at all. The smelting could affect you because, you are learning, certain acids are released into the air, but as long as this is done in a sensible manner *that* is [not harming] you. If you are harmed in any manner at all, it would be due to the acid content, and that would cause the red cell structure to alter in [its] size and shape, and cause the red cells to become more abundant. This is a condition that is true in any area; it is true in the area you have come from. Because of pollutants this factor was true. You probably have cleaner air and cleaner water than you have had in years where you are now.

November 6, 1987: **You have other questions, ask.**

*"Thank you, Aka. [18-541-2…Albuquerque, New Mexico] asks, 'Being under your care, will my mother's liver return to normal? If so, how long will it take?'"*

Yes, we see your need, and we shall answer your question in this manner. Time is a fleeting thing. There is never enough of it. Yet, you count it and you cherish it.

We should answer your question in saying, it shall take whatever time it shall take. You will think that we're being harsh with you, yet we are not. We're answering you in a truthful manner. For it is not all one-sided, this healing. The other side must come from he who seeks it.

December 4, 1987: **You have other questions, ask.**

*"Thank you, Aka.* [1-409-1...El Paso, Texas]*, and she asks, 'Will my vertigo go away?'"*

**The question is yes, it shall go.**

# 1988 Health Readings

January 29, 1988: **You have many questions, ask.**

*"Thank you, Aka. [18-544-3, who is here this evening, and resides in _____, New Mexico] asks, 'What will it take to heal my mother's lungs? I feel she is a good person and has the faith. Please help me to understand.'"*

**You must understand that her condition is not one of a single thing, it is one of a multiple thing. The lungs in themselves became damaged because of the virus, and so did the muscles of her throat. These shall be healed, but she must put the faith within herself that this [may] come about.**

**We say unto her, go unto the *Rose without Thorns* and read of the healing well. But we say unto her, look unto the faith of her granddaughter, and be as a mirror.**

January 29, 1988: **You have other questions, ask.**

*"Thank you, Aka. [18-544-1, who is also here this evening, and lives in Las Vegas, Nevada] asks, 'Will my baby be a healthy boy or girl, and will I deliver before or after my due date of May 25, 1988?'"*

**This child shall be long remembered, as the earth shall tremble at the time of its birth. We shall say unto you, it shall be a girl. And it shall be much beloved.**

January 29, 1988: **You have other questions, ask.**

*"Thank you, Aka. [18-544-2, who is also here this evening, and resides in Las Vegas, Nevada] asks, 'about [18-544-4], my husband, how and to what extent is it going to get before it gets better?'"*

**We see your need. But we cannot violate the freedom of choice of another person. But for your own sake and for the good of your own soul, we should answer your question in this manner. If it is possible, bring him unto soul Ray. There's many kinds of healing, but the greatest healing is the healing of the soul. If you were to move a mountain, the first step in moving the mountain is to pick up the first stone. Speak unto soul Ray unto these words, and he shall have more to tell you.**

January 29, 1988: **You have other questions, ask.**

*"Thank you, Aka. [18-533-1, who is also here this evening, and resides in Albuquerque, New Mexico] asks, 'My sister is very ill. Is there anything that I can do to help her?'"*

You can only help those who would help themselves. But sometimes, even death is an extension of life, for it is the total cycle. It can only begin again by allowing it to pass through. But for those who would throw their life away and not care for it, it the same as committing suicide. For them, their journey back is more [hardship].

Soul Ray has been conducting classes in your study groups on the between life. It is something you should know about.

March 18, 1988: **You have other questions.**

*"Thank you, Aka. [10-384-1] who is here tonight asks, 'I want to know if the disease, muscular dystrophy, is curable?'"*

**We say unto you, all things are curable. But if you cut off your hand, the Lord has given you knowledge to replace the [hand]. But if you cut away the brain and place that of synthetic proportions of the pineal gland known as the aldophine** [*"adolphine"*(a synthetic methadone)?, acetylcholine? dopamine?] **back into the brain, the disease shall stop. These things shall be done. But even after this is completed the brain must be stimulated and fed in what you know as the Magellic [Magellan] region of the brain. Come unto soul Ray and ask in the awakening state. The knowledge has been placed there.**

April 8, 1988: **You have other questions, ask.**

*"Thank you, Aka. In February you asked, you said to ask again. [12-419-6] requests a life reading."*

**At the present time, we would suggest that this question be asked at a different time.**

*"Thank you. Aka. [18-549-2] would like to know, what does the future hold for her, and what about her health?"*

**We see your need, and we shall answer your question in this manner. If you take the necessary steps that we have placed before you, your health shall improve. Your destiny, until now, of that of the future, is one of free choice. And being so, your past has been your present. And until you make the decision to change, so it shall be your future.**

**To elaborate in detail could bring embarrassment to you at this time. But we say unto you, there are many beautiful flowers around you, and these flowers are relations which you seek out, and have sought you out. Allow yourself to go unto these. If you do so, seek them with love and give it love. You shall find that love shall be given back in proportion that you give.**

April 8, 1988: **You have other questions, ask.**

*"Thank you, Aka. [18-544-3] asks, 'My brother, [18-549-3] has many problems with heart palpitations. Is it truly a heart problem or is it just tension and stress? He is in his early 30's and has always been a healthy person.'"*

We will try to answer your question in this manner and in this way, not to violate the rights of the individual, and that individual being your brother, for he has not asked or given permission. So then we must speak in generalities. But we should answer your question by saying that stress is the number one factor in heart problems.

April 15, 1988: **You have other questions, ask.**
*"Thank you, Aka. [18-550-4…Houston, Texas] asks, 'What will happen to me in my 33rd year in this body?'"*
(Chuckle.) **We see [her] need. And we shall answer you in this way. You have looked into the body and not seen it as a temple, and you have abused the temple and not made it a righteous thing before God. Remember that life is a gift, and as a gift it should be treated as such, with great respect. You have thought of that of suicide, and we shall say unto you, seek out counseling. Do not cast stones at the temple of God.**

May 6, 1988: **You have other questions, ask.**
*"Thank you, Aka. [18-532-1] who is here tonight asks, 'I am greatly concerned about my sister, [18-551-1]. I am seeking your help in finding her and your advice on how to help her if she lets me.'"*
**We have before us the body, the soul, the spirit, and we say unto you, normally we would not be allowed to interfere between one soul and their free choices. But we say to you, this person seeks, wants help.**

**In what you call your Roosevelt Estate region you will find her. By morning she will be back in what you call Claypool with her friend. She is running from herself. She is afraid she cannot fulfill your expectations or your parent's. She know not what to do with her husband or her children. She needs help. She needs mental help. If there is something or some way — one moment, please. Yes, we see this, yes. We shall answer in this manner. We shall place in your mind this night the direction and picture and we shall do so in dream state that will allow you to find her. We shall place that also in soul Ray's mind that he may help you.**

May 6, 1988: **You have other questions, ask.**
*"Thank you, Aka. [18-547-1] asks, 'I would like to ask the reason for my husband, [18-551-6], having chest pains sometimes. Does [18-551-6] have angina or any kind of heart problems? If so, what should he do about it?'"*
**We have before us the body, soul, the spirit and the immortal body and we say unto you, we cannot violate the freedom of will of one person unto another. We can answer questions given to us by a person. We see that your need is from love and concern, and we shall answer your question in this manner.**

**Come unto soul Ray and we shall place the answer, therefore, in his mind that he may help you and you may receive the information that**

you need to assist your husband. The angina pains are [due] to the narrowing of the blood vessels from the heart. If this narrowing continues it could be very dangerous.

June 3, 1988: **You have other questions, ask.**
*"Thank you, Aka.* [18-547-1…Houston, Texas] *asks, 'I would like to ask Aka the reason for my eleven-year-old son,* [18-552-1], *having frequent headaches lately, accompanied by much vomiting – also what to do about it?'"*

Yes, we see your need, and we shall answer your question. Your son has the problem of an intestinal flu, or a virus. The second part is your son has come into contact with toxic waste from the area. We would suggest the using that of the [dock] herb in all of his drinking water, diluting it one-half ounce to the gallon. This should correct his problem.

We would also suggest that the son seek out the advice of soul Ray.

June 10, 1988: **You have many questions, ask.**
*"Yes, Aka.* [11-405-4] *who is here tonight asks, 'Could you please tell me the seriousness of my father's physical condition?'"*

Yes, we see your need. We may not violate the freedom of choice of another human being or a soul, but since you ask from love we will tell you these things.

If your father had truly wished you to know he would have told you himself. But since you should worry, we should say unto you, your father's condition is not so severe that he will not be with you for a while, for he shall. He has listened to a lot of your words. With small encouragement, he will come unto soul Ray for healing. And this might be an answer for both of you.

But because of your asking as a loving daughter, more can be done.

June 10, 1988: **You have other questions, ask.**
*"Thank you, Aka.* [18-553-2] *who is also here tonight asks, 'What is causing the pressure pain in the back of my head?'"*

Yes, we see *your* need, and we shall answer your question, that the pressure pain was created from a combination of things – first, the lack of hormones; second, a hypoglycemic condition; third, that of the migraine or restriction of the blood flow; and [fourth], you had what we call, you have a condition within yourself, a psychic ability which is unschooled as yet. You are now finding ways of turning it loose and beginning to use it. As you do, your life shall become happier and fuller. Because of this, prolonged conditions, scar tissue grew in the brainstem area. This, hopefully, is being removed by the procedures now taken.

July 8, 1988: **You have questions, ask.**

*"Thank you, Aka. Please, Aka, can you give us information on the health and life of the new baby, [18-554-1]?"*

**Yes, we see thy need. We should say unto you, for in soul Ray's mind he has asked unto the Lord for life for both the mother and the child.**

**And he went unto the mountain and he prayed for them, and he spoke unto the Lord, thy God, and he did promise unto the Lord. And he did give offering unto the Lord. Therefore, that that he has offered has been accepted. And the mother and the child shall live. Be patient.**

**And we say unto the mother, be patient, for what you have prayed for has been given. But give it time now. Allow the child to mature in your womb.**

July 8, 1988: **You have other questions, ask.**

*"Thank you, Aka. [18-554-3] who is also here this evening asks, 'I would like to know if my son, C____ R____ [18-554-3], will walk again and have better health?'"*

**Yes, we see thy need and we shall say unto you, [18-554-3] shall walk again, and his health shall be better, but it shall not come in a one time. For in five times you shall bring him unto this land. And five times you shall take him as here for treatment and then unto the water of the Healing Springs and bathe him in this water. But he must continue in body and soul and mind in the healing process.**

**Each person who is here tonight is here for a reason.**

July 29, 1988: **You have other questions, ask.**

*"Thank you, Aka. [18-555-4] who is also here tonight asks, 'Will my son [18-555-5]'s back get well without an operation?'"*

**We see your needs. And we say unto you, bring him unto soul Ray. Allow him to see; allow him to touch; and allow him to speak unto you, and then an answer shall come. But allow those things to happen which need to happen, for there is more than the physical body that should seek healing.**

August 26, 1988: **You have other questions, ask.**

*"Thank you, Aka. [18-557-3] who is also here tonight asks, 'Will my son [18-557-4] get his surgery completed safely and successfully?'"*

**We see thy need. All things that you speak of shall not be as the way you expect – but it shall be in the end for the best. We know that we sound as if, that we are not answering that question in full. Should you stop and look you shall see that we are.**

September 2, 1988: **You have other questions, ask.**

*"Thank you, Aka. [18-523-4] seeks your guidance."*

Yes, we see thy need. And we have before us the body, the mind, the soul, the spirit, and the immortal body of the same. And we say unto you, we see what is in your mind and your heart. We find goodness. We see that you want what is best for both the spiritual development of your children — and we shall answer your words in this way.

Give unto that of your husband time, time that he may find himself if it is that that he shall do. But in finding himself he must also find God in truth. Give him time to know of this. Give yourself the time. Put a time period upon this and say, "I shall give six months, or four months, or three months." But have a home up there ready, before you rush across the land and act as a whim.

This has already been done, and what was good and clear to you has become confused. You have the responsibility unto yourself for happiness. You have the responsibility for the spiritual growth of your children. Take these into consideration. You also have a winter that is about to come upon you. To go into the land that you have chosen would be a very difficult thing at this time — not impossible, but difficult. Then think unto yourself, "I must have a home that is warm and secure for my family."

Take these things that we have said, read them carefully, and know these things that we say unto you. The Lord is with you, for you are Lot of Lot and of Lot. We know you shall be confused at what we have just said. Take the time and you shall understand what we have said.

The greatest of all things is the time to do nothing and the knowledge to do it. There is a time for action and a time for waiting.

It is hard for you, for you wish to sink your roots deep[ly] and become a part of all things. We may not answer that part of your question, for that must come from within you. That decision cannot be ours, but yours. But take the things we have said, weigh them carefully, and make your own decision. And know this, that wherever you are, whatever decision you make, the Lord is with you. And if you wish, open your heart and mind and for the next five days, as you open your door, we shall enter. But know this, the Lord is with you. Know this as a truth.

October 28, 1988: **Now, we say unto you, you have many questions, ask.**

*"Thank you, Aka.* [18-559-1] *who is here tonight asks, 'How can I help my wife become well and healthy again?'"*

We say unto you, give unto her the dignity and respect and the love that she deserves. But give unto her faith, and allow that which has been brought before her to come into fulfillment.

You are saying unto us, "Why do you not rise her and heal her?"

And we say unto you, we have given you the tools that are needed. But you shall receive more than a healing before you leave.

October 28, 1988: **You have other questions, ask.**

*"Thank you, Aka.* [18-554-3…Chihuahua, Mexico], *he asks, 'I wanted to know if I will walk again?'"*

**We say unto you, we have already answered your question, and you *shall* walk again. You shall not only walk, but you shall run.**

# 1989 Health Readings

March 24, 1989 [in Philosophy]: **You have other questions, ask.**

*"Thank you, Aka.* [18-556-1 says], *'I have been taking Ray's supplements for ten months now and my health is a little better, but I am still plagued with my any allergies and depression and hormone imbalance. Can you give Ray some insight about what else I might need to take for this or is it just a matter of being on the supplements a little longer?'"*

**We shall answer your question at this time. The greatest potion of all potions is that which is in the heart of man, the heart of the soul. We have given you a parable and the parable [is] one of depression [and] one of hope.**

**We say unto you, within the *Rose without Thorns* you shall find the journeys of the spirit[s] of God. Bring [these] forth, not by yourself, but with others; study and learn from them. Know the meaning of what it is and what is said.**

**You have been given many parables and much knowledge in many ways. The cup is before you; drink from it.***

*Editor's note: A second book, the book given to ministers upon ordination, is also called, *A Rose without Thorns*; the book given to teachers is *The Cup and the Rose*.]

March 24, 1989 [Also in Philosophy document]: **You have one more question, ask.**

*"Thank you, Aka.* [12-424-2] *asks, 'I desire to have acute hearing. Will you help me to accomplish this? Thank you.'"*

**We understand thy need; we also understand thy want.**

**But we should say unto you, look into the time of Daniel and study the prophecy therein, and bring it forth into today and look at it and see of it, and you shall begin the journey you wish to begin.**

August 30, 1989 [in Philosophy]: **But we will tell you this parable. It is of the [ ] shooting star that you see.**

**For once man looked upon the heavens and saw this star. He thought in his own mind, if he could only be as the star, [he could] only be through time and space at such a speed. So man went out and he built a great spacecraft, and he hurled himself through space. And he went faster and faster. And one day, he not only broke the time and light barrier, but he exceeded life in itself.**

**And he thought unto himself, "Where shall I go? I now can visit**

the universes upon universes. Which one shall I seek upon my own?"

He thought very long and hard upon it. He thought, "I guess I should ask my God." And so, he went forth unto his own private place, and he spoke into the Lord, and he said to the Lord, "Forgive me, Lord, but I should speak unto You, for I do not know what to do. I have [gone] and taken Your knowledge unto its limits, yet I know there is more. What shall be Your will, oh Lord?"

And the Lord spoke back unto him and said, "LET THINE WILL BE DONE. BUT REMEMBER, THERE ARE PLACES TO GO, AND THINGS TO SEE, BUT HAVE YOU SEEN ALL THOSE THINGS UPON YOUR OWN PLANET? ARE YOU READY NOW TO LEAVE IT BEHIND YOU? OR HAVE YOU YET MORE TO LEARN FROM IT? HAVE YOU TOUCHED ALL THINGS UPON YOUR EARTH, THAT YOU ARE SO READY TO LEAVE IT FOREVER?"

And the Lord went by.

And he thought upon this. And he went out into his garden and he saw all its beauty there in [it], and it multiplied tenfold. And he went unto the smallest of things upon the Earth and saw [them], and the greatest of things upon the Earth and saw that. Yet he knew that he had not seen enough, or tasted, or drank, or touched, or felt, or sensed all of the things there was on this Earth. He had yet to take the time to be able to smell the roses, for he was so busy in trying to reach the universes. He did not give up his space travel altogether, to have always returned back to the Earth that he loved.

Now we say unto you, so it is with soul Ray. He has taken you to the outer boundaries. Now he is taking the time to smell the roses. He will reach into the outer boundaries with you many times, but he will do this in his own way. He now can take you to the light in *his* way. His way, you will find, is quite different than you might have experienced. For his [own] time, he has been a teacher many times. Yet each time he has moved aside to allow us to speak, to talk, to touch and feel. He has allowed, at all times he has moved aside to allow his brother, who he prepares the way for, to speak, and to be heard and to be seen. He has made *him* the most important part of his life.

Now, he shall begin to lead his own life, to touch these things of Earth, and smell his own flowers. If he is to live − he is an eagle − let him be free. For we have known this. This is why we have freed him, so he *could* live, because he was dying. And he *will* die if you do not free him.

[It's not meant] to be because of his health. [It's] not meant [to mean] that we cannot continue to heal him. But he needs his own time, his own space. He needs to be his own person.

*Allow* him; give him these things.

You have seen him reach for them, and you have thought him angry and insane. Have you not seen a person that was starving, a person [that] did not have water and was dying of thirst? He reaches for it. This is why he is now fighting. Even the eagle [can] be free. He is reaching for his freedom, for his right to exist as a person. Give him that. If he has that, that time to himself, he may heal and mend. If he does not, he will die.

August 30, 1989: **In your mind you have had many questions. We have answered some of these. Now we shall answer others.**

**In your own mind, you have asked the nature of his illness. We would call it, stress syndrome, which has aggravated, a rheumatoid arthritis condition which was created a long time ago when he was involved in 1965 in a wreck.*** 

---

*Editor's note: Ray was diagnosed in the late 1980s with systemic lupus erythematosus, which many people developed who drank the water in South Tucson in the 1950s that was contaminated by solvents that seeped into the groundwater that were to clean aircraft engines. Like many others there, Ray later developed a brain tumor. It was successfully removed, partially by surgery and partly by radiation of the inoperable portion in the brainstem.

---

**It was like a time bomb waiting to go off. He's known this and he's lived with it. He [knew] that he was living on borrowed time. He has never asked us for additional time; he never asked us for anything, but to be able to do his work.** [See the February 14, 1976 reading.]

**You** *have* **to realize that when the brain stem is damaged, a malfunction occurs in both the biochemical [and] emotional supporting, and the muscular reaction of the same; for both [are] necessary electrodes and neutrons within the brain, throughout [emotion], therefore, within the same. His mind [has been] without, but he has kept control. We have warned him before that should he reach too far to his limits, this could happen; he knew it. He has known this for some time.**

**But he did not know that when the prostatectomy was preformed, before the prostatectomy, that which occurred to cause the infection in the hemorrhoid area, the lesion of the rectum removed, was, as you would know, a form of cancer. He asked us at that time for help, and it was given it. When the prostatectomy was performed there were errors made in the surgery. Instead of the sperm entering into the bladder and it being expelled, it is entering, and being contaminated as it goes into the body; therefore, it is attacking his body as his own immune system is fighting it. In the process of doing this, the body [creates] your [immune symptoms] such as a kind of anger, or sometimes even in joy, but mostly of anger. There are other parts that can [create] it. The adrenal system can even speed it up, and be aggravating and aggravate the [injury in] itself.**

**Soul Ray at the present time has [the formula] in his mind that he is about to prepare to bring about the possibility [that it] will buy him time, the time he needs for this. You can help him greatly by bringing forth the seed and the leaf and [the pulp] of the different species of yucca that he wishes. He will show you these species. He will show you [the] seed form. There will be other plants that he will show you. Gather them**

for him. Before he leaves this Earth, it is *his* choice and *his* wish [ he has discussed], that he has asked the Lord, thy God, that he will be able to leave upon the Earth a cure for your AIDS, for your cancers, and for the type of rheumatoid arthritis that is now possessing his body at such a rapid rate. The chemotherapy [which] he is taking will aid to help control this. But the true healing will come from his own work.

You must understand that because of his great pain that he does not share with you – most of the time you do not know he has it – it shall make him irritable at times; it will almost seem as though his personality will be changed. Sometimes it is very difficult to act, to work as a calm person when inside your body is being torn apart and your nervous system is failing.

Now, we must say unto you, our time is short.

Now is the time of the cherubim.

# Epilogue

*"Thank you, Aka. [10-380-3] asks, 'The book I wish to write on Ray, I'd appreciate your comments and advice.'"*

Yes, we see thy need; we shall answer in this manner. Look into the man deeper and you shall find the complexity of the same, and the versatility of the same. But you shall also find his humor, if the book is to succeed that you desire.

We would say unto you, none of us may violate the freedom of choice of another, nor can soul Ray. Within your mind you wish to know why one would live and one would die. And you say in your mind, "If he saved all of them, if he walked on water for all of them, then the whole world would look upon him and know of our presence and our purpose. In some ways, this is true. But we may not interfere in the ultimate plan of God and man of life and death. We may give life back only where life is truly desired. But when the time has come for renewal, and the choice has been made, there is little we can do to change that person's mind. All we can do is still the pain within. For death within itself is a form of healing. Within this you have only looked at one side, as you have only looked at one side of the compassion that lies within the man.

You asked why he should manufacture the vitamins, and how they differ. That the vitamins may be marketed, they must be called vitamins, or your laws would not allow them to be called or be sold. So his decision to keep them as such has been wise.

Yet there are those who should come unto him who can neither afford of his service or the vitamins themselves. Therefore, the necessity within him that each shall get their equal share shall be part of the balancing factor in his never-ending search for the improvement of man's health. We have watched as man has tried to stop our progress and the progress of our instrument. He has not succeeded. Flowers are planted in the stranger places upon the Earth, but the wisdom of our Father to plant them so they can multiply has been greater than man's.

Once again you say unto us, "He has spoken as into riddles." And we say unto you, nay − for if you shall see this man, it shall take patience and fortitude.

*Aka, April 14, 1978*

August 30, 1989, was the last time Ray's failing health allowed him to give a reading. Yet healing others was the passion of his life.

On October 5, 2000, Ray passed on during the Jewish high holy Days of Awe. This is after the new year (Rosh Hashanah) begins, during the ten days when one looks within and repents, as he or she asks God for forgiveness. This is before the Day or Atonement (Yom Kippur) which some call, Judgment Day.

**There are many types of healing, and for those who should grieve, remember our Father has many mansions.**

*Spiritual messengers of God, January 7, 1977*

Yet, the gift the one with more love in his eyes than anyone, who gave him back life 30 years before, lives on. And the work of the spiritual messengers of God who spoke and healed through him continues today.

.

And we shall say again, for hark. For those who have ears to listen, and for those who have faith, both in their selves and in God, our Father, let them bring the bread that is needed, and the bread shall be the body of the same. And let them pray over it, and ask for healing of the same. And the healing shall be given, for as we have said before, we shall furnish the wine that is needed, and we shall turn the bread into yeast, that the healing may grow outward and inward.

From this day forward, your medical readings shall not be needed, for those who come in faith shall be given the healing that is needed.

*Aka, January 1, 1972*

Yes, we shall answer that question in the mind of one. "For what purpose have you been brought unto this small town?"

And we say unto you, you are part of a whole. You are part of God's plan. You have been brought here to visualize and see with your own eyes, for you shall become, all of you, a part in the preparation for the coming of the Messiah. Take both the healing gift as it has been given and that that shall be added and give it wings. The healing that has been given unto your bodies is only a part. The greater part is the linking of the hands in true friendship and in true understanding that this work may go on.

Now is the time of the Cherubim.

*Spiritual messengers of God, July 22, 1977*

# A new BOOK with Wings

You can read all of the words of the spiritual messengers of God, Aka, that were recorded from 1970 to 1989 as they spoke through A. Ray Elkins, who left his body to stand with God each time so they could enter to speak in words that we can hear, so that we could receive these messages.

This knowledge, they call the BOOK with wings, is now available for you in three parts, as the spiritual messengers of God requested.

You have just finished reading the medical or health readings: *Angels "See Our Needs: the Health Readings.*

Another part of the healing offered to individuals is written as Aka read the akashic or records of time, the life readings: *Angels Give a Glimpse through All Time: the Past-life Readings.*

Healing of the soul (mind) and spirit is also lovingly shared in teachings, prophecies and personal guidance by the spiritual messengers of God called the philosophy: *Universal Philosophy.*

The parables were also gathered from the philosophy because some people enjoy learning from them: *Angel Messages: Parables of Wisdom for the Thirsting Soul.* These are duplicated in a second series of shorter ebooks: *Angels Tell Parables for Today.*

You can find all of these books in paperback or in kindle ebooks at createspace.com in the store, or at amazon.com. Just enter the titles.

May you be blessed by this knowledge the spiritual messengers of God have freely given to us.

We are here but for one purpose; that purpose is the preparation of the coming of the Messiah. Let those who have eyes to see, let them see. For those who have ears to hear, let them hear. But we say unto you, glory be the name of the Lord.

*Spiritual messengers of God, December 2, 1977*

Your question is that of the coming of the Messiah.

And we should answer first in this manner. Within your mind is the name of the one known as Jesus, and that of the preparation for the entry of those who have reached the Christ state into this one. As we have said before, there are many who have reached the Christ state. And through the combination of these shall be the new Messiah.

You asked that he should come walking from the clouds? And we shall answer your question in this manner. When he should first appear unto the Jewish people, and they shall see him first, he shall be standing upon a cloud. And the Jewish nation in their despair shall kneel before him. This was meant so that that that had been written should be fulfilled. And as we have said before, written upon the clouds, written upon the sky, our Father shall make known of this entry in this way. [See *Acts* 1:6-11, *The Revelation of John*, 7:2-12, chapter 10, 14:1-5, 14:14-16, 15:2-4, 19:1-16, 21:1-7, 22-27, 22:1-7, *Zechariah*, chapters 12-14.]

But he should come unto the body form, for is it not written also that that that does not know of earth can not know of heaven? And those who do not know of heaven can not know of earth? For he should come to lead you through your thousand years of peace upon your earth. [See *John* 3:1-21 and *The Revelation*, chapters 19-22.]

The spirit was left that it may flow through all mankind. As we have said before, we have come but for one purpose, and that is for the preparation for the coming of the Messiah. And we say unto you, all of you, open your door that we might enter, and therefore, there can be a place prepared within each of you for his coming. [See *John* 14:1-5, 14:15-26, 15:26-27, 16:7-15, 16:19-24, and chapter 17.]

But from a mother's womb, so shall he be born. Look within your book of *Revelation*, and you shall see of the same. [See *The Revelation of John*, chapter 12.]

But hark unto these words. Our Father has written only upon the Tablets. Man has written upon your pages and your paper; therefore, many things have been extracted from, taken away from that that inspired the men in the beginning to write of the same, and some has been added to by others. We have come, not to change the Laws, but to fulfill the prophecies of the same. We have come not to change that that was given within Moses' time. We have come not to change that that was given unto Isaiah. We have come not to change that that was given, and the gift that was given, in the one known as Jesus. But hark unto these words. We have come for this time.

We have come from those who should make their entry. We have come from those who did say unto our Father, "Send those who know You best to prepare a way for our coming, that our Father's words should not be misinterpreted." [See *John* 14:15-26, 15:26-27, 16:7-15, and 16:19-24.]

*Spiritual messengers of God, December 29, 1972*

**New words shall be written upon the sky, but they must be written in men's hearts first.**

*Spiritual messengers of God, December 1, 1972*